Animal
FEED TECHNOLOGY

Animal
FEED TECHNOLOGY

Dr. S.S. Kundu
Dr. S.K. Mahanta
Dr. Sultan Singh
Dr. P.S. Pathak

Indian Grassland and Fodder
Research Institute (ICAR), Jhansi (U.P.)

SATISH SERIAL PUBLISHING HOUSE
403, Express Tower, Commercial Complex
Azadpur, Delhi-110033 (India)
Phone : 011-27672852, Fax : 91-11-27672046
e-mail : info@satishserial.com, hkjain1975@yahoo.com
Website : www.satishserial.com

Published by :

SATISH SERIAL PUBLISHING HOUSE
403, Express Tower, Commercial Complex, Azadpur, Delhi-110033 (INDIA)
Phone : 011-27672852 Fax : 91-11-27672046
E-mail : info@satishserial.com, hkjain1975@yahoo.com

Reprint, 2021

ISBN : 978-81-89304-06-2

Composed, Designed & Printed in India

ABOUT THE EDITORS

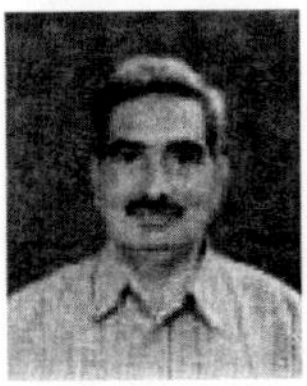

Dr. S.S. Kundu is currently Principal Scientist and Head, Plant Animal Relationship Division at IGFRI, Jhansi (U.P.). He has over 28 years of experience in the field of ruminant nutrition research. He was instrumental in initiating and shaping the work on feed technology, developing the feed block technology and feed microscopy for quality assurance. Dr. Kundu has undergone advanced training in the field of ruminant nutrition at the Netherlands and U.K. He is pioneer worker in the field of carbohydrate, protein fractionations of animal feeds in the country. In addition to books on "Buffalo Production Under Different Climatic Regions, Animal Feed Technology, Complete Feed Block (Bulletin)", he has more than 150 research publications in the Journal of National and International repute. He has guided many post graduate and PhD. students at NDRI, Karnal. He is Vice President (Animal Nutrition Society of India), and also life member of eight scientific societies.

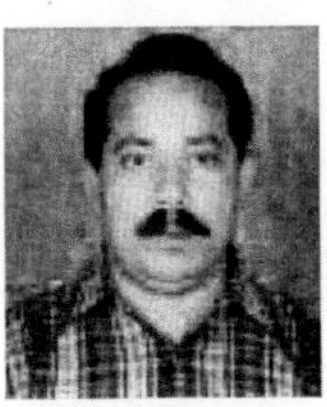

Dr. S.K. Mahanta Scientist (Animal Nutrition), PAR Division, IGFRI, Jhansi has 10 years of research, extension and training experience in farm animal nutrition and feeding. He specializes in forage evaluation and development of forage based feeding system for different categories of ruminants. He has over 40 research papers of national and international repute. He is also in editorial board of two national journals and an active member of many scientific societies.

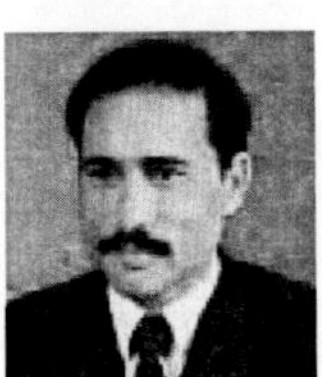

Dr. Sultan Singh is a Scientist (Animal Nutrition) in PAR at IGFRI, Jhansi (UP). His main areas of research in last 12 years are rumen metabolism and microbiology and evaluation of feeds and fodders. Transinoculation a mean of rumen manipulation and standardization of technique for in vitro dry matter digestion are accredited to his accomplishments. Recipient of two awards viz. ICAR Team Award (1994-96), for outstanding research in Agriculture and allied sciences and ICAR Young Scientist Award (1997-98) for his outstanding contribution in field of Animal Nutrition. He has over 50 research papers published in National and International journals and 3 Technical bulletins to his credit.

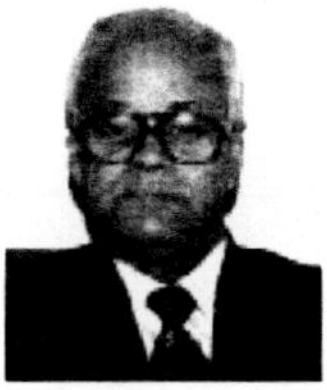

Dr. P.S. Pathak after studies at Banaras Hindu University, Varanasi, started his career as a lecture and has 36 years of research experience in the field of Agroforestry, Agrosilvipoastoral systems, Silvipastoral systems, Growth and production modeling of trees, Wasteland reclamation and development, Range management. He served as Assistant Director General (Agro forestry), ICAR, New Delhi from 1996-2000. Dr. Pathak coordinated the TPN-2 network project on agroforestry and soil conservation of CCD of the United Nations where 5 institutes of ICAR were involved.

He was associated with the development of an IDRC, Canada supported project proposal on Silvipastoral Systems of Production for Development of Degraded lands in Bundelkhand region. He is President RMSI and Portfolio Holder of a number of scientific societies and fellow of National Institute of Ecology and National Academy of Agricultural Sciences. Dr. Pathak visited 16 countries for attending international meetings, workshops and field trips related to Agroforestry, Multipurpose Trees and Shrubs(MPTS) development, Grassland management, Development oriented research in agricultural and development of degraded lands.

He is recipient of ICAR Team Research Award for outstanding research in the area of agricultural sciences (Natural Resource Management) in the year 2002. He has almost 265 research publications including 16 books (edited) and 2 books authored to his credit. Currently, as Director of Indian Grassland & Fodder Research Institute (IGFRI), Jhansi. He is guiding and managing research in the area of forage production and its utilization in the country since July 2000.

PREFACE

Both livestock and human population have attained an increasing streak in the post independent era of the country. India has registered a marked growth in the development and diversification of industrial sector. Livestock rearing has undergone a metamorphosis that has put the India on the top position in the milk production. To cater the need of increasing population for animal origin food, sustainability coupled with higher livestock production is of paramount importance. There are several obstacles in maintaining the pace of livestock production to match the increasing demand of food of livestock origin, but supply of feed and fodders and poor genetic makeup are the most critical. The present supply of compound feed from feed manufacturing sector is only 10 million tones. There is ample scope to boost the animal feed manufacturing industries that needs a cohesive interaction and coordination among the researchers, engineers, policy makers and feed manufacturers. The editors of the book "Animal Feed Technology" have made an attempt to organize and synthesize the information contributed by engineers, nutritionists, feed manufacturers in their respective areas of expertise. Subject matter of the book comprises of cereal processing, pelleting, protected nutrients technology, probiotics, feed resources, feed quality standards, gelatinization, extrusion technology, anti-quality factors in feeds, liquid feed handling, feed microscopy, feed purchase procedures, codex alimentarius, agro-industrial byproducts, processing techniques etc. Thus the compiled information in the book will provide the complete scenario of the Indian feed industry specially in terms of present scientific know how on machinery, processing techniques, compound feed quality, feed supplementation and future thrusts of animal feed science and technology aspects. The editors extend special thanks to contributors for their contribution in form of different chapters.

The encouragement and blessings poured by honorable Director General, ICAR and Secretary DARE, Dr. Mangala Rai ji; Dr. G. Kalloo, Deputy Director General (Crop Sciences); Dr. V. K Taneja, Deputy Director General (Animal Sciences) and Dr. S. N. Shukla, ADG are gratefully recorded. It's pleasure in extending thanks to Department of Science and Technology and especially to Dr. V. P. S. Tomar and Dr. J. K. Sharma advisors for their financial support to enable us to arrange this workshop to discuss different aspects of the subject.

It is our duty to thank the advisors namely Dr. K Pradhan, Dr. S. K. Ranjhan, Dr. V. K. Singh, Dr. V. D. Mudgal Dr. S. M. Ilyas, Dr. N. N. Patahak for their advice in finalizing the contents of the book.

It is pleasure in extending the thanks to our colleagues namely Dr. N. C. verma, Dr. B. K. Bhadoria, Dr. A. B. Majumdar, Dr. L. K. Karnani, Dr. B. P. Kushwaha, Dr. A. K. Mishra, Dr. S. B. Maity, Dr. N. P. Singh, Dr. K. K. Singh, Dr. A. K. Samanta, Dr. M. M. Das, Dr. G. H. Pailan, Dr. S. K. Nag and students/ staff especially Dr. Ranjan Kumar, Chanderbhan and Sudheer for their help at different stages in preparing the book.

S. S. Kundu
S. K. Mahanta
Sultan Singh
P. S. Pathak

LIST OF CONTRIBUTORS

Dr. Ambalkar
Irrigation and Drainage
Engineering Division,
Central Institute of Agricultural
Engineering, Bhopal (MP)

Dr. A.K. Tyagi
Dairy Cattle Nutrition Division
National Dairy Research Institute,
Karnal - 132001 (Haryana)

Dr. A. Thulasi
Scientist
National Institute of
Animal Nutrition & Physiology,
Adugodi, Bangalore-560 030

Dr. Anil Kumar
Scientist
Indian Grassland and
Fodder Research Institute
Jhansi-284 003

Dr. Arun Varma
Assistant Director General
ICAR (Retd.)

Dr. B.M. Bhanderi
Animal Nutrition and
Feed Technology Laboratory
Productivity Enhancement Group
National Dairy Development Board
Anand 388 001 (Gujarat)

Dr. B.S. Tewatia
Research Officer
Department of Animal Nutrition
CCS Haryana Agricultural University,
Hisar (INDIA)

Dr. Brijesh K Bhadoria
Principal Scientist
Indian Grassland and
Fodder Research Institute,
Jhansi

Dr. D.D. Sharma
Dairy Consultant, Formerly Head,
Department of Dairy Cattle Nutrition
National Dairy Research Institute,
Karnal - 132001 (Haryana)

Dr. D.M. Bhandarkar
Irrigation and Drainage
Engineering Division,
Central Institute of Agricultural
Engineering, Bhopal (MP)

Dr. D.M. Hegde
Directorate of Oilseeds Research
Rajendranagar, Hyderabad – 500030

Dr. G.V.N. REDDY
Professor
Acharya N. G. Ranga
Agricultural University,
Rajendranagar,
Hyderabad-500 030, India

Dr. Jai Singh
Project Director & Coordinator
Doon (PG) College of Agriculture Science
and Technology, Dehra Dun

Dr. K.K. Singhal
Principal Scientist & Head
Dairy Cattle Nutrition Division
National Dairy Research Institute,
Karnal 132 001 (Haryana)

Dr. K.T. Sampath
Director
National Institute of Animal Nutrition & Physiology, Adugodi, Bangalore-560 030

Dr. K.R.Yadav
Professor & Head
Department of Animal Nutrition,
CCSHAU Hisar-125004

Dr. M. Parthasarathy
Professor
Department of Animal Nutrition
College of Veterinary Science
TIRUPATI - 517 502, A.P., INDIA

Dr. M.R. Garg
Animal Nutrition and
Feed Technology Laboratory
Productivity Enhancement Group
National Dairy Development Board
Anand 388 001 (Gujarat)

Dr. M. Chandrasekharaiah
Scientist
National Institute of
Animal Nutrition & Physiology,
Adugodi, Bangalore-560 030

Dr. Mukesh K. Raikwar
Plant Animal Relationship Division
Indian Grassland and
Fodder Research Institute
Jhansi-284003, U.P., INDIA

Dr. Nand Kishore
Associate Professor
Department of Animal Nutrition,
CCS Haryana Agricultural University,
Hisar-125004

Dr. N. N. Pathak
Ex. Director, CIRB, Hisar

Dr. Nitin Tyagi
Dairy Cattle Nutrition Division
National Dairy Research Institute,
Karnal - 132001 (Haryana)

Dr. P. Prakash
Irrigation and Drainage
Engineering Division,
Central Institute of Agricultural
Engineering, Bhopal (MP)

Dr. Ram Singh
Scientist
Indian Grassland & Fodder Research
Institute, Regional Research Centre
CSKHPKV, Campus,
Palampur-176062

Dr. R. Bhar
Senior Scientist
Indian Veterinary Research Institute,
Izatnagar 243122, UP

Dr. R.K. Gupta
Director
Central Institute of Post Harvest
Engineering & Technology
PAU, Ludhiana

Dr. S.S. Thakur
Principal Scientist
Dairy Cattle Nutrition Division
National Dairy Research Institute,
Karnal 132 001 (Haryana)

Dr. S.K.Tomar
Senior Scientist
Dairy Cattle Nutrition Division
National Dairy Research Institute
Karnal-132001 (Haryana)

Dr. S.K.Sirohi
Senior Scientist
Dairy Cattle Nutrition Division
National Dairy Research Institute
Karnal-132001 (Haryana)

Dr. S. S. Kundu
Principal Scientist & Head
PAR Division,
Indian Grassland and
Fodder Research Institute,
Jhansi (U.P.)

Dr. S. K. Sirohi
Senior Scientist
Dairy Cattle Nutrition Division,
National Dairy Research Institute,
Karnal-132001 (Haryana)

Dr. S.K. Tyagi
Director
Central Institute of Post Harvest
Engineering & Technology
PAU, Ludhiana

Dr. S.S. Kundu
Principal Scientist & Head
Indian Grassland and Fodder Research
Institute, Jhansi-284 003

Dr. S.B. Maity
Senior Scientist
Indian Grassland and Fodder Research
Institute, Jhansi-284 003

Dr. S.M. Ilyas
Director
Central Institute of Post Harvest
Engineering & Technology
PAU, Ludhiana

Dr. S.K.Mahanta
Plant Animal Relationship Division
Indian Grassland and
Fodder Research Institute
Jhansi-284003, U.P., INDIA

Dr. Subir K. Nag
Plant Animal Relationship Division
Indian Grassland & Fodder
Research Institute,
Jhansi-284003, U.P., INDIA

Dr. S.K.Tomar
Senior Scientist
Dairy Cattle Nutrition Division,
National Dairy Research Institute,
Karnal-132001 (Haryana)

Dr. T. K. Dutta
Senior Scientist
Central Institute for Research on
Goats Makhdoom, Farah, Mathura,
UP-281 122

Dr. T.K. Walli
Principal Scientist
Dairy Cattle Nutrition Division
National Dairy Research Institute,
Karnal 132 001 (Haryana)

Dr. Y. Ramana Reddy
Asstt. Professor
Acharya N. G. Ranga Agricultural
University, Rajendranagar,
Hyderabad-500 030, India

CONTENTS

1
STATUS OF FEED INDUSTRY

D.D. Sharma

India is the richest in livestock wealth (201 million cattle, 98 million buffaloes) and is the largest milk producing country in the world. The annual milk production has crossed 88 million tones this year and expected to produce 150 million tones by the year 2020, but milk produced by individual lactating animal is just at the bottom. The low productivity of livestock, which is a matter of great concern, in the country is due to unsustainable breeding, uncomfortable housing, inadequate feeding and inefficient herd management systems. Efforts have been made in several Research Institutes as well as Agricultural Universities to develop new technologies to improve productivity in cattle and buffaloes. Most of the techniques are still on laboratory premises but few have percolated in developing cattle feed industry as well as management of dairy animals.

Indian Cattle Feed Industry

Feed Industry in India is just four decades old and mainly caters to Dairy and Poultry, but more recently to Aquaculture also. The development in this sector initiated after the formation of Compound Livestock Feed Manufacturers' Association (CLFMA) during June, 1967 with 180 members on roll. The primary focus of the Feed Milling Industry in the present era is to firmly position into food chain and assure to the consumers to produce products that are friendly to animals, consumers and environment. Out of total cattle and buffalo population, hardly 10 million crossbred cows, 15 million improved cows and 36 million improved buffaloes require good quality compound feed. In India, the present demand of total feed by a conservative estimate is 45 million tones. However, presently, only 10 million tones of feed is produced by different agencies (Members of CLFMA, Members of State Cattle Feed Manufacturers Association, Government Institute Farms, Progressive Dairy Farms). Some of the demand is met through on farm mixed feed. The remaining lot gets feed in the form of single feed ingredient available locally (either oil cake or wheat grain or bran). Even the improved animals kept on compound feed, also gets additional supplement as top feed available at home.

The perspective of dairying and its potential in India has changed with time. Earlier milk production was considered to be only for home consumption but slowly and slowly specialized dairy farms are coming up though with restricted number of animals and anxious to feed animals as per recommended nutrients requirement (Table 1). Now the quantity and quality of animal products such as milk and meat are getting the attention of consumers and becoming a major concern due to liberalization and globalization of Indian economy. In recent past, emphasis has also been shifted from basic and general aspect of livestock production to sustainable animal production. If the dairy production is to be commercially viable, the animals maintained should produce at least 3000 litres of milk per lactation.

Table 1. Daily nutritional requirement of lactating cows using absorbable protein

Live wt. (kg)	Fat (%)	Milk yield (kg)	Live wt. change	DMI (kg)	TDN (kg)	Protein UIP	DIP	Minerals Ca	P
400	4.5	8.0	0.220	10.14	6.44	511	753	44	28
400	4.5	14.0	0.220	12.66	8.48	710	1052	65	41
400	4.5	20.0	0.220	14.91	10.51	880	1355	85	54
400	4.5	26.0	0.220	16.94	12.54	1026	1662	106	67
400	5.0	8.0	0.220	10.36	6.60	526	778	46	30

* Intake at 100% of the requirement for maintenance, lactation and weight gain, (NRC, 1989)

UIP : Undergraded intake protein

DIP : Degraded intake protein.

The compound feeds produced scientifically having all the nutrients required for optimum production play a vital role to develop the developing dairy industry. The majority of the farmers have still not left the traditional way of management and feeding of their animals. The animals are mainly kept on available fodder resource (mainly crop residues, little green fodder or grazing) and very little concentrate ingredients (wheat grain/wheat bran/pulse churi etc.) if the animals yield up to 5 kg milk per day. They also supplement up to 500 g oil cake if the animals produce still higher quantity of milk. As a result, the animals are not getting nutrients even to keep them healthy and acquire common problems like low conception rate, prolapse, retained placenta, milk fever, anaemia, etc. The productive potential of crossbred and animals of improved breeds could not be harvested until they are fed on appropriate quantity of well balanced cattle feed.

Changing Scenario of Feed Industry

During the last decade, dairy industry has taken a significant turn. The strength of progressive dairy farmers is coming up though at a slow rate. The population of crossbred cows and improved cattle and buffalo is also on the increase. Simultaneously, the demand for compound feed is pressing hard on Cattle Feed Industry, though the increasing cost of raw material is a major depressing factor. Of the total required feed, now 25 per cent is produced by the industry. Leaving aside the members of CLFMA, most of the other feed manufacturers did not comply the quality norms and lose the confidence of consumers. Very recently, feed manufacturers have started their move towards quality feed. Many have registered with Bureau of Indian Standards (BIS) and many have adopted BIS specifications. Many hurdles are still on their way, i.e., the ingredients are not available as per BIS specifications, cost of ingredients is not under control and experiencing lack of technical manpower with them. Every individual is not prepared to bear the expenses of Quality Control Laboratory and they don't have that much load to engage the workers for analytical work.

BIS have laid down specifications and guidelines for the feed manufacturers on the basis of levels of crude protein, crude fat, fibre and acid insoluble ash (Table 2). The cost of feeds prepared as per such specifications of BIS do not suit to farmers owning low yielding animals. Looking into the practical difficulties of feed manufacturers and also at the level of end users, the Compound Livestock Feed Manufacturers Association of India and Govt. of Karnataka have proposed specification for cattle feed (Table 3). Few specifications are lower than the BIS specifications but suits to low yielding animals. The CLFMA also prepared specifications for some of the common feed ingredients which could be adopted as such. The members of CLFMA are producing feeds which are nutritionally equal as well as superior to BIS specifications. The challenging rations for high milk producing cows and buffaloes having high quality protein ingredients with high by-pass protein, high energy concentrate with higher level of oil/and or with high bypass fat are also produced by the feed industry. Levels of structural and non-structural carbohydrates have also been maintained in such formulations. It appears that feed industry is conscious to face the challenges of high yielding animals. Few examples of feed formulations prepared by feed industry have been listed in Table 4.

Looking into the upward progress of feed manufacturers, the supplementary industrial units have also come up to assist them. The products like vitamin pre-

Table 2. Specifications of Bureau of Indian Standards for cattle feeds

	Type I IS:2052, 1979 Re-affirmed 1990	Type II IS:2052, 1979 Re-affirmed 1990
Moisture, % max.	11	11
Crude protein, % min. *	22	20
Crude fibre, % max.	3	2.5
Crude fibre, % max.	7	12
Acid insoluble ash, % max.	3	4

*Except moisture, all on dry matter basis.

Table 3. Specifications for cattle feeds

	Govt. of Karnataka Type of cattle feed				CLFMA Type of calle feed			
	I	II	III	IV	Dairy special	I	II	III
Moisture, % max.	11	11	11	11	12.0	12.0	12.0	12.0
Crude protein, % min.	20	18	16	10	22	20	18	18
Fat, % min.	2.5	2.0	1.5	1.0	3.0	2.5	2.5	2.0
Crude fibre, % max.	7	12	16	20	7	7	12	14
Sand silica, % max.	4	4.5	5	10	3.5	4	4.5	5

Table 4. Concentrate formulations

Ingredients	Quantity (kg)			
	I	II	III	IV
FFS	5	–	–	–
Soymeal	7	8	–	–
Cottonseed cake	4	–	–	–
Mustard oil cake	18	14	20	12
Groundnut oil cake	–	12	13	–
Sunflower cake	–	4	5	3
Maize gluten	–	–	–	–
Guar Korma	7	–	–	–
Maize	10	8	8	10
Barley	10	8	–	–

Ingredients	Quantity (kg)			
	I	II	III	IV
Wheat	5	7	6	–
Rice kani	5	7	7	–
Rice polish	–	5	7	16
Deoiled rice bran	20	18	24	18
Phak	–	–	–	28
Urea	1	1	1	1
Mineral mixture	2	2	1	0.5
Common salt	1	1	1	2
Calcite powder	–	–	1	1.5
Molasses	5	5	6	8
CP %	22	22	22	16
TDN %	74	74	72	69

mix, mineral mixture, protected protein, protected amino acids, protected fat, toxin binders, pellet-binders, herbal complex, flavours, pesticides, etc. are useful supplements which have not only increased quality of the feed, but also improved animal performance. The improved feed processing technologies have also increased feed quality and quantity at reasonably low cost.

Protected Feed Nutrients in Feed Industry

Recently the protected feed nutrients are taking its entry into feed formulations, though at slow rate. Energy is the first limiting nutrient affecting the productivity of animals. Higher levels of grains in the ruminant diet have been found to reduce fibre digestion and in many cases cause acidosis which further effects functioning of rumen and alters physiological function in the animal body. Concurrent to this, the energy utilization from cereal grains is improved when it is digested post-ruminally, is an encouraging one. Several methods have been recommended from time to time to bring a shift in the site of digestion of such feeds without altering the rumen function. Some success in this direction has been achieved by treatment of grains with formaldehyde. The formaldehyde forms cross linkages with starch which prevent swelling of starch granules or there may be a formation of protein matrix which become resistant to microbial action. Thus protecting the underlying starch granules. Formaldehyde treatment at 1 per cent level increased fibre digestion in the rumen and also availability of glucose in the intestine which favoured higher production. Maize and sorghum grains have higher level of naturally protected starch than Barley grains. The total tract digestibility of starch in barley, maize and sorghum were reported similar but their ruminal digestion was 93, 73 and 66 per cent, and hence the amount of rumen escape starch was 7, 27 and 34 per cent in barley, maize and sorghum, respectively. Actually, non-structural carbohydrate include starch, sugar and fructan. The energy reserve in grain is mostly in the form of starch. Wheat has the highest content of starch for the grains (77%), followed by corn and sorghum (72%) and then by barley (57%), and oats (58%).

The densified source of energy to ruminants is through fat. BIS recommended 2.5 to 3.0 per cent fat in concentrate feed. However, recent reports indicated that there should be at least 5 per cent fat in total mixed ration beyond that depression in milk yield may occur. Higher levels of fat decrease fibre digestibility in the rumen. However, protected or prilled fat could be incorporated up to 9 per cent in the diet. The optimum recommended level of fat content varies from 4 to 6 per cent of the total diet of high yielders which may be 1/3rd from natural feed, 1/3rd from oil seed and 1/3rd from by-pass source.

In early lactation period, particularly of high yielders and in growing animals where growth rate is rapid, the microbial protein synthesized in the rumen is not adequate to meet the total amino acid requirement and so it has to be supplemented with the by-pass protein. Formaldehyde treatment (1.2 g per 100 g protein) may be effectively applied to oilseed meal during or after manufacture, or to milled feeds during mixing or prior to pelleting. The treated material may be held in plastic bags or silos for several days before feeding. The protected protein escape ruminal degradation and digested in abomasum and small intestine. The ruminal undegradability of protein in selected feeds is presented in Table 5.

The quantities of total amino acids leaving the abomasum and absorbed from the intestines are markedly increased when fed on formaldehyde treated protein. Roasted soybean, soybean meal (extruded) and soybean oil cake are rich blend of both by-pass protein as well as bypass fat (Table 6). Supplementation of ruminally protected methionine and lysine to high yielders also increase milk production, fibre digestibility as well as acetate level and acetate:propionate ratio improved. The success in lactational output depends on how fast feed industry adopt these techniques and incorporate protected feed nutrients into feed formulations.

Table 5. Rumen undegradability of protein in selected feeds

Feed	Crude protein %	Undegra-dability	RDP (g/kg DM)	UPD (g/kg DM)
Babul seed meal	15.9	0.42	92	67
Coconut cake	25.4	0.44	142	112
HCHO		0.62	97	157
Cotton seed cake	38.2	0.47	202	180
Cotton seed extraction	41.0	0.60	164	246
Gingely oil cake	36.9	0.45	203	166
Groundnut cake	42.9	0.26	317	112
HCHO		0.52	206	223
Guar meal	43.4	0.17	360	74
Kranja cake	33.4	0.45	184	150
Mustard seed cake	34.1	0.12	300	41
HCHO		0.69	106	235
Niger seed cake	32.0	0.39	195	125
Rape seed meal	36.6	0.21	289	77
HCHO		0.79	77	289
Safflower cake	32.3	0.29	229	94
Soybean meal	50.7	0.46	274	233
HCHO		0.69	157	350
Heat		0.64	183	324
Extrusion		0.59	208	299
Sunflower cake	30.1	0.46	163	138
HCHO		0.63	111	190
Soybean full fat	38.0	0.26	281	99

Table 6. Chemical composition of soymeals

Proximate analysis	Soymeal (extruded)	Soymeal (expeller)
DM	93.0	94.0
Crude protein	38.0	46.0
Crude fat	18.0	7.0
Crude fibre	5.2	5.5
Ash	4.5	5.3
Undegradable protein (% CP)	65.0	52.0
Free fatty acids	1.0	0.5
Linoleic acid	9.0	4.5
Linolenic acid	2.0	0.9
Lecithin	0.7	0.2
ME Mcal/g	4.14	3.43
TDN (%)	107.0	88.0
NDF (%)	12.0	11.0
ADF (%)	11.0	10.0

Concept of Complete Feed in Feed Industry

Feeding of total mixed ration or complete feed to dairy animals is a departure from conventional feeding system. In case of conventional system, the concentrate requirement is worked out separately. It may be fed individually or mixed with dry roughage. In this case, animals may have more access to concentrate than the roughage. However, the green fodder is offered separately. In case of complete feed system, the chaffed roughages whether dry or green are evenly mixed in a proper proportion with the desired amount of concentrate and fed to animals according to their requirement as such (mash form) or converted to cubes/pellets or blocks. In this case, the animals cannot have selective eating and there is energy sparing action from the forage, particularly low grade roughages (Table 7).

Various feed processing techniques are applied for manufacturing complete feed in the form of total mixed ration:

Table 7. Saving of energy through the concept of complete feed system

Total available crop residues	300 MT
Crop residues used by dairy animals (40 % of total)	120 MT
Available TDN to dairy animals (40 % TDN)	48 MT
Expected increase in TDN on complete feeds (10 %)	60 MT
Net saving of energy (TDN)	12 MT

(a) Mash mix

Roughages whether green or dry or in the form of silage are finely chaffed and evenly mixed with the ground concentrate prepared for this purpose.

(b) Pellets/cubes/blocks

The mash mix is compressed and densified into different shapes or sizes, such as pellets/cubes or blocks with the help of specific machines designed to present in a desired shape.

Changing the physical form of the feed has reflected on the performance characteristics of the animals. The total mixed ration is widely fed in large dairy operations and feed lots of the United States, Israel and United Kingdom where green roughages, silage, hay, straw and concentrate are mixed mechanically in a trolley having blending arrangement. The mixed ration so obtained is allotted to animals as per their needs. For additional requirements to the high yielding cows, a supplementary concentrate mix is offered separately. In such combination, the level of concentrate may vary from 50 to 60 per cent of the diet. In the developing countries where green fodder availability is negligible, only crop residues are being used as roughage source. It has been reported that pelleting increased DM intake but depressed the digestibility. It has been reported that cubes or pellets of dried grass passed through the digestive tract more quickly and had a lower digestibility than the long material. For diets based on silage, the particle length of chopped forage of 10 to 20 mm ensures uniform mix with cereals and other ingredients.

The pellet mill operated with 5 HP electric motor has the capacity of pelleting 150 kg feed per hour on fresh basis. For preparation of pellets, dry tree leaves or chopped fodder and concentrate mixture in the ratio of 40:60 mixed manually. Water is added to maintain the moisture at 50 per cent level. The moist mixture is then passed through the pellet mills. The pellets obtained are dried under the sun. The cost of pelleting works out to be Rs.15 per 100 kg complete feed.

However, the production of complete feed blocks using hydraulic compressing machine has been standardized with a capacity of 60 blocks per hour (weight of each block 14 kg). It has been tested commercially that available crop residues (wheat straw/paddy straw/jowar, bajra, maize stovers/sunflower straw/ cotton straw/mustard straw etc.) mixed with balance concentrate mixture and converted into compacted blocks had the potentials to sustain 20 kg milk production in the crossbred cows. The nutrients requirement of animals differ as per stage of lactation. Therefore, dietary specifications also differ (Table 8).

Table 8. Specifications for total diet of animal

	Far-off dry cow	Closeup dry cow	Early lactation	Mid-late lactation
Crude protein (%)	12-13	14-15	17-19	15-17
Rumen undegraded protein (% of crude protein)	-	-	36-40	32-36
Acid detergent fiber (%)	28-32	22-26	19-21	21-22
Neutral detergent fiber (%)	38-42	30-34	28-32	32-36
Non-fiber carbohydrates (%)	32-34	34-36	37-40	34-37
Fat (%)	2-3	2-3	3-7	3-6

The concept to prepare complete feed blocks emerged from National Dairy Research Institute, Karnal during early 90's and were commercially prepared for the first time in the country by M/s. Anmol Feeds Pvt. Ltd. at Bulandshahr (U.P.) under the guidance from experts of that Institute. The product was marketed in Delhi and Bombay. Later on, the concept was adopted by M/s. Poshak Feeds (India) Pvt. Ltd. at Karnal (Haryana) during the year 2000 again under the expert guidance of NDRI. M/s. Poshak Feeds marketed the products of 10% CP and 14% CP successfully for cattle yielding 12 kg and 18 kg milk per day in different states in the country.

The "Hydraulic Machines "Employed to Densify Complete Feed Blocks were prepared by M/S Advance Hydrau-Tech Pvt.Ltd., New Delhi. The Machines were continuously updated by that company and improved the output from 20 Blocks to 75 Blocks of 14 kgs weight Per Hour. Now another Agency, "Indian Fodder Care & Technologies Pvt. Ltd". New Delhi has taken up responsibility to provide facilities to "Densify Fodder" on turn -key Basis.

Punjab Agricultural University, Ludhiana has also recently (year 2004) worked on TMR and suggested to feed a combination of 55 kg green fodder and 10 kg concentrate of 18% CP to cows yielding 30 kg milk per day and a combination of 40 kg green fodder, 2 kg wheat straw and 2 kg concentrate of 18% CP to cows yielding 10 kg milk per day. M/s. Godrej Agrovet at Khanna (Punjab) has also recently (year 2004) taken initiative to produce and market complete feed blocks. Certain feed manufacturers at Khanna/ Kurukshetra have started work towards commercial approach to produce complete feed pellets. The guidelines for preparing own TMR using compound concentrate mixture and crop residues have been given in Table 9.

Table 9. Guidelines for preparing feed mix

Upto 10 kg milk production Mix 42 to 45% concentrate mixture of 22% protein and 55 to 58% crop residues
Upto 15 kg milk production Mix 48 to 50% concentrate mixture of 22% protein and 50 to 52% crop residues
Upto 18 kg milk production Mix 55 to 58% concentrate mixture of 22% protein and 42 to 45% crop residues

This is just a small deviation from concentrate feed production to complete feed production. This momentum is to be encouraged so that our livestock get wholesome and balanced feed. The success of these projects depends upon the availability of cost effective and efficient compacting machines. Crop residues as roughage source are deficient in protein, non-fibrous carbohydrates, minerals and vitamins, it must, therefore, be substantiated with high quality protein as well as oil resource for producing productive complete feed blocks. The American Soybean Association in India has given a slogan to use roasted soybean, soymeal extruded or soymeal expeller in cattle feed formulation since the by-pass protein of such product is above 50 per cent and it is also an effective source of by-pass fat. The new concept has not only provided opportunity for effective utilization of crop residues of the country but has revolutionized the feeding system of dairy animals. Even illiterate dairy farmer can provide balanced nutrition to their animal.

Constraints towards Future Development

1. Control on Quality

All the suggested specifications for feed formulations demand revision since new concepts for feeding high yielding animals have recently emerged (level of by-pass protein/by-pass fat/ NDF/NFC etc.). Feed cannot be prepared of desired quality unless ingredients used are of desired specification. BIS should prepare and enforce standards for feed ingredients both on sellers and buyers. Also should enforce each feed manufacturer to maintain a quality control laboratory having facilities to analyse at least proximate principles of feed ingredients as well as finished product of the factory (Table 10).

Table 10. Principal parameters to be considered in different feed ingredients for analysis

Feed Ingredient	Moisture	Protein	EE	CF	AIA	Ca	P	Others
Maize and other cereal grains	✓							Mycotoxins
Ragi	✓			✓	✓			
Sorghum	✓							Tannins
Rice bran and rice polishings	✓	✓	✓	✓				Iodine number
DORB	✓	✓		✓	✓			
Salseed meal	✓	✓						Tannins
Soybean, full fat	✓	✓	✓	✓				Urease activity
Soybean meal	✓	✓		✓	✓			Urease activity
Groundnut meal	✓	✓	✓	✓				Nonprotein nitrogen
Groundnut meal extraction	✓	✓		✓				Nonprotein nitrogen
Sunflower meal	✓	✓	✓	✓				Mycotoxins
Copra meal	✓	✓	✓	✓				Mycotoxins
Mustard meal	✓	✓	✓	✓				Mycotoxins
Guar Meal	✓	✓	✓	✓				Mycotoxins
Safflower Meal	✓	✓		✓	✓			Mycotoxins
Cottonseed meal	✓	✓		✓				Gossypol
Dicalcium phosphate	✓				✓	✓	✓	Loss on ignition
Rock phosphate	✓				✓	✓	✓	Magnesium Fluorine
Calcite powder	✓				✓	✓		
Oil	✓		✓					Iodine number
Molasses	✓							Sugar brick test

2. Availability of Feed Stuffs

Country is short of protein as well as energy resources. Protein is made available through oil seed meals. Despite demand from domestic feed industry, India exports large quantities of solvent extractions, mainly soybean meal to earn foreign exchange. The maximum export is for the high class protein source, which should immediately be checked.

The food grain production was 212 million tonnes during the year 2003, major share goes to wheat and rice. The grains which are commonly used for feed production are maize, barley, wheat, sorghum, millet, broken rice, etc. Maize grain is used in bulk which is also shared by starch industry as well as for human consumption. Hardly half the produce is available for animal and poultry feed Barley grain is also shared by brewery industry. Sorghum and millets are also shared by starch industry and human consumption. The grain on neglect storing and handling are declared unfit for human consumption, and ultimately takes its entrance in animal feed industry. Such products, even if used at lower level in the feed, certainly reflect on animal health as well as production. Even the broken rice as such is not spared for animal feed. It is further graded, the better one is used as adulterant in wheat flour and the second quality pushed to feed industry. All the cereal grains are graded, the second quality goes to feed industry.

3. Import/Export Policy

Instead of importing oil, we should import oilseeds. It shall keep the extraction plants to work for full capacity and oil seed meal be available for feed industry. Thus, instead of exporting feed ingredients, we shall be able to export compound feed.

From April 2000, imports have been allowed under the open general licence. But with 15 per cent duty and grain inspection fee, there is no price priority. Under such constraints, it is difficult to import maize. Emphasis should be laid on export of milk and milk products so that farmers get remunerative price for milk and, in turn, be prepared to use more compound feed.

4. Regulations on Animal Feed Industry

Bureau of Indian Standards (BIS) has published animal feed standards as guidelines. Industry has also framed guidelines in their own way. There should be common consensus and the specifications updated. There should be offical compulsion on the industry to strictly follow it.

In some states, sales tax of 4 per cent has been imposed on animal feeds which is ultimately a burden on the consumers. Since dairying is a developing sector, so, it requires more support from the government by which the sale price of the feed is reduced rather to increase it by putting tax on it.

Overhead charges on feed production which include labour on processing, electricity, maintenance of equipment, packaging, technical personnel, laboratory expenses, transport, margin of the owner etc. varies from Rs.80 to Rs.160 per quintal. The ingredients.procurement price is also exaggerated. There should be some common consensus to work out such charges so that the sale rate should be most competitive.

The feed industry should be liberal to import animal feed supplement or additives and these items should be placed under free category for import. On the import of essential amino acids (analogue), government has reduced import duty to 10 per cent but countervailing duty (CVD) is still there. To promote animal husbandry, government should delete all such duties.

5. Emphasis on Diversification of Cropping Pattern

The production of wheat and rice has already reached certain height and now there should be a shift on the specific cropping pattern so as to put more area under oilseed crops and selected cereal crops like maize and barley. The oilseeds production has declined in the last 4 years from the level of 24.7 million tonnes in 1998-99 to 18 million tonnes in 2002-03. The yield of the crops is hardly 60 per cent of the world average. Similarly, yield of maize and barley is also low compared to the developed countries. The productivity of oilseeds and cereal grains could be increased manifold either by the import of productive seed or strengthening the research inputs to evolve high yielding varieties in the country.

6. Anti-nutritional Factors in Protein Meals

The anti-nutritional factors present in the oil meals are well known (Table 11), some are destroyed during heat processing and few got degraded by the rumen microflora. Unhealthy storing of oil seed meals and grains promote fungal growth and development of mycotoxins. For taking preventive measures, the feed manufacturers should use toxin binders in their formulations. Controlling the mycotoxin contamination should be given top priority as it not only affects the livestock health but also the human due to the residues in the products.

The success of animal feed industry depends upon :

- To secure the confidence of consumer towards quality product.
- To supply him the cost effective product.

For achieving above, the feed manufacturers should adopt the following points on priority:

1. Educate consumer on the quality of product.
2. Use healthy raw material.
3. Formulate the product on the basis of currently available concepts and technologies.
4. Claim only one margin, i.e., on sale of the product, leaving the other margin, i.e., on purchase of ingredients to the dairy farmer.

Table 11. Anti-nutritional factors of Asian protein meals

Ingredients	Anti-nutritional factors
Soybeans meal	Protease inhibitors*, allergens*, oligosaccharides, phytin, lipoxygenase*, lecithins*, saponin
Rapeseed meal	'Erucic acid, glucosinoloates, sinapine, tannins, pectins, oligosaccharides
Canola meal	Gossypol, cyclopropenoid fatty acids, tannins
Sunflower meal	Clorogenic acid, fibre
Fish meal	Oxidised fat, high minerals, biogenic amines
Peanut meal	Mycotoxins, tannins, oligosaccharides, protease inhibitors*, lecithins
Copra meal	Fibre, mannans
Palm Kernel meal	Fibre and sharp shells, galactomannans

*Destroyed during heat processing.

2
DESIGN AND DEVELOPMENT OF FEED PLANT

D.M. Bhandarkar, Prakash P. Ambalkar and Jai Singh

They demand of high valued aqua/poultry/dairy/processed meat and products of animal origin is increasing rapidly in domestic as well as export market. For strengthen and consolidation of agrarian economy, tapping of tremendously vast potential of natural wealth of animal planet of India seems to be the panacea as income/ employment generation source of Indian farmer/ rural youth. Scientific, systematic and planned adoption of practice like combination of crop/livestock/ fishery farming system horizontally (complementary activities) and vertically (as agribusiness) at small and large scale. The biggest advantage for farming community micro level from this will be the by product use and improved space utilization. However integrated system may depend in part on the use of agro-industrial products such as commercial inorganic fertilizer balance with organic manure and consumption of nutritionally complete or formulated pelleted feed.

Integrated system will help in meeting availability of quality feed in acceptable form, which is a major constraint as an essential technological input for the success of profitable commercial aquaculture/ animal husbandry ventures. Though the hatchery and feed plant models have been installed in India but their engineering designs and models are not still available. Therefore, there is a need to develop indigenous designed models of feed plants to reduce the dependency on foreign countries for import of formulated feed for fish growers/ animal rarer of commercial values. Initially from capacity utilization point of view for economic modeling and development of feed plant, it is better to assess the aqua/poultry/ dairy scenario of the country. Further, design and development of the feed plant can be segregated on the basis availability of based on demand of pelleted feed area (geography) / income / demography and education/ socio-cultural market segments.

General Assessment Of Existing Potential Of Aqua/ Poultry / Dairy Animal Planet In India

If we look Indian scenario at aquaculture production front, data reveals information that at present, India's inland annual fish production is about 2.82

million tonnes. However, the estimated inland potential based on the present levels of productivity is about 4.50 million tonness. If modern states of art technologies, are used there is a vast untapped potential, which can be exploited. With nearly 250 million potential consumers, there is a tremendous potential in domestic market. The fish exports from India are rising. The export earnings, which were Rs 51170 million in 1999-2000, have increased to Rs 63000 million in 2000-1. The major export is of shrimp (almost 70% in value terms).

As far as poultry sector of India is concerned there is annual growth rate of 8-10% in egg and 12-15% in the broiler industry. With the annual production of 33 billion eggs, India is the fifth world's largest egg producing country. It also produces 530 million broilers per year. Poultry provides employment to about 1.5 million people. The annual per capita consumption in India is only 33 eggs and 630 grams of poultry meat. This is much lower as compared to the world average of 124 eggs and 5.9 kg meat. The National Committee on Human Nutrition in India has recommended per capita 180 eggs (about one egg on alternate day) and 10.8 kg meat .To meet this target, it is estimated that by year 2010, the requirements will be 180 billion eggs and 9.1 billion kg poultry meat while the estimated production may only be around 46.2 billion eggs and 3.04 billion kg poultry meat. This shows that there is a tremendous scope for growth with rapid urbanization and increasing demand from the present 250 million economically strong, consumer market base (which is likely to go up to 350 million by year 2010).

Similarly in dairy sector with an estimated 86.8 million tonnes of annual milk production from animals managed by nearly 70 million farmers, India is the top-most milk producing country in the world. The average annual growth is about 5.6%. Per capita milk availability is about 214 gm per day as against the recommended requirement of 250 gm. Milk is one of the most important items of common vegetarian diet of Indian people. With rapid industrialization, economic growth and 250 million potential economically strong domestic consumers of milk and milk products, there is a very strong potential for future growth of the industry. Milk yield has been targeted from the current low level of 500 l/annum/ per cattle due to inadequate feeding and mismanagement to 1000-2000 l/annum in the short term to 2400-3000 l/annum/per cattle in the long term.

Methodology for Design of Feed Plant

It is generally agreed that mass production is justified only when production quantities are large and product variety small. The ideal situation for mass production would be when large volumes of formulated pelleted feed (without any change in design set up of feed plant) are to be produced continuously for an extended period of time to cater the need of aqua/ avian/ bovine/ goat/sheep and angora rabbit culture etc. Here, in feed plant design the rate of consumption of feed (or demand) as compared to the rate of production of feed needs to be balanced. This can be done through continuous production where no change in design of plant is required only replacement of die in pellet mill and screen of grinder will serve the purpose of continuity in production process.

Demand Forecasting and Measurement of Capacity Requirement of Proposed Feed Plant

It is based on demand function; a comprehensive formulation, which specifies the factors, that influences the demand for the nutritionally complete or scientifically formulated pelleted feed can be exercised as follows:

Dx = D (Px, Py, Pz, B, W, A, E, T, U)

Here, Dx, stands for demand for pelleted feed
Px, per kg price of feed,
Py, per kg price of substitutes like unprocessed mixture of raw feed ingredients

Pz, the price of it's complements like raw materials, fuel, electricity and labour

B, the income (budget) of the consumer i.e aqua / avian/ terrestrial animal culture farmer

W, the wealth of the consumer (farmer) as animal rarer ,

A, the advertisement and wide publicity of the feed

E, the price expectation of the producer

T, the price expectation of feed consumer and

U, all other factors such as socio-cultural and environmental impact.

It is based on above demand analysis, which seeks to identify and measure the forces that determine the sale of feed. It reflects the market conditions for the feed produced from the plant. Once the demand analysis is done, the alternative ways of creating, controlling or managing demand can be inferred for planning and creation of capacity, which always requires investments. Capacity is the limiting capability of a feed plant unit to produce within a stated time period, normally expressed in terms of output in units per unit of time. However, the limiting capability of feed plant also depends on the intensiveness of use of the scientifically formulated and processed feed in the form of pellets. Since here feed plant produces relatively homogeneous feed for animal culture hence it's capacity can be measured in number of units of output per unit of time as feed produced in q/h can be set as an standard example for design and development of modules of multipurpose feed plant. One such plant of 01q/h capacity production for aqua feed is designed and installed at CIAE, Bhopal. The scope of the aqua feed pilot plant was further augmented for production of feed for avian/ bovine farming.

The Plant (Fig 1 and 2) constitutes following unit operation processing machines.

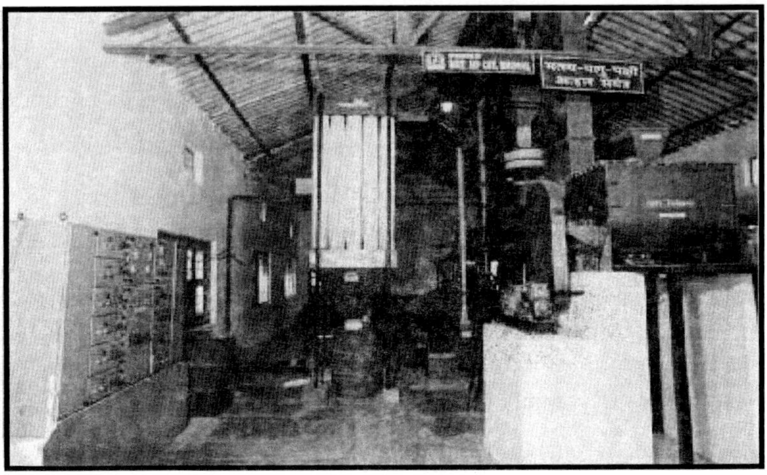

Fig.1. Aqua Feed Plant, Front View

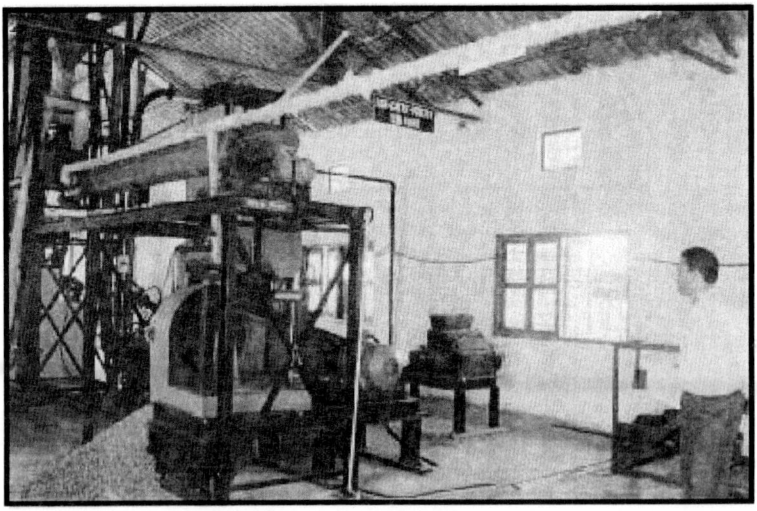

Fig.2. Aqua Feed Plant, Rear View

Pre- Mixer

It is a horizontal mixer used for dry mixing of various feed ingredients. It comprises spiral clamped alloy steel shaft, feeding hopper, and discharge slide gate into elevator, 3 hp, 1440-rpm electric motor, gearbox, sprocket and chain.

Bucket-Elevator

It is used to lift the mixture of ingredients supplied from pre-mixer up to the top most height of plant (9.7m) from the floor level and transfers it to a material holding hopper to regulate the flow of mixture according to the capacity of grinder installed below. The bucket-elevator comprises 15 cm rubber belt, boot pulley, 100 x 100 mm bucket, 1hp motor (1440-rpm) & worm reduction gear.

Gyro Screen

The material received from bucket elevator gets ground here. It is a swinging hammer type miracle (hammer) mill used to grind mixture of de- oiled (DO) rice bran/ wheat bran, DO soya cake, DO mustard cake, maize, fish meal etc. into desirable mesh size. The machine comprises 3-hp, 1440 rpm motor, screen and holding hopper, V-belt/coupler leading to outlet of dust suction system.

Dust Collection System

The discharged ground material from grinder having finer dust particles get sucked through suitably matching pipe/ duct which is ultimately collected into the dust bags. Dust collection system comprises aspirator, ducts and dust bags. The unit is operated by 2 hp, 1440-rpm electric motor.

Gyro (Vibro) Screen Shifter

The material left out after separation of fine particles needs to be screened, graded and shifted to paddle –conveyor-mixture as standard particle size required for pelletization. The coarse and oversize material is shifted from outlet to premixer for re-grinding or discarded. The screen shifter machine vibrates in horizontal plane as well as in the circular vertical direction. It is driven by 0.5hp, 1440-rpm motor.

Molasses Pump

The hot molasses from the molasses tank gets sucked through this unit and is supplied to moisten the ground material discharged from the gyro screen outlet in to paddle-mixer- conveyor. It comprises of 3 hp, 1440 rpm motor, control valve, spray nozzle in-let, out-let & by-pass piping.

Steam Generator (Boiler)

The coil type water tube steam boiler is installed to supply steam at 100^0 C and above, with steam output capacity of 100kg/h and steam pressure of 10.5 kg/cm^2 fired by light diesel oil or furnace oil (gross combustion value 10,250-10,700 kCal/kg). Steam is supplied by1.5 hp motor to the jacket of paddle-mixer-conveyor for cooking /conditioning of feed material.

Paddle-Mixer-Conveyor

It is used to mix, moisten (14-18 % moisture content) and heat up the milled material received from gyro-screen with hot molasses and provided with jacket for hot/ cold water/ steam to optimize the cooking process for different feeds. It is driven by 2hp, 1440-rpm motor with worm gear with chain and gear drive.

Steam Conditioner

The moistened mix from the paddle-mixture-conveyor is delivered into the conditioner where steam treatment is given to condition the mixed material before pelletization. Here, steam adds moisture, liberates natural oils, acts as disinfectant and in some cases gelatinize the starch ingredient of feed.

Pellet Mill

Conditioned material is discharged into the mouth of the pellet mill. The pellet mill is provided with a pair of stationary rollers and a revolving die. During operation the roller press the conditioned material through die to form pellets. A set of two cutters has been provided to produce pellets of desired length ranging between 12 mm to 30mm. Choosing the die of 3/4/6/8/10 mm size can change the pellet diameter. The mill is driven by 30 hp motor, 1440 rpm with shear pin arrangement as protection device due to overload.

Pellet Crumbler

The cooled dried pellets from pellet mill will be taken to pellet crumbler, if required to break pellets into desired size pieces fit for the mouth opening of cultured species like prawn, fingerling and poultry breeder etc. It comprises of two engraved rollers with adjustable gap where roll pressure is mechanically created by helical rings. It is driven by 1hp, 1440-rpm motor.

Sieve Separator

A power operated mechanically balanced reciprocating sieve is provided to separate the pellets from pellet dust and mesh powder form during pelletization.

It is also used to grade the crumbled pellets in to fine, medium and coarse grain sizes as per the size of species cultured. It is driven by 0 .5hp, 1440 rpm motor.

Electric Control Panel

Electric controls for different power units have been combined on a single panel for convenient operation of the entire plant and it's maintenance. All power points are connected through cables, safety fuses, illuminated indicators and switchgears.

Structure, Platform - Walkways

The structure made of angle iron, iron channels, steel ladder and chequered plates have been provided to support, position and easy approach for maintenance of the different units/ machines as well as to provide walking space for the operator and service engineer.

Space Requirement Of The Entire Installed Plant

The plant is installed in shed (ACC roof) of 12 m length x 8 m width x 5.7 m height. The ceiling height is further raised 4m above the truss ridge in the form of a box of 5.3 x 3m to accommodate elevator, grinder, hoppers and gyro screen along with working platforms.

Total Connecting Power Requirement

A connecting electrical load of 45 hp (33 kw) is required for the entire plant. However, the running electrical load comes around 30 hp (22.5 kw).

Storage Equipment & Facility

In a manufacturing business of feed one can encounter stores of raw materials or feed ingredients, small consumables such as single phase coils, couplings, bearings, belt, chain and sprocket and swinging bars of hammer mill and buckets of elevator and nut-bolts, washers and lubricants (List of spare parts given by manufacturer). Tools such as spanners, screw wrenches, pliers, safety fuses, indicator lamps etc. need to be stored. Goods in course of production such as ground maize, fishmeal and feed in mesh form and finished feed in pellet form may be stored with different racks in one separate storage compartment. It is preferable to keep raw ingredients and finished feed in their own separate stores. Small consumable material, parts and tools are often housed in a further separate store, but are sometimes to be found in a separate section of the main raw materials stores.

The fixing of maximum and minimum levels of raw ingredients of feed in store reliable source of supplier, supplier's delivery time and premonition of scarcity of essential ingredients etc. Stocks should be reordered when the reorder level is reached, which may be fixed at or somewhat above the minimum stock level as circumstances warrant. In CIAE feed plant the raw ingredients and finished feed are stored in metallic bins 08 nos. and 02 nos. resp. (10 quintal capacity each). The tools and spares are also housed in small steel cabinets / racks for efficient and easy retrieval in the store section. For packaging material and packed finished feed is stored in 3.3X 3.3 m separate racks.

The continuous progress of feed production from feed plant is dependent on it's ability to optimally and judiciously allocate and utilize it's basic resources, technology, skill and knowledge such as money (capital resources), machine (feed plant machinery and equipment), men (human resources skilled/ semi-skilled and unskilled), material (raw feed ingredients), motive power (light diesel fuel and electrical energy), meters (space or premises to install the feed plant), method (production of pelleted feed through pellet mill), minutes (time scheduling of feed production to fulfill the accepted demand) and management (effective, innovative and imaginative management to reduce wastage and enhancement of quality production). This undertaken so as to provide desired quality products and/ or services in the form of feed production as complete ration at the right time, place, price, quality and quantity to the fish grower/ animal rarer community.

Modular design and development of feed plant may be recommended on the basis of scale- up and downsizing of feed plant designed and established at CIAE, Bhopal, the feed so produced will not only be nutritionally complete, palatable, digestible, durable, acceptable and easy to transport but also would be economical. However, this requires the need for adopting scientific, systematic and integrated approach to work design so as to have more production and less waste.

The proper planning and design of the housing of raw feed ingredients, storing equipment such as bins and racks, and material handling equipment such as iron trolley in store system is important for the efficient and smooth operation of the feed plant since, raw material constitutes the major fraction of cost i.e. 60 to 80 percent of total feed production cost. The CIAE feed plant store is designed for keeping raw material, spare parts and tools section adjacent to the plant pre-mixer unit and then the finished feed and packaging material is housed next to raw material storage (3mx3m) section in compartment with proper racks and material handling devices.

Techno-economic feasibility of the feed plant at CIAE, Bhopal for manufacturing feed for aqua/ birds/ bovine rearing was carried out. The Break Even Point (BEP) on output unit of 281 tons of aqua feed production, the BEP on selling price @ Rs.10/- is found Rs. 28,12,500/- for 100kg/h capacity. The Pay Back Period is 4.63 years on 11.8% net profit margin or also it is 2.73 years on 20% net profit margin. On the basis of pay back period, 4.63years, the Internal Rate of Return (IRR) is found to be of 18.9%. The total capital investment on equipment and shed incurred is Rs. 13.30 lakh, wherein working capital (operational expenditure) for 3 months is Rs. 10.30 lakh. Since the IRR is higher than the interest rate used to work out the cost of funds, the techno-economic feasibility study on feed plant suggest that the economic viability signifies investment prudence on feed plant in rural sector.

Further, stores management is concerned with carrying the right kind of materials in right quantity, neither in excess nor in short supply, providing it quickly as and when required, keeping it safe against any kind of deterioration, pilferage or theft, and to carry out the efficient performance of all these functions at lowest possible cost.

Bibliography

Course MS-5 (2001), Work & Job Design, Volumes III , Management of Machines and Materials, MBA programme from Indira Gandhi National Open University, New Delhi, pp 06-& 26.

Course MS-9 (2001) Demand Decision, Volumes II, Managerial Economics, MBA programme from Indira Gandhi National Open University, New Delhi pp- 77 to 100.

Edwards Peter, 1994, A Systems Approach for the Promotion of Integrated Aquaculture, Integrated Fish Farming International Workshop, Wuxi, People's Republic of China pp 1-7.

Instruction Manuals (2000) of aqua feed plant and installation of plant established at CIAE, Bhopal.

Kaulgud Aruna (2003), Entrepreneurship Management, Vikas Publishing House Pvt. Ltd.,

576, Masjid Road, Jangpura, New Delhi- 110 014 pp-182.

Singh Jai and Singh G. (2000) Brochure on Aqua Feed Pilot Plat, CIAE, Bhopal.

3
AQUA FEED PLANT-OPERATION AND MAINTENANCE

D.M. Bhandarkar, Prakash P. Ambalkar and Jai Singh

Operation means process of changing resource inputs into some useful form of outputs. The optimal solution to produce output of desired characteristics defines operation research. Choosing optimal (best under the circumstances and for the purpose) process of conversion system is an important decision concerning choice of technology, equipment and machines. Therefore, the output of an operation (or production) system may be in terms of desired end product for example conversion of raw feed ingredients into aqua feed pellets with quality specifications viz. nutritionally balanced, economical, digestible, palatable, acceptable, water stable, minimizes waste output & effect on water quality, produces desirable final product which is also found durable (to withstand rigors of handling and delivery of bulk supply of pellet s), attractive and safe.

The aqua feed production system follows straight flow characteristics. Facilities are arranged according to sequence of processing operations where the output of one stage becomes the input to the next stage(flow chart). However, major operational management problems in mass production of aqua feed are- alignment and balancing of production/ assembly lines, unit operation machine maintenance and to ensure timely supply of raw materials.

Process operational planning pertains to careful detailing of processing technology of resource conversion required and their sequence. Maintenance becomes important because if any production stage is under breakdown it will block the whole line unless quickly restored back into operational effectiveness. Raw material to first stage is important to avoid shortage and subsequent starvation of the whole line.

Methodology

Under Alignment and Balancing of Production/ Assembly lines

For cost effective feed production first the procurement of raw feed ingredients is ensured based on practical considerations such as - ingredients price and availability, anti-nutritional factors, pelletability of mixture and storage and handling requirements. Here planning is required for material procurement actions through development of reliable sources of supplies so that the demand of product can be satisfied reasonably well without having to stock (in inventory) too much of material so as to avoid pilferage, wastage and storage losses.

Various solid raw ingredients as per formulation suitable for species cultured (for fish and prawn feed given in Table 1 and 2 respectively) are fed into the horizontal mixer. After mixing it gets discharged into the bucket elevator. From bucket elevator the mixed feed material is fed into the hopper. The material will be discharged from the hopper into the hammer mill i.e. grinder. The rate of flow into the hammer mill is controlled by slide gate below the hopper. After the grinding the material will be discharged into collecting hopper for temporary stay and smooth fall here aspiration system and dust collection chamber is provided to reduce the dust problem.

Each process under unit operation as segment of production line is depicted below

Flow Chart

Raw Materials/ Ingredients Planning (Inventory Evaluation)

↓

Raw Material/ Components and Spare Parts Procurement

↓

Pre- Mixing

↓

Elevator

↓

Temporary Holding Through Hopper

↓

Grinder

↓

Temporary Holding Through Collection Hopper

↓

Gyro Screening — Coarse Material (back to Pre- Mixing)

↓

Molasses → Paddle- Mixture-Conveyor → Cooking through Hot Water Jacket

↓

Steam Generation & Supply → Conditioner

↓

Pelletization and Pellet Ejection

↓

Pellets Cutting as per desired Pellet Length

↓

Pellet Sieving for powder separation, if any

↓

Pellet Crumbling (size reduction for small specie like Prawn)

↓

Form of Feed

Feed in Mesh Form | Crumbled Feed | Pelleted Feed for Fish | Pelleted Feed for Cattle

↓

Feed Packaging & Transport

Each above process is required to be properly balanced with mutual alignment in the entire set up of assembly line for smooth and trouble free operation.

Table 1 Formulation of fish feed and its cost.

S. No.	Details of Raw Feed Ingredients	Percent content ingredient per kg feed (%)	Protein % ingredient (gm/kg	Per kg cost of ingredient (Rs)	Percent cost of ingredient (Rs)
01	De- Oiled Rice Bran	20	28	4.50	0.90
02	De-Oiled Soya Cake	40	184	7.00	2.80
03	Fish Meal	25	135	15.00	3.75
04	Molasses	08	6.4	9.00	0.72
05	Maize	05	2.5	7.00	0.35
06	Soya Oil	02	0.4	50.00	1.00
	Sub Total of Protein and Raw Ingredients Cost	100	353.1		9.52
07	Processing Expenditure on Fuel, Electricity, Labour, Repair and Maintenance, Interest, Depreciation, Insurance, Wastage and Handling				1.48
08	Net Profit Earned per kg of Fish Feed				Rs. 1.00
09	Price of Feed Produced at Plant Site				Rs 12.00/kg
10	The Packaging and Forwarding Charge is Rs 50/quintal for minimum order of 02 quintal.				

Table 2 Formulation of prawn feed and its cost.

S. No.	Details of Raw Feed Ingredients	Percent content ingredient per kg feed (%)	Protein % ingredient (gm/kg	Per kg cost of ingredient (Rs)	Percent cost of ingredient (Rs)
01	De- Oiled Rice Bran	10	14	4.50	0.45
02	De-Oiled Soya Cake	40	184	7.00	2.80
03	Fish Meal	40	224	15.00	6.00
04	Molasses	08	6.4	9.00	0.72
05	Soya Oil	02	0.4	50.00	1.00
	Sub Total of Protein and Raw Ingredients Cost	100	433.0		10.97
07	Processing Expenditure on Fuel, Electricity, Labour, Repair and Maintenance, Interest, Depreciation, Insurance, Wastage and Handling				1.53
08	Net Profit Earned per kg of Prawn Feed				1.50
09	Price of Feed Produced at Plant Site				Rs 14.00/kg
10	The Packaging and Forwarding Charge is Rs 50/ quintal for minimum order of 02 quintal				

All the mixed and ground material from collecting hopper is fed into the vibro screen. The vibro screen is provided to separate the coarse and oversize material from powder material containing standard particle size. Standard powder material is fed into the paddle mixture conveyor arrangement. Here mixing with 8 per cent molasses and 2 per cent cooking oil is followed. Flow of steam is provisioned in the jacket attached to the conveyor to circulate hot or cold water for cooking/ conditioning. Here common drive is provided for paddle conveyor with feed conditioner where conveyed material is fed for steam conditioning. Slide gate is provided at outlet of paddle conveyor to control the feed rate. For steam cooking and conditioning boiler of recommended steam output and pressure is fitted with aqua feed processing plant which is to be connected at specified electrical load and recommended fuel for it's operation is light diesel oil or high speed diesel mixed with @ 0.1 percent lubricating oil with gross combustion value (GCV) 10,250-10,700 kcal/kg supplied at specified oil pressure.

From feeder conditioner the conditioned material is fed into the pellet mill. Conditioning is accomplished by the addition of controlled amount of steam; molasses and natural oil help in lubrication of pellet die. In the pelleting unit the conditioned feed is forced through perforation of 04 mm diameter in the die by roller pressure and gets compressed and forms into pellets. Adjustable knives cut pellets into desired cutting length. From the pellet mill pellets are collected manually and pellets will be taken to the reciprocating pellet sieve to remove the powder/ dust if any formed with pellets. After screening the full pellet with 8-12 mm length can be directly fed to cultured specie of size of adult fish or otherwise it may be taken if necessary to pellet crumbler for further size reduction which can be used to feed animals like fry, fingerling and prawn, Fig. 1 and Fig. 2 for Prawn and fish feed respectively.

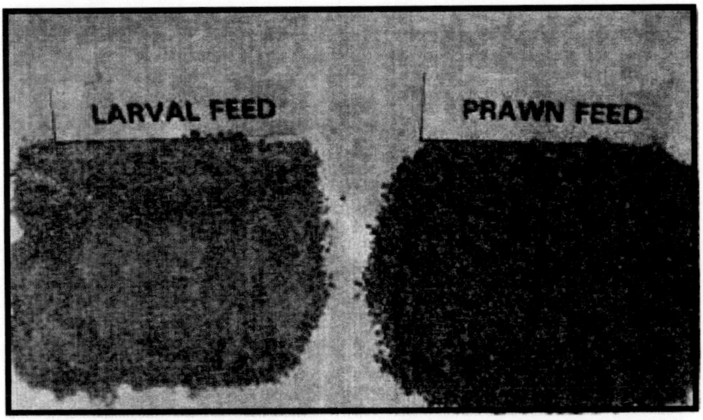

Fig. 1. Aqua Feed for Larvae and Prawn

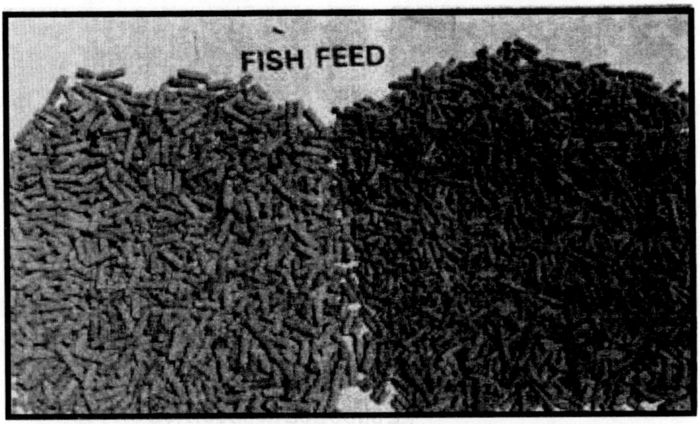

Fig. 2. Aqua Feed for Fish

Unit Operation Machine/ Aqua Feed Plant Maintenance

It is always safe and beneficial for plant operator to keep ready the inventory of essential spares/ parts/ tools of plant machinery first and foremost. As per plant installation following measures segmented as per ease of engineering personnel can be categorized -

Civil Maintenance

i) Construction procedure, level, height of the foundation as per foundation and general assembly drawing needs to be maintained. Hang all the foundation bolts vertically by means of base plate (supplied along with machine) such that about 5.5 inch-threaded lengths will protrude above the ground level. Now for easy detachment apply grease to the threaded portion of the foundation bolts.

ii) Sufficient ventilation, illumination and dehumidification should be facilitated within the premises of aqua feed production plant to save the feed from aflotoxin effect.

iii) Below the ground level rat/ crab nuisance sometimes dig small holes or develop cracks disturb the floor balancing if such possibility exists proper cement concrete jelly is to be applied for complete filling of the holes/ cracks.

Mechanical/ General Maintenance

i) Regular monitoring and check of the nut and bolts of the entire plant machinery. Especially on the contact part of the machine and rotor where looseness may be they're due to vibration.

ii) Tightness of chain and belt is to be observed if it is loosening get it tightens, so as to keep chain/ belt in center position while running.

iii) Proper and timely lubrication is to be monitored. Always use branded and correct grade of lubricant viz. ISO VG 320 recommended for oil and EP-2 for grease.

iv) Apply greasing in the bearings, chain and sprocket of the chine once or twice a week depending on the working hours of the machine. Apply greasing in the motor bearings, once a period of 3 to 6 months, depending on the working hours. The bearings are greased by opening the bearing cover. Ensure free movement of bearing and correct alignment of machine pulley and motor pulley should be in one straight edge. Check the mobile oil in the worm gear box if it is below the marking level refill it for lubricating gears. Apply lubricant on input and output of the shaft.

v) Screen of the screening and sieving machine must be cleaned regularly to avoid closing. Clean rolls by steel wire brush once a week or so for easy movement .

vi) Provide general cleaning and de-dusting of machines, corridors and passages for clear observation and clean environment. Less noise and vibration control is required to be assured along with facilitating availability of safety devices/ equipment like goggles, belts, aprons, shoes and rubberized gloves etc. First aid box and fire fighting equipment will also be an added advantage for operator.

vii) If anywhere leakage of oil is found due to oil seal/ packing damage replace with new oil seal/ packing. If it is due to looseness of drain plug then immediately tighten it. Insert washers/ gaskets wherever necessary.

viii) It is always safe to use pre-cleaned raw feed ingredients to avoid damage to components due to heavy metals or entry of foreign material this also helps in removing light impurities from the feed as product. Ensure proper falling of the material without any kind of deviation on either side due to misalignment of pulley.

ix) Initially always ensure that the required speed is achieved before feeding the material. Ensure that the initial feeding be in smaller quantity and then gradually increased to full capacity. Now onwards do not over/underfeed otherwise operator will get poor performance of the operation with plant machinery. Always ensure correct feeding as per the specified capacity of the machine.

x) For trouble free operation with steam generator always monitor cleaning of nozzle in burner. First by removing it from assembly and then cleaning it's all parts by using kerosene. Check the electrode gap and porcelain insulators are clean and the spark gap is correctly set. Check that no other part of the burner assembly gives spark with any of the electrodes, when ignition is switched on. Keep photoelectric relay (Photocell) viewing glass clean. Take great care not to touch transparent cover of head with hands. Clean only with a lint- free cloth and spirit. Do not use oil smudges as it decreases the sensitivity of the photocell. Observe the raw water, soft water and diesel oil sufficient in their respective tanks.

Electrical Maintenance

i) When installation is complete the plant is ready for operation. Connect and ensure correct electrical supply and complete wiring on control panel with the each individual motor of every unit operation machinery by starting empty machine initially for some time. Check the direction of rotation of every unit operation machine. If it is found wrong then correct it by interchanging the electrical phase.

ii) Ensure proper gap by correcting angularity/ eccentricity errors through feeler gauges between two coupling halves of motor and gearbox. Ensure free rotation of coupling by hand.

iii) After all electrical wiring is completed it is must to ensure that the required plant speed is achieved before feeding operation commence. No where leakage of current is felt for that proper earthing with body of induction motor. However, in case of power failure or tripping, through the cycle once more and ensure idle running before feeding.

iv) Higher rated power capacity motor needs to be protected through over load protection device such as safety fuses, indicator lamps and shear pin etc.

v) Ensure immediate tightness to electrical connections wherever sparking/ flickering of lamps/ bulbs and other electrical devices on single phase/ three phases are observed.

vi) Rodent nuisance damage the insulation of electrical cables and wires. It is therefore safe to provide sand base in underground channels of cable/ conduit pipe base for protection.

Still for any further information/ doubts on repair and maintenance work plant operator may refer to instruction manual of the plant erection, commissioning and operational procedures and literature.

Timely Supply of Raw Materials

Since materials constitute an extremely important and costly resource to a production system, an improvement in materials productivity will lead to overall improvement in systems performance and cost reduction. Therefore, our materials planning system, should be such that we are able to ensure adequate supply of materials to meet anticipated demand pattern with the minimum amount of capital blocked in inventories in a non- productive manner through development of reliable sources of supplies to have 'just in time ' supply of cost effective and quality raw ingredients having sufficient nutritional values and pelletability properties of mixture for aqua feed production.

In a production line consists of the series of processing centers, if due to misalignment and/ or machine/workload is uneven/ unbalanced then the most bottle- necked production stage will negatively govern the whole output rate. This will result in increased throughput time and poor capacity utilization thus contributing to low productivity in terms of manpower, material, energy and end – product i.e. aqua feed. Further improved capacity utilization and up keep of aqua feed plant and machinery productive and available for use every time as and when require. In addition to that a well coordinated and integrated approach involving decision making with respects to cost effective and quality materials that apart from storage also through development of reliable sources of supplies to have ' just in time ' supply will reduce uncertainties in demand and supply and therefore may lead to 15- 20 % anticipated cost reduction. Further wherever the production technology has got developed, in those places most management now saw maintenance efficiency as a factor that can affect the all mass business effectiveness and risk-safety, environmental integrity, energy efficiency, product quality and customer service and not contained only to plant availability and cost.

By scientific and systematic planning of operational and maintenance work through and execution on alignment and balancing of production/ assembly lines, unit operation machine maintenance and proper storage of essential spare parts and required tools, lubricants etc. and to ensure apart from storage ' just in time' supply of cost effective and quality raw materials from reliable sources having sufficient nutritional values and pelletability of mixture will help in achieving control over failure or aqua feed plant breakdown which could create problems such as a loss in production time, rescheduling of production, wastage of materials, which could possibly damage components, failure to recover overheads because of loss in production hours, need for overtime, need for subcontracting work and temporary work shortages etc. will conclude in substantial saving in cost, time, energy, direct and indirect labour and material input and product as well.

Bibliography

CourseMS-1 (2001) Operations Management- An Overview, Volumes IV, Management of Machines and Materials, MBA Programme from Indira Gandhi National Open University, New Delhi, pp 05-16.

Course MS- 5 (2001) Operational Planning and control, Volumes IV ,Management of Machines and Materials , MBA Programme from Indira Gandhi National Open University, New Delhi pp- 77 to 100.

Instruction Manuals (2000) of aqua feed plant and installation of plant established at CIAE, Bhopal.

Kaulgud Aruna (2003), Entrepreneurship Management, Vikas Publishing House Pvt. Ltd., 576, Masjid Road, Jangpura, New Delhi- 110 014 pp-186.

Singh Jai and Singh G. (2000) Brochure on Aqua Feed Pilot Plat, CIAE, Bhopal.

4
FEED INDUSTRY IN SOUTHERN INDIA

K.T.Sampath, M. Chandrasekharaiah and A. Thulasi

There are a large number of compound livestock feed manufacturers in Southern India. The list of some of feed manufacturers is given state wise in Table 1. Feed Industry in Southern India is fairly well organized. A good number of the feed manufacturers come under the umbrella of compound livestock feed manufacturers association of India (CLFMA). However, still a large number of fee manufacturers are there outside this umbrella.

Quantity of Feed Produced

The quantity of cattle feed, poultry feed and other feeds produced by the organized sector in four southern states during the year 2001-02 and 2002-03 is given in Table 2. As can be seen from Table 2, the quantity of poultry feed manufactured occupies the highest position followed by that of cattle feed and other feeds. The major portion of other feeds is aqua feed followed by lab animal feed and rabbit feed. Among the four southern states, the highest quantity of livestock feed is produced and sold in Tamil Nadu followed by Karnataka, Andhra Pradesh and Kerala. In the states of Tamil Nadu, Karnataka and Andhra Pradesh, the quantity of poultry feed produced is much higher than that of cattle feed.

The quantity of cattle feed produced and sold in Karnataka and Andhra Pradesh is much lower as compared to other two states. The quantity of cattle feed produced is almost negligible in the state of Andhra Pradesh. The reason for this state of affairs in those two states is that most of the dairy farmers in these states follow traditional system of feeding locally available feed ingredients mainly brans and oil cakes. However, in Tamil Nadu and Kerala farmers have become much accustomed to the feeding of compounded cattle feed. The percentage of farmers feeding compounded cattle feed is much higher in the state of Kerala as compared to other three states.

Table 1 Certain Feed industries in Southern parts of India.

Karnataka

Agro Therm Pvt Ltd
Aims Feeds Pvt Ltd
Amarnath Enterprises
Asha Feeds
Bhaskar Bio Industries
Bramhappa Tavanappanavar Pvt Ltd
Encee Feeds Pvt Ltd
Godrej Agrovet Ltd
Gokul Agro Industries
Goldmohur Foods & Feeds Ltd
(Hindustan lever)
Government of Karnataka
Hassan Feeds
Hulkoti Cooperative
Cattle Feed Processing Society
International Fisheries Ltd
Kamadhenu Feeds
Karnataka Cooperative Milk Producers' Federation
Karanataka State Agro Corn Products Ltd
Komarla Feeds
Kwality Animal Feeds Pvt Ltd
Laxmi Feeds & Exports Ltd
Mysore Feeds Ltd
Nandini Feeds
Nav Maharashtra chakan Oil Mills Ltd
Nutri Feeds Pvt Ltd
Panaje Agro Industries
Pashukpriya Feeds Pvt Ltd
Paichur Oil Complex
Ravi Vegetable Oil Industries
Sangemeshwar Trading Co
Shubha Mangala Industries
Sudarshan Feeds
Sujay Feeds
Tijbetan Feeds
Tirumala Feeds (Pvt)Ltd
Venkateshwara Feeds
Viswa Adgro En terprises Ltd
Yarana Feeds & Farms

Andhra Pradesh

Adoni Proteins
Feeds
Andhra Pradesh Dairy Dev
Cooperative Federation Ltd
Avanti Industries Ltd
Balaji Foods & Feeds Ltd
Balaji Poultry & Cattle Feeds(P)Ltd
Coromandel Agro Products & Oils Ltd
Crown Aqua Feed Pvt Ltd
Essen Enterprises
GP Cotton & Oil Products Ltd
Godrej Agrovet Ltd
Goldmohur Foods & Feeds Ltd
(Hindustan Lever)
Guntur Dist Cooperative Milk Producers Union Ltd
Haji Mohamed Husain Traders
Hindustan Livestock Feeds
Janaki Feeds Pvt Ltd
Kwality Feeds Pvt Ltd
Maheshwara Industries
Markfed Feed Mixing Plant
Metta Feed Specialities
Nandyal Agro-Vet Industries Pvt Ltd
Poshak Feeds Ltd
Saptagiri Feeds
Sri Satya Sai Chemicals & Feeds(P) Ltd
Srinivasa Poultry &Cattle Feeds Pvt Ltd

Tamilnadu

AVM Cattle & Poultry Feed
Mfg Industries
Amajin Agro Exports Ltd
Annam Feeds Ltd
Arafath & Adrafath Associates
CP Group
Coimbatore Chemicals &
Fertilizers Pvt Ltd
Feeds India
Godrej Agrovet Ltd
Goldmohur Foods & Feeds Ltd
(Hindustan Lever)
Indian Commercial Syndicate
KRV Agencies
Kaveri's Bio Proteins Pvt Ltd
Kerala Solvent Extractions Ltd
LSP Fats & Feeds
Pe Pe Feeds
Periyar Dist Cooperative Milk
Producers Union Ltd
RG Sundar & Co
Rohini Poultry Feeds Pvt Ltd
Ruhsa Animal Feeds and Foods
Sakthi Feeds Pvt ltd
Sakthi Soyas Ltd
Selvi Feeds
Shunmugamohan Trading Co
Shunmugarajeswaran Trading Co.
Tamil Nadu Cooperative Milk
producers federation
Thirunirai Products
Vangili Feeds
Viswa Agro Enterprises Ltd
Walfars Feeds Pvt Ltd

Kerala

Higashimaru Feeds(India)Ltd
Kerala Cooperative Milk
Marketing Federation Ltd
KSE Ltd
Kerala Trading Corporation Koyenco
Feeds Ltd
Prima Agro Products Ltd
Vijay Feeds &Farms Touns Pvt Ltd

Pondichery

Aurofo Ltd
Government of Pondichery
Cooperative Milk Producers Union

Table 2: State wise production (in tonnes) of cattle, poultry and other feeds by CLFMA members during 2002-2003

ANDHRA PRADESH

S. No.	Name of the members	Cattle Feeds		Poultry Feeds		Other Feeds		Total	
		2001-02	2002-03	2001-02	2002-03	2001-02	2002-03	2001-02	2002-03
1	Balaji Foods & Feeds Ltd.	-	-	7500.00	-	-	-	7500.00	0.00
2	Bhavani Feeds	-	700.00	14160.00	13390.00	-	-	14160.00	14090.00
3	Chalimeda Feeds	-	-	18807.00	17540.00	-	-	18807.00	17540.00
4	Godrej Agrovet Ltd	3329.00	4503.00	19408.00	13630.00	6888.00	3870.00	29625.00	22003.00
5	Gold Mohur Foods & Feeds Ltd.	1442.20	1764.22	49208.00	49273.07	108.00	1806.85	50758.20	52844.14
6	Janaki Feeds Pvt. Ltd	-	77.00	34726.00	21831.00	-	-	34726.00	21908.00
7	Poshak Feeds Ltd Hyderabad	300.00	400.00	17850.00	20600.00	-	-	18150.00	21000.00
8	Srinivasa Food & Feeds Pvt.Ltd	-	-	8564.00	14665.00	-	-	8564.00	14665.00
9	Suguna Poultry Farm Ltd.	-	-	-	24449.00	-	-	0.00	24449.00
10	Tirumala Foods & Feeds Pvt.Ltd.	-	-	2050.00	-	-	-	2050.00	0.00
11	Venkateshwadra Hacheries Ltd.	-	-	12620.00	-	-	-	12620.00	0.00
	Total (Andhra Pradesh)	**5,071.20**	**7444.22**	**184893.00**	**175378.07**	**6996.00**	**5676.85**	**196960.20**	**188499.14**

KARNATAKA

S. No.	Name of the members	Cattle Feeds		Poultry Feeds		Other Feeds		Total	
		2001-02	2002-03	2001-02	2002-03	2001-02	2002-03	2001-02	2002-03
1	Agro Therm Pvt.Ltd.	14200.00	-	453.00	-	-	-	14653.00	0.00
2	Asha Feeds	197.00	-	5972.00	-	-	-	6169.00	0.00
3	Bhaskar Bio Industries	6300.00	4215.00	3080.00	5050.00	-	-	9380.00	9265.00
4	Godrej Agrovet Ltd.	-	8752.00	-	33314.00	-	36.00	0.00	42102.00
5	Gold Mohur Foods & Feeds Ltd.	11287.34	7907.92	16237.49	19759.41	1709.43	32.60	29234.26	27699.93
6	K.S.E.Ltd	12294.00	10090.00	-	-	-	-	12294.00	10090.00
7	Komarla Feeds, Bangalore	2447.00	1695.00	30424.00	3155.00	-	-	32871.00	4850.00
8	Nutri Feeds & Farms Pvt. Ltd.	19300.00	862.00	-	16747.00	-	-	19300.00	17609.00
9	Pranav Agro Industries Ltd	24600.00	1486.00	1600.00	29659.00	960.00	426.00	27160.00	31571.00
10	Samruddhi Feeds Pvt. Ltd.	-	-	6000.00	-	-	-	6000.00	0.00
11	Sandur Hatcheries Pvt. Ltd	51.00	-	7239.00	-	-	-	7290.00	0.00
12	Suguna Poultry Farm Ltd.	-	-	-	96801.00	-	-	0.00	96801.00
13	Veda Feeds Pvt. Ltd	1336.00	-	3670.00	-	-	-	5006.00	0.00
14	Yarana Feeds & Farms	1000.00	-	6980.00	5100.00	-	-	7980.00	5100.00
	Total Karnataka	**93012.34**	**35007.92**	**81655.49**	**209585.41**	**2669.43**	**494.60**	**177337.26**	**245087.93**

S. No.	Name of the members	Cattle Feeds		Poultry Feeds		Other Feeds		Total	
	KERALA								
		2001-02	2002-03	2001-02	2002-03	2001-02	2002-03	2001-02	2002-03
1	Godrej Agrovet Ltd.	-	27913.00	-	-	-	-	0.00	27913.00
2	Higashimaru Feeds (I) Ltd	-	-	-	-	9868.00	7660.00	9868.00	7660.00
3	K.S.E.Ltd.	100321.00	110720.00	2712.00	-	-	-	103033.00	110720.00
4	Koyenco Feeds Pvt. Ltd.	10215.00	9536.00	0.00	-	-	-	10215.00	9536.00
5	Prima Agro Ltd.	13954.00	18532.99	3964.00	-	-	-	17918.00	18532.99
	Total (Kerala)	**124490.00**	**166701.99**	**6676.00**	**0.00**	**9868.00**	**7660.00**	**141034.00**	**174361.99**

S. No.	Name of the members	Cattle Feeds		Poultry Feeds		Other Feeds		Total	
	TAMIL NADU								
		2001-02	2002-03	2001-02	2002-03	2001-02	2002-03	2001-02	2002-03
1	Gold Mohur Foods & Feeds Ltd.	-	-	-	-	10697.57	8956.63	10697.57	8956.63
2	Godrej Agrovet Ltd.	24918.00	27175.00	30326.00	31872.00	2237.00	5500.00	57481.00	64547.00
3	Gold Mohur Foods & Feeds Ltd.	6241.65	16637.41	47127.40	54491.29	-	14.48	53369.05	71143.18
4	Kerala Trading Corporation	6872.00	8092.00	-	-	-	-	6872.00	8092.00
5	Komarla Feeds, Bangalore	-	151.00	10260.00	13834.00	-	-	10260.00	13985.00
6	Pe Pe Feeds	195.00	-	12575.00	-	-	-	12770.00	0.00
7	Pioneer Feeds Pvt. Ltd.	98.00	-	137716.00	-	-	-	137814.00	0.00
8	Shunmugarajes waran Trading Co.	1069.00	-	-	-	-	-	1069.00	0.00
9	SKM Animal Feeds & Foods (India) Ltd.	57424.00	67580.74	125359.00	108715.26	-	-	182783.00	176296.00
10	Suguna Poultry Farm Ltd.	-	-	-	120238.00	-	-	0.00	120238.00
11	K.S.E.Ltd.	39967.00	51533.00	-	-	-	-	39967.00	51533.00
	Total (Tamil Nadu)	**136784.65**	**171169.15**	**363363.40**	**329150.55**	**12934.57**	**14471.11**	**513082.62**	**514790.81**

Quality of feed produced

The feed manufacturers in Southern India produce fairly a good quality feed. There has been a gradual improvement in the quality of the feed produced in organized sector in these states. In early eighties although a large number of feed manufacturers followed the specifications of Bureau of Indian Standards (BIS), some of them resorted to produce market driven demand of certain feeds, which was lower than that of BIS specification. This lead to quality control measures by the Government in some of the states. The argument of the feed manufacturers that there has been demand for type of feed outside the BIS specification such as type I and type II to meet the requirement of low yielding animals and also to meet the requirement during natural calamities like drought, lead to the formation specification for compounded livestock feed by certain state governments which included more types of feeds than specified by BIS. Meanwhile, compound livestock feed manufacturers association (CLFMA) of

India also came out with specifications for different types of livestock feeds. The specifications of BIS, Karnataka Government and that of CLFMA for different categories of feeds are given in Table 3a, 3b and 3c.

Most of the feed manufacturers in the organized sector in Southern India follow any one of the specification mentioned above.

Table 3a: Specifications of Bureau of Indian Standards for Cattle Feeds

	Type I IS:2052,1979 Re affirmed 1990	Type II IS:2052,1979 Re affirmed 1990
Moisture, % max	11	11
Crude Protein, %min	22	20
Crude fat, % min	3	2.5
Crude fibre, % max	7	12
Acid insoluble ash, % max	3	4

Table 3b: Specifications of Government of Karnataka for Cattle Feeds

	Cattle Feed Type			
	Type I	Type II	Type III	Type IV
Moisture, % max	11	11	11	11
Crude Protein, %min	20	18	16	10
Fat, % min	2.5	2.0	1.5	1.0
Crude fibre, % max	7	12	16	20
Acid insoluble ash	4	4.5	5	10

Table 3c: CLFMA Specifications for Compounded Feeds for Dairy Cattle and Buffaloes (1995)

Item	Types of Feed			
	Dairy Special	I	II	III
Moisture, % max	12.0	12.0	12.0	12.0
Crude Protein, %min	22.0	20.0	18.0	16.0
Undegraded Protein (%min)	8.0	-	-	-
Crude fat, % min	3.0	2.5	2.5	2.0
Crude fibre, % max	7.0	7.0	12.0	14.0
Acid insoluble ash (%max)	3.5	4.0	4.5	5.0

Role of Co-Operative Sector

Co-Operative sector mainly under state milk federations form the large share of cattle feed produced in Southern India. As the milk federations follow a system of semi integration like procurement of milk, providing health care to the dairy animals etc, the private feed manufacturers face a stiff competition from the co-operative sector in these states.

Problems faced by feed Industry

The compound livestock feed industry has been facing multiple problems each year. The demand for poultry feed was drastically reduced during last few years due to bird flue scare and also due to low broiler cost. Further, the integration system followed by certain firms and the self compounding of feeds by certain of poultry farms has reduced the demand. The high cost of molasses due to failure of sugarcane crops on account of drought during last 3-4 years has lead to increased cost of production of compounded feed. The low production of groundnut in the country leading to lesser availability of groundnut cake and export of soyabean meal due to lower production of soyabean in some western countries severely affected the domestic market during recent years.

Requirement for new specification for compounded cattle feed: Judicious utilization of available feed resources is the need of the day. Majority of dairy farmers in India who maintain 2 or 3 cows or buffaloes yielding small quantities of milk cannot offered to pay high costs for cattle feeds. At the same it is essential to have high energy compounded feeds with good quality proteins to exploit the genetic potential of high yielding animals. It is also essential to exploit the potential of non-conventional feed resources and agro-industrial byproducts for incorporation in livestock feeds. Looking into these aspects and the need to satisfy the nutrient requirement of different categories of cattle, it is desirable to have specifications for multigrade compound cattle feed.

Need for Uniform Specification and Nodal Agency:-It is evident from the comparative analysis of specifications prescribed for cattle feeds by different agencies that there is wide variations in these specifications which is resulting in difficulties in regulations and implementation. Therefore, it is desirable to have a nodal agency on the lines Agricultural Research Council of United Kingdom and National Research Council of United States. This agency may be entrusted with the responsibility of fixing nutrient requirements for different categories of livestock, fixing specifications for livestock feed and periodical review and publication of standards. The nodal agency may also look into the needs for specifications in respect of vitamins, probiotics and other feed additives. It is also desirable to have region- wise/state -wise reference laboratories for analyses of feeds.

Bibliography

BIS (1979). Indian Standard: Specification for compounded feeds for cattle. Bureau of Indian Standards.

CLAFMA (1995). Compound Livestock Feed Manufactures Association. Bombay.

5
OIL CAKES – QUALITY AND AVAILABILITY

D.M. Hegde

In the agricultural economy of India, oilseeds are important next only to food grains in terms of area of production and value. India is the third largest producer of oilseeds after the USA and China. Currently, India accounts for 12-13% of world oilseed area, 6-8% of world oilseeds output and 5-7% of world oil meal production (Tables 1-2). India also exports oil meal mostly soybean earning valuable foreign exchange (Table 3). India has agro-ecological conditions favourable for producing all the annual oilseeds, seven edible viz., groundnut, rapeseed – mustard, soybean, sunflower, sesame, safflower and niger and two non-edible viz., castor and linseed. In addition, India has favourable environment for producing tree oilseeds like coconut and oil palm besides large number of oilseeds of tree origin, which are mostly found in forest and waste lands. Vegetable oils are also obtained from several unconventional items including rice bran, cotton seed, maize gluten etc.

Table 1: Area, production and productivity of oilseeds in India and world (2003)

Oilseed	India Area ('000 ha)	World Production ('000 t)	Yield (kg/ha)	Area ('000 ha)	Production ('000 t)	Yield (kg/ha)
Groundnut	5953	4363	733	26417	37058	1403
Rapeseed- Mustard	4482	3842	857	25241	37012	1466
Soybean	5866	4558	777	83614	189525	2267
Sesame	1385	431	311	6681	2765	414
Sunflower	1638	902	550	20709	26086	1260
Safflower	350	157	450	795	731	920
Linseed	459	173	376	2428	2054	846
Castor	585	428	732	1146	1154	1007
Niger	425	106	250	-	-	-
Total	**21144**	**14960**	**708**	**167029**	**296384**	**1774**

Table 2: Oil meal production in India and World ('000t)

Oil meal	**India**		**World**	
	2002	**2003**	**2002**	**2003**
Soybean	3301	3644	128451	133493
Cotton	3213	3235	15928	14961
Groundnut	2281	2434	7205	6319
Sunflower	388	468	8769	10134
Rapeseed	2666	2038	20036	19198
Sesame	240	223	1028	978
Linseed	163	173	1211	1145
Copra	256	265	1763	1856
Palm kernel	-	-	2719	2944
Total	**12508**	**12480**	**187110**	**191028**

Table 3: India's exports of oil meals

Oilcake/Extractions	**2002-03**	**2003-04**		
	Quantity ('000t)	**Value (Rs. Crores)**	**Quantity ('000t)**	**Value (Rs. Crores)**
Soybean	1333	1280	2684	2684
Rapeseed- mustard	456	214	447	250
Groundnut	15	13	127	95
Castor	93	20	86	23
Others	6	4	18	11
Total	**1903**	**1531**	**3362**	**3063**

There has been a sea change in the Indian oil seeds scenario, form a net importer in the 1980s to a net exporter status during the early 1990s. Again, it is back to net importer status importing more than 40% of its annual edible oil needs. The main contributors to such transformation up to early nineties have been (i) availability of improved oilseeds production technology and its adoption (ii) expansion in cultivated area (iii) price support policy and (iv) institutional support, particularly establishment of Technology Mission on Oilseeds (TMO) in 1986. The TMO scored a remarkable success in the first eight years of its career (1986-94). This was facilitated by relatively protectionist umbrella of higher import duties in the import of edible oil of the order of 65% on palmolein, the commonly imported oil.

India's distinct position in the world in terms of richness in diversity and enhanced production through varietal improvement in the nine commercial annual oilseeds crops and also the domestic achievements in oilseed production are unparalleled. The latter being particularly so when are observe that a 5 time increase in oilseed production could be achieved during the period 1950 to 2004 under the rainfed agro-ecological situations, which is even higher than the corresponding production increases in total food grains. It is worth recording that four time increase in production in total food grains was achieved with the highest national priorities to this commodity group and also that such production jump was recorded under relatively much more favourable farming environments, particularly the irrigated lands.

Oilcakes in Animal Nutrition

Improving efficiency of feed use is critical to raising the productivity and profitability of livestock. The cost of feed accounts for 50-60% of the total cost of production in ruminants and 65-80% in non-ruminants under intensive production system. The significant impact of improved nutrition on animal productivity in the developing countries has repeatedly been highlighted (ILRI, 1995). Crop residues and other cellulosic materials are stable ruminants feeds in India. The low nitrogen and mineral content, along with high lignin and silica contents of roughage, leads to its row digestibility. To achieve productive levels in the animal consistent with their genetic make up, the straw –based rations need protein-rich oilseeds and oilcakes as supplements. This is important in the countries such as India that have large livestock populations and shortage of feed in relation to requirements (Krishna, 2003).

Oilcakes Availability and Quantity

Oilseeds are rich source of energy. The residues left after extractions of oil from oilseeds are rich source of nutrients, specially protein (Table 4) and other valuable feed nutrients for livestock. About 85% of the oilcakes produced in the country serve as animal feeds. The protein content of the oilcakes ranges from 25 to 55%. Hence, they are important sources of nutrition to animals. Oil is extracted from oilseeds by using pressure to force out the oil, or by using an organic solvent, usually hexane to dissolve oil from the seed. Seeds such as groundnut, cottonseed, sunflower and safflower have a thick coat or husk, rich in fibre and of low digestibility, which lowers the nutritive value of the material. This husk may be completely or partially removed by cracking and riddling, the process being known as decortication. Removal of the husk lowers the crude fibre content (Table 5) and improves the apparent digestibility of other constituents. Generally, the residual oil content of the cake is higher in screw-pressed cakes than in solvent extracted meals. The method of extraction, dehulling, temperature at the time of extraction etc. will have major influence on the composition of cake (Tables 6, 7 and 8).

Table 4: Compositions of oilseed (%).

Oilseeds	Moisture	Protein	Oil	Carbohydrates	Crude fibre	Ash
Groundnut (seed)	4-13	21-36	36-54	6-25	2-3	2-3
Mustard	4-9	42-44	38-41	12-21	10-11	3-5
Sesame	6-7	20-28	48-55	14-16	6-8	5-7
Sunflower	6-9	14-19	36-43	7-9	16-27	2-3
Niger	4-8	10-30	30-43	7-18	10-11	4-5
Safflower	5-8	19-29	28-32	18-24	14-18	5-7
Soybean	5-8	39-42	12-18	21-28	8-11	5-6
Castor	4-9	12-16	40-55	3-7	17-23	2-3
Linseed	6-10	20-24	37-42	15-29	5-9	2-4

Table 5: Chemical composition of oilseed cakes

Cakes	Crude protein (%)	Oil (%)	Crude fibre	General remarks
Groundnut cake				Low in lysine, arginine, histidine and S-containing amino acids
Expeller-pressed	48	8	7	
Solvent extract	51	1	10	
Rapeseed-Mustard				Palatability problems due to pungent odour
Expeller-pressed	37	5	10	
Sesame cake				-
Expeller-pressed	40	8	7	
Linseed cake				-
Expeller-pressed	29	8	10	
Solvent extract	33	1	9	
Cottonseed cake (Decorticated)				Low in Ca, Zn, Mn. Effect of gossypol in greater in monogastric animals
Expeller-pressed	41	5	12	
Solvent extract	42	1.5	16	
Safflower cake (Decorticated)				
Expeller-pressed	48	5	15	-
Coconut cake				
Expeller-pressed	22	6.5	12	-

Table 6: Chemical composition of palm kernel cake/meal obtained by different methods of extraction

Constituent (% of dry matter)	Expeller extracted	Hydraulically extracted	Solvent extracted
Dry matter (%)	89-92	88	91
Crude protein	14.9-20.4	15.8	17.5-18.6
Ether extract	8.3-8.8	23.0	1.0-1.7
N free extract	56.6	27.8	38.2
Crude fibre	9.0-17.2	29.7	14.9-37.0
Ash	4.6-5.7	3.7	3.9-4.7
Ca	0.32	0.21	0.28-0.31
P	0.77	0.47	0.80-0.85

Table 7: Effects of dehulling and the method of oil extraction on the composition (%) of sesame flour/cake.

Sesame seed and processing	Moisture	Fat	Protein	Ash	Crude fibre	Ca	P	Oxalic acid
Flour	5.2	49.8	19.1	5.7	4.1	1.2	-	2.3
Expeller-pressed flour	6.6	10.7	41.4	8.7	6.8	1.7	-	3.7
Expeller-pressed cake	8.1	13.5	35.1	8.9	5.3	1.8	0.8	3.0
Alcohol –extracted cake	8.6	3.1	38.2	9.4	5.9	2.0	0.9	3.5
Hexane –extracted cake	8.6	0.8	39.6	9.7	6.1	2.1	1.0	3.6
Dehulled seeds								
Flour	4.1	60.2	22.1	3.2	3.1	-	-	0.1
Expeller-pressed flour	5.8	10.0	54.4	6.2	5.1	0.3	-	0.2
Prepress solvent-extracted flour	6.0	0.4	56.1	6.1	4.9	0.4	1.0	0.4
Expeller-pressed cake	8.3	12.7	41.3	4.8	3.1	0.4	1.1	0.5
Alcohol –extracted cake	8.9	3.4	45.8	5.0	3.1	0.5	1.2	0.5
Hexane –extracted cake	8.8	1.1	46.7	5.2	3.2	0.4	-	0.3

Table 8: Effect of various degrees of heat treatment on composition and nutritive value of coconut meal

Treatment temperature (°C)	Protein content (%)	Available lysine (g/16g N)	Coefficient of true N digestibility	Net protein utilization
40	25.3	3.29	77.7	45.9
90	25.8	3.09	78.3	41.0
105	26.3	2.81	74.6	36.1
120	25.6	2.34	73.3	35.8
135	26.4	1.63	68.2	33.9
150	26.3	1.12	56.1	17.1

India also has many unconventional oilseeds of which only a small proportion is presently exploited (Table 9). They are also rich source of protein and other nutrients, but their use in the livestock industry is limited by the presence of one or more undesirable nutritional factors (Table 10). These, however, can be used in concentrate mixture in varying proportions depending on their chemical composition.

Table 9: Unconventional oilmeals/cakes available for animal feed

Source	Availability of oilseeds ('000t)	By-product availability ('000t)	Extraction rate (%)	By-product
Sal seed meal	5504	4806	88	Meal
Mahua seed	2176	1414	65	Cake
Neem seed	418	334	80	Cake
Rubber seed	336	117	35	Cake
Karanj	111	81	73	Cake
Kusum	105	70	67	Cake
Undi, Mahua	102	59	40-75	Cake
Khankan				
Tobacco				
Mango seed	1000	500	50-55	Meal/kernel

Source: AIRCP on agricultural by-product and industrial wastes for livestock and poultry feeing, ICAR, New Delhi.

Table 10: Chemical composition, toxic factors and safe level of inclusion in the concentrate mixture of unconventional oilcakes

Extraction	Crude protein (%)	Crude fibre (%)	TDN	Toxic factors	Level of inclusion in diet
Mahua seed cake	20	13	50	Mowrin (19%)	20% in CM of cross bred calves
Karanj cake	34	4.5	62	Karanjine, pongamol, Glabrin	15% in CM of growing and lactating cows
Kusum seed cake	22	5.7	79	HCN (2.4 mg/100g DM)	35% in CM of cross bred calves and 17% in broiler chickens
Sal seed cakes	9-20	2-4	40-58	Tannic acid (8-10%) Glucosides (3.83%)	10% in CM of milch cattle
Kokam cake	16	4	70	-	15% in CM of cross bred calves
Castor cake	35	33	-	Ricin (0.22%)	Only detoxified meal at 10% in CM of sheep
Neem seed cake	17	42	57	Nimbia, salamin	Only detoxified cake at 10% in CM of adult animals
Mango seed kernels	6.1		70	Tannins (5-6%)	10 % level in CM of milch cattle
Rubber seed cake	18.6		66	HCN (9 mg/100g)	25-30% in CM of calves and milch cattle

Source: AIRCP on agricultural by-product and industrial wastes for livestock and poultry feeing, ICAR, New Delhi.

The quality of a protein in oilseed is relatively constant, but may vary in the cake or meal, depending on the technique employed for the extraction of the oil. As mentioned earlier, generally, the residual oil content of the cakes generally higher in screw-pressed cakes than in solvent extracted meals. High temperatures and pressure of expeller processing may result in the lowering of the nutritive value. For ruminants such denaturation may be beneficial, owing to an associated reduction in degradability. High temperatures and pressures also degrade some delicious substance such as gossypol. Solvent extraction does not involve processing, temperatures are comparatively low and protein value of meals is almost the same as that of the original seed. The oilseed cakes may make a significant contribution to the energy content of the diet, particularly when the oil contents are high.

Antinutritional factors

Some oil meals contain certain antimetabolites or other antinutritional factors which when consumed may be toxic to animals. Some of the important antinutritional factors found in different oilseed cakes/meals are trypsin inhibitors, haemagglutinis ricin, goitrogens, saponins, phenolic compounds, oxalates, phytates, cyanogenic compounds, allergens, unusual fatty acids, oligosaccharides and mycotoxins (Table 11). These factors may affect the absorption of dietary nutrients in the digestive tract as a result of toxic action on some organ or tissue, or production traits. Some of these factors also affect human health. Detoxification of some factors is possible by treating a particular ingredient. Some of these treatments are simple whereas others are cumbersome. It is however, necessary that whenever such ingredients containing toxic factors are mixed in the feed, their inclusion levels should be such that an animal can tolerate them without any adverse effect on their productivity/ performance. Toxic factors can be of two types, intrinsic and extrinsic. Intrinsic factors are usually of plant origin such as tannins, trypsin inhibitors, giotrogens, cynogenic glucosites, saponins, hemagglutinins, gossypol, lathyrogens and nimba and its derivatives. Extrinsic factors are those produced by the attack of pathogens on feed ingredients, i.e. Aspergillus spp. causing aflatoxicosis.

Table 11: Antinutritional factors in oilseeds/plant protein meals

Meals	Antinutritional factors
Soybean	Protease, inhibitors*, allergins*, oligosaccharides, phytin, lipoxygenas*, lectins*, saponin, citrinin, hemagglutinins, goitrogenic factors
Rapeseed	Euric acid, glucosinolates, sinapine, tannins, pectins, oligosaccharides, isocyanates
Canola	Glucosinolates, sinapine, tannins, pectins, oligosaccharides
Cotton seed	Gossypol, tannins, cyclopropenoid fatty acids
Sunflower	Chlorogenic acid, high fibre, achratoxin
Groundnut	Mycotoxins, tannins, oligosaccharides, protease inhibitors*, aflatoxins
Copra	Fibre, mannans
Palm kernel	Fibre and sharp shells, galactomannans
Sesame	Phytase, oxalate
Sal seed	Tannins
Linseed	Prussic acid
Castor seed	Ricin, ricinine, ricinus allergens
Neem seed	Nimbin, nimbinin, nimbidin, nimbosterol

* Destroyed by heating

Critical Amino Acids in Oilseed Meals

Oilseeds cakes and extractions are the most important source of essential amino acids. In general, oilseed proteins have low cysteine and methionine content and a variable but low lysine content (Table 12). As a result, these cannot adequately supplement the cereal proteins with which they are commonly used. The gross protein value of some oilseeds such as cotton, groundnut and soybean is high; their chemical composition does not favour their greater use. Cottonseed also has the disadvantage of a low cysteine, methionine and lysine conternts, with lysine being the first limiting amino acid.

Different oilseed meals are degraded at varying rates in the rumen of livestock. Since high yielding cattle and fast growing goats and sheep need higher levels of undegradable dietary protein, it is possible to select desirable components of protein meals and formulate rations for differential levels of productivity (Sudhakara Rao et al., 1992).

Table 12: Important limiting amino acid (%) contents of commonly used oil meals

Source	Arginin	Lysine	Tryptophan	Methionine	Cysteine
Groundnut	4.4	1.3	0.4	0.6	0.7
Soybean	3.0	2.6	0.5	0.8	0.7
Sesame	3.7	1.2	0.6	1.4	0.4
Safflower	3.8	2.0	0.6	1.6	0.7
Cotton seed	3.4	1.4	0.5	0.8	1.0
Mustard	6.1	5.8	0.5	2.0	0.2
Sunflower (Dehulled, sol)	8.1	6.8	1.1	1.4	0.6
Castor (sol)	5.3	1.2	0.4	0.7	0.2
Neem (sol)	-	1.0	-	0.5	0.1

Limitations to the Use of Oilseed Cakes

The problem of aflatoxins in the animal feeds is being debated at length. The use of groundnut, which is very susceptible to fungal infection and aflatoxin contamination, has drastically decreased recently despite the superiority of its protein. Improver harvesting, transport, processing and storage all contribute to aflatoxin contamination. Preventive measures during crop production and post harvest handling of seeds would greatly reduce the level of contamination in feeds. Drying the produce quickly to less than 8% moisture and storing them at low humidity levels help in reducing mycotoxin contamination and levels. Creating awareness among farmers about aflatoxins would help in increase groundnut meal use in animals feeds. While soybean meal is not normally found to contain detectable amounts of aflatoxins, the incidence of these metabolites has bean on the rise recently.

Sunflower meal is very rich in many essential amino acids, but its use has been restricted owing to its high fibre content. Decorticating the sunflower seeds prior to expelling/solvent extraction produces oil with less gum content, better clarity and a meal with low fibre. However, the economic viability of the process has to be established. Similar problems limit the use of other meals such as sunflower meal, and niger seed meal in animals feeds.

Bibliography

International Livestock Research Institute (ILRI), 1995. Global agenda for livestock research (Gardiner, P. and Devendra C. eds.). Proceeding of a Consultation, ILRI, Nairobi, Kenya.

Krishna, N. (2003). Unconventional feed resources. Various approaches for their optimum utilization. Feed Processing Technology, ANGRAU, Rajendranagar, Hyderabad, pp. 20-35.

Sudhakara Rao, M., Krishna, N. and Prasad, A. (1992). Determination of effective protein degradability of some unconventional protein sources in cattle by nylon bag technique. Indian Journal of Agricultural Sciences, 52: 280-281.

6
PROCESSING OF OILSEEDS FOR CAKES

S.M. Ilyas, R.K. Gupta and S.K. Tyagi

The quantity of vegetable oil production, both for edible and industrial uses, depends on yield of oilseeds. The major oilseeds are: groundnut, rapeseed/mustard, linseed, sesame, castor, soybean, sunflower and safflower. The cottonseed and coconut are other important oil bearing sources being grown in various parts of the world. The production of major oilseeds in the country is 20.80 million tonnes (Table 1).

Table 1: Oilseed production (million tonnes) in 2001-2002.

Oilseed	Production (million tonnes)
Groundnut	7.20
Soybean	5.86
Rapeseed /mustard	5.04
Sunflower	1.04
All remaining oilseeds	1.66
TOTAL	**20.80**

All other oilseeds namely sesame, castor, niger, safflower and linseed account for 8% of the total oilseeds production excluding cottonseed (5.14 million tonnes). The percent production of four major oilseeds is given in Table 2.

Table 2: Percent production of major oilseeds (2001-02)

Oilseed	% of total production
Groundnut	36%
Soybean	28%
Rapeseed /mustard	23%
Sunflower	5%

(Source: Statistics 2002-03. Central Organization for Oil Industry & Trade, New Delhi)

Proper handling and storage of oilseeds is important for their processing into quality products including oilcakes since oilseeds are prone to auto-catalytic and deteriorative processes, enzymatic action, microbial spoilage, etc. Immature seeds, harvested before their enzymes have become dormant deteriorate more rapidly than normal seeds during storage. Aflatoxin produced in oilseeds by strains of Aspergilus flavus comes out partly in the expressed oil and the rest remain in the residual cake. Such oil requires further refining for removal of its aflatoxin which render it unsafe for human consumption and as such the deoiled meal unless fully detoxified is unsafe for even animal feed.

Methods of oil extraction and production of oilcakes

Oil from oilseeds is mostly extracted with the help of :

- Traditional animal drawn ghanies
- Power ghanies,
- Hydraulic press
- Mechanical expellers
- Solvent extraction units

However, solvent extraction techniques are extensively used for recovery of oil from soybean, rice bran and pressed cakes. The oil cake is obtained as a by-product during oil extraction process.

Present practice for the production of various oilcakes and their use as livestock feed.

Groundnut cake

Groundnut meal, a by-product of oil industry, is rich in protein. Because of its dark colour due to the presence of red skins and bitter taste because of saponins presents in the hearts i.e., germ of groundnut, the cake despite of high protein value is not considered fit for human consumption and is mainly used as cattle feed and partly as manure.

Groundnut cake is a valuable livestock feed containing about 2-7% oil, 45-55% protein and 4-10% fibre depending upon the method of extraction. Solvent extracted cake has low oil content than the expeller cake. High oil content cake is often used for live stock feeds. But cake with oil content of 2% or less if produced under hygienic conditions can be ground into flour for human consumption. The composition of groundnut meal varies widely according to the method of extraction, variety and location of growth. A good quality groundnut meal is comparable with soybean meal in its feeding value. When used in poultry diets, lysine and methionine must be added or supplied by components of the ration.

Solvent extraction has been employed successfully to remove aflatoxin from groundnut meal. Aqueous solution of dimethyl ether (methoxymethane) has been tried to extract groundnut oil and aflatoxin from groundnut meal (Desai, 1999). The dimethyl ether can be continuously recycled and the resulting meal is free of solvent. When the groundnuts are crushed for oil the major portion of the aflatoxin is concentrated in the groundnut cake. Aflatoxin in oilseed meal can also be inactivated by treating them with sodium hydroxide, methylamine, hydrogen peroxide and sulfur dioxide. The commercial use of these chemicals is however, limited due to solvent cost, deleterious residues or decrease in nutritional value of the groundnut meal.

Cottonseed meal

Due to acute shortage of edible oil and increased demand of cake, the cottonseed crushing has increased and the practice of feeding whole seed to cattle has been reduced considerably. In view of the realization of feed value of cottonseeds cake, farmers prefer to use cake as an animal feed. They also prefer that cake should be produced by expelling of decorticated cake. However there is need to motivate the farmers to the great extent by convincing them that the decorticated cake is superior in protein content than the un-decorticated seed cake. For this, the Ministry of Commerce and Industry, Government of India has appointed a committee which as recommended the following,

(i) Develop suitable balanced animal feed utilizing decorticated cottonseed cake, hull, salt, rice bran etc.,

(ii) Popularize the same among the farmers by way of publicity giving salient features of such products and its plus points by through radio, TV and other mass media. Beside it was also suggested to provide means of supply of decorticated cake at tax free, reasonable price to the farmers at the milk supply centres. These efforts have helped in increased use of decorticated cottonseed cake in animal feeding in the country.

Cottonseed meal has been found as one of the best protein concentrate feeds for milch cattle. Animal fed on cottonseed-meal ration showed better growth and performance. Normally 2.5 kg cottonseed meal is fed to mulch cattle per 450 kg live weight.

Cottonseed hulls are used as roughage in the animal feed. Hulls can be fed up to 8 kg per day per adult animal. The best way of feeding hulls to cattle is to mix with salt and other grains or meal in the form of slop or gruel. Comparative nutritional trials on cottonseed, sarson and toria cakes showed higher digestibility coefficient for fat and fibre for cottonseed cake than for the others (Lander and Dharmani, 1977). Similarly, there are few more studies reported on feeding of whole cottonseed meal to cattle although these studies give conflicting information.

Use of cottonseed cake in ration for livestock and poultry

Cottonseed cake or meal is an excellent cattle feed and is very rich source of protein. It is fed to cattle as concentrate along with fodder or roughage. Cottonseed meal/cake contains about 60% high quality protein and rich in essential amino acids. Cottonseed cake is one of the best feeds to cattle and milch cows.

The major problem with the use of cottonseed meal/cake in the diet of non-ruminants (single stomach animals such as poultry, swine, rabbits) is the presence of a number of toxic pigments such as gossypol and other pigments. These pigments cause darkening in the meal and also making amino acids unavailable. However, several processes have been developed where gossypol and related pigments can be reduced to a very low level without adversely affecting the quality of protein. The cake containing negligible gossypol can be fed to non-ruminants without any problem.

Improving protein quality of cottonseed cake

The most important factors for nutritive value of cottonseed cake are the percentage of protein, its quality and free gossypol content. Numerous studies have been conducted for improving the protein quality and nutritive value of cottonseed cake. The major objectives of such studies have been to maintain the quality of protein and keep the free gossypol and bound gossypol within accepted limits without adversely affecting the quality of cake protein and yield of oil. The free and total gossypol of this meal varied from 0.02 to 0.04% and from 0.08 to 0.95%, respectively. At constant moisture level and after raising boiling temperature from 93-110^0 C, free gossypol content showed lower value. Higher temperature cooking up to 137^0 C reduced the free gossypol. In view of this, cooking of meal at lower temperature (93^0 C) is advocated to give better quality products, which can be fed to chicken and ruminants. It may be mentioned that small amount of free gossypol present in the meal can be removed by boiling with water. The gossypol level in the cake obtained by extracting the cottonseed employing various extraction methods is given in the Table 1.

Table 1. Gossypol (free and total) in various types of meal, (%)

Type of pressing	Free gossypol	Total gossypol
Expeller	0.02-0.08	0.75-1.38
Hydraulic press	0.09-0.34	1.0-1.38
Solvent extraction	0.24-0.40	1.06-1.08

Source: (Pandey, 1998)

Mustard cake

Mustard defatted meal is used as a feed supplement for pig, poultry and cattle. The residue that remains after the oil extraction usually is high in protein content but has undesirable principles such as glucosinolates, phenolics, tannins and phytates. The high amount of erucic and eicosenoic acid present in mustard cake is deleterious to the health. Likewise, the presence of glucosinolates and phytates limit the utilization of cake due to pungency and poor digestibility causing various nutritional disorders and even toxicity in animals. The mustard meal has protein (35 to 45%), fat (10 to 14%), fibre(6 to 8%) and minerals(6 to 9%). However, the value of rapeseed mustard meal as protein source for human feeding is limited due to presence of sulpher containing compounds called glucosinolates. The presence of isothyocynate and their toxicity is not desirable in the protein meal. A considerable amount of work is in progress for modification of the milling process and on removal of toxic components for better use of protein meal.

Sunflower meal

The deoiled meal/cake of sunflower is used as animal feed. Functional test data show that sunflower cake and concentrate have high salt solubility, oil absorption and oil emulsification. High weight gain in rat feeding was obtained for sunflower blends fed with legume and animal proteins suggesting their applications in milk and meat extenders and in soybean based infant formulas. Heat treatment, mechanical agitation and emulsification are reported to be effective in stabilizing 80% of sunflower proteins. Sunflower cake blended with other cereal and legume gives better results as animal feed (Table 2).

Table 2. Protein nutritive values of sunflower cake blends with cereal, legume, animal proteins and lysine tested with rats

Protein Source	Feed consumption (g/rat)	Weight gain (g/rat)
Casein	264	72.8
Sunflower cake		
+Wheat flour	241	36.4
+Peas	342	101.7
+ Lysine	339	116.7

(Source: Sosulski,1979)

Safflower meal

The major problems in the utilization of safflower meal for animal feed purpose is the presence of high fibre in meal and a strong bitter flavor which can be reduced by dehulling of the seeds and pre-treating the meal. The removal of the hull affects the chemical composition of the safflower meal. The effect of dehulling is highly significant on reducing crude fibre content in ghanies pressed and solvent extracted meal. Effect of dehulling on chemical composition of safflower cake obtained by extracting the safflower seed employing various extraction methods is given in the Table 3.

Table 3. Effect of dehulling on chemical composition of safflower meal, (%db)

Type of meal	Crude protein (Nx6.25)	Crude fat	Crude fibre	Ash
Un-dehulled ghani/ expeller crushed	41.8	12.5	16.6	6.6
Dehulled ghani/ expeller crushed	55.4	13.2	3.9	4.2
Un-dehulled solvent extracted	54.2	2.0	19.6	7.2
Dehulled solvent extracted	59.9	2.1	4.3	5.9

(Source: Kulkarni et al.,1988)

Linseed cake

The linseed meal is normally obtained from ground un-extracted seed (35% oil), ground linseed cake (10% oil) and linseed meal (3% oil) from a solvent plant. Rich oil content can affect texture and flavor of meal. Immature linseed contains the enzyme linasi which releases prussic acid from glucoside linamarin. To avoid poisoning of cattle, linasi must be inactivated by heating the meal at 90°C for 10 minutes.

Losses in oilcakes during storage

The losses during post harvest operations are net losses and cannot be compensated, whereas, growth loss of crops is partially compensated by increasing yield from surviving plants. Losses in storage include loss in weight, quality, nutritive and market value. Each of these types of losses may have different significance, which varies with people, time, and place and also with existing loss assessment methods and techniques. Storage losses caused by insect infestation in food grains including the oilcakes are as follows:

1. Quantitative or weight loss
2. Qualitative losses
3. Damage to storage containers.

Qualitative losses in oilcakes during storage

Apart from physical loss in weight, there are qualitative depletions in nutrient profile, calorific value, and other adverse transformation during storage that must be considered. The growth of insects, moulds, and mites in stored oil cakes also results in development of toxins and allergens. Qualitative losses are further divided into following groups:

(i) Loss of nutritive and caloric values

Infestation by insects degrades nutritive and calorific values of oilcakes. The nutritional quality of the oilcakes is adversely affected by a number of factors. Deterioration of the cake initiates immediately after fertilization and embryonic development of the caryopsis or cotyledons by the disturbance of the enzyme sequence. Development of artifact in the biosynthetic process that could be induced by environmental stress, xenebiotics, abnormal levels of growth, regulatory compounds, infection by fungal, bacterial, and viral agents.

(ii) Chemical changes in cakes content

During storage insects infestation takes place either inside or on the surface of cakes resulting biochemical degradation. Biochemical changes in cakes take place are discussed below:

(a) Changes in protein

The deterioration of nutritive value of oilcakes is assumed to be associated with change in protein solubility and digestibility by pepsin and trypsin enzymes.

(b) Changes in fats

The residual oilcake fats and oils are changed either by hydrolysis, which may result in free fatty acids. If only flour is kept in storage for short time, it will give some foul odor even at low moisture content. Fat hydrolysis is faster as comparatively carbohydrates and proteins.

Processing of oilseeds for quality cake

For better oil recovery and good quality cakes, pre-treatments of the oilseeds has to be done while, oil is being extracted using mechanical expellers. The following pre-treatment are suggested:

- grading of oilseeds
- decortication
- instant addition of moisture
- moisture addition 24 h prior to expression
- size reduction
- steaming, etc.

Cleaning and grading of oilseeds

Normally, the oilseeds are get mixed with a variety of foreign materials such as sand, stones, stalks, weed seeds, foliage etc., during harvesting, handling and transportation. It is advisable to clean oilseeds before putting in the store, which can be used for further processing later on particularly oil extraction. Proper cleaning of oilseeds can increase crushing capacity of oil expelling units, oil recovery, and energy consumption, reduction in plant maintenance and improvement in the quality of oil and cake. Hence, pre-cleaning of oil is advisable for getting quality cakes.

Shelling/decortication

Most of the oilseeds hulls are not fit for direct oil expression and as animal feed therefore, removal of hulls of seeds like groundnut, sunflower, safflower, castor including cotton seed is necessary for higher oil recovery and better quality cakes. The diversity of machines used for the dehulling process is dependant their different shape and structures and differences in physical and mechanical properties of the kernels and hulls. In brief, presence of hull i.e. about 20-30% depending upon types of oilseeds causes the following;

- rapid wear of the moving parts of the expeller
- reduce total oil yield
- transfers yields pigments from the hull to the extracted oil
- consumption of high specific energy.
- yielding cake of poorer quality

Moisture addition/steaming of the oilseeds

The optimum levels of moisture content of oilseeds required for the appropriate physico-chemical changes during pressing which in turn increases the oil recovery and yield the cake having less residual oil in it. Moisture also works as heat transfer medium so that total heat generated by worm during pressing might be fully transferred to the individual fat globules which results in break down of the emulsion form of the fat and helps in releasing more oil droplets. The most important steps in oilseed preparation for extraction of oil is steaming or hydrothermal treatment of the ground or flaked oilseeds. The steaming temperatures may vary in the range of 70-110°C, depending upon the type of oilseed and expression process. This unit operation serves different objectives such as; rupture the oil globules for ease of oozing out of oil, increase the flowability of the oil, render cell walls more permeable to oil flow, increase plasticity of crushed seed for fast and efficient pressing, inactivation of anti-nutritional constituents such as trypsin inhibitor and toxic substances like gossypol, aflatoxin, etc., de-activation of the lipase that release free fatty acids and increase refining losses, destruction of enzymes which are detrimental to oil and meal quality(Shukla et al., 1992).

Almost all the oilseeds yield oil more readily if cooked adequately prior to their mechanical expression and or solvent extraction. The cooking process destroys moulds and bacteria to improve microbiological as well as keeping quality of oilcakes. Further the process destroys the heat labile anti-nutritional factors to improve the nutritive value of protein rich oilseed meals. Heat supplement work of water in cooking meal and also in coagulating albuminoids. The cooking temperatures and its duration period for most of the oilseeds range between 105-130 °C and 30-120 minutes respectively.

Provision of cooling during extraction

Mostly oilseeds are crushed in mechanical expeller oil extraction. During the process of extraction, cake as discharged from press is at high temperature, (around 90-160 °C) and low moisture content of 1-4% (wet basis) due to the frictional heat developed by pressure in the press barrel. It may continue to heat and begin to smolder if accumulated in heaps or if immediately ground into meal and stacked hot. To lower the temperature, cake should be quickly passed through a cooler, which tumbles the cake about in a cold air blast. Cold water may also be sprayed on the cake conveyor ahead of the cooler and at the exit. Adding water in several stages permits better absorption and produces equilibrium between the cake and atmospheric humidity, reducing the amount of moisture lost in milling. Cooled, humidified cake may be stored for longer period without spoilage and ground when convenient in hammer mills/attrition mills for further use.

Hence, for getting good quality cakes, pre-treatments to the oilseeds have to be applied while oil is to be extracted using mechanical expellers. The cooking/steaming process destroys moulds and bacteria to improve microbiological as well as keeping quality of oilcakes. Further the process destroys the heat labile anti-nutritional factors to improve nutritive value of protein rich oilseed meals. A typical process for production of quality oilcake has been suggested below;

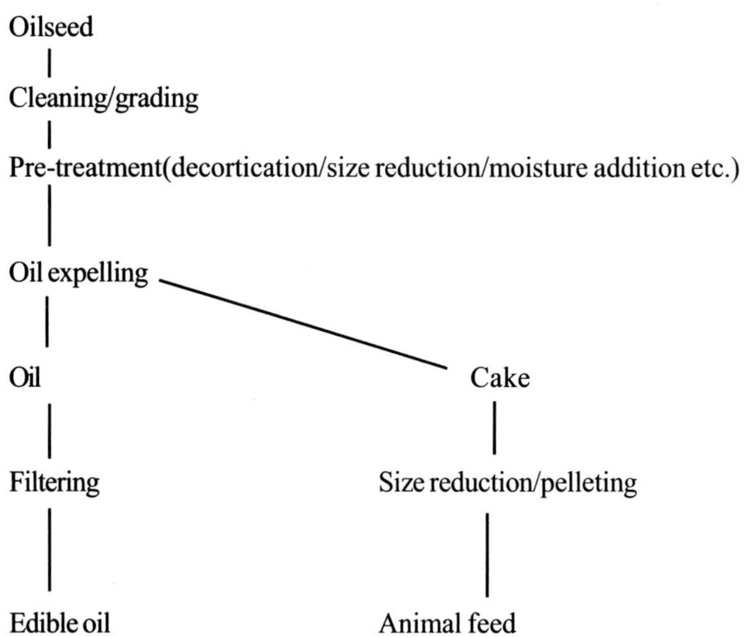

Fig. 1. A typical process for production of quality oilcake

Suitable storage structures and methods

The oilcakes can be well protected by using various types of improved storage structures.

(A) In-door bins

i) Domestic metal bins: the capacity of these bins ranges from 3-30 quintals. These are indoor bins. These bins are prepared from galvanized iron sheets. These are found suitable for storage of all types of grains including oilcakes.

ii) Pucca kothi: this is made up of burned bricks plastered with cement mortar. The structures is constructed in two compartments and 1 metric tonne of material can be stored.

iii) Paddy straw-mud ring bin: this is made from paddy straw rope plastered on both sides with specially prepared mud. The outer surface is further plastered with mud to prevent moisture. Capacity of such structures is about 400 kg.

(B) Out-door bins

i) **Storage bin:** There basis quite popular in rural India. These bins are either circular or square with storage capacity ranging from 1 to 15 quintals.

ii) **Pusa bin:** The design of pusabin consists of two brick walls of 10 cm thick each using sun dried bricks with polythene sheet sandwiched in between. The structure is constructed on masonry plat form plastered with cement mortar. A mud slab is provided at the top on a wooden frame structure. The polythene sheet is also provided at the top and the base to make the structure completely moisture proof and air tight.

Surface treatment and fumigation techniques with suitable material may be used in oilcakes to avoid fungus growth during storage.

Recommendations

1. The oilseeds have to be cleaned properly before oil extraction. Proper cleaning of oilseeds can increase crushing capacity of oil expelling units, oil recovery, and energy consumption and reduces in plant maintenance and improve the quality of oil and cake
2. Most of the oilseeds hulls are not fit for direct oil expression and as animal feed therefore, removal of hulls of seeds like groundnut, sunflower, safflower, castor including cotton seed is necessary for higher oil recovery and better quality cakes.
3. For getting better oil recovery and good quality cakes, pre-treatments such as grading, size reduction, moisture addition, etc. to the oilseeds has to be applied before extraction by mechanical expellers.
4. The provision for cooling arrangement of oil cakes immediately after extraction should be done for its longer storage period without spoilage.
5. Appropriate storage structures and methods should be adopted for enhanced storage life of oilcakes and to insure its quality during storage.

The livestock play an important role in the agrarian economy of most of the developing countries and more so in India because of small land holding and a substantial proportion of rural population possessing no land. Much progress has been made in the livestock improvement as is reflected from the increase in milk, meat, egg and broiler production. Still the productivity of the livestock in India is relatively lower as compared to those in agriculturally advanced countries. However, considering the efforts put in for their genetic improvement, the feed resources available, tropical heat and disease problems they are to face. A major limitation in production is the non-availability of adequate quantity of quality feed. The livestock in India are fed, on crop residues, poor quality natural vegetation, cereal and oilseed milling waste and other industrial by products. There is serious shortage of feed concentrates, dry and green fodder and the livestock have to obtain greater part of their nutrients from agricultural and industrial by products. The meal remaining after oil extraction from various oilseeds is also being used as livestock feed. Proper handling and storage of oilseeds is important for their processing into quality products including oilcakes since oilseeds are prone to auto-catalytic deteriorative processes, enzymatic action, microbial spoilage, etc. Aflatoxin produced in oilseeds by strains of Aspergilas flavus comes out partly in the expressed oil and the rest remain in the residual cake. Such oil requires further refining for removal of its aflatoxin and render it unsafe for human consumption and such oilcakes unless fully detoxified is unsafe for even animal feed. Apart from physical loss in weight, there are qualitative depletions in nutrient confronts, caloric value, and other adverse transformation in oilcakes during storage. The growth of insects, moulds, and mites in stored oilcakes also results in development of toxins and allergens. The storage life of various oilseeds cakes could also be increased with use of proper post harvest techniques and pre-treatments. For getting better oil recovery and good quality cakes, pre-treatments to the oilseeds has to be done while oil is being extracted using mechanical expellers. Almost all oilseeds yield oil more readily if cooked/steamed adequately prior to their mechanical expression and or solvent extraction. The cooking/steaming process destroys moulds and bacteria to improve microbiological as well as keeping quality of oilcakes. Further, the process destroys the heat labile anti-nutritional factors to improve nutritive value of protein rich oilseed meals.

In this paper, prevalent practice for production of oil cakes from various oilseeds has been described. The use of various pre-treatment and a typical process for production of quality oilcake has also been suggested. Apart from this, qualitative losses in oilcakes during storage have been listed and the optimum storage conditions and improved storage structures to over come these losses have also been mentioned hoping that with technology intervention, oilcakes could be made up to high quality protein source for livestock.

Bibliograhy

Desai, B.B., Kotecha, P.M. and Saunkhe, D.K.1999. Science and technology of groundnut: Biology, Production, processing and Utilization. Published by Naya Prokash, 206, Bidhan Sarani, Calcutta:524-545.

Kulkarni, D.N., Rao, M.S.N. and Ingle, U.M.1988. Nutritional and processing aspects of edible grade meal from available cultivars of sunflower. Proc. National Seminar on Strategies for making India self reliant in vegetable oils, DOR, Hyderabad

Pandey, S.N.1998. Cottonseed and its utilization. ICAR Publication, New Delhi

Shukla, B.D., Srivatava, P.K. and Gupta, R.K.1992. Oilseed Processing Technology. CIAE, Bhopal, India.

Sosulski, F.1979. Food uses of sunflower proteins. J. Am. Oil Chem. Soc., 56: 438-42.

Statistics 2002-03. The Central Organization for Oil Industry& Trade, New Delhi.

7
LIVESTOCK SITUATION AND CEREAL DEMAND

Anil Kumar, S.S. Kundu and S.B. Maity

The livestock production system is undergoing a radical change in India. The traditional agricultural sector, which provides employment to about 75% of the rural working population, can no longer support any additional employment. With arable land under cultivation remaining stagnant and more of agricultural machinery and implements being employed, there remain limited scope for more employment in agriculture. Livestock on the other hand, has been providing succor to rural people through employment and income, in addition to the help rendered in agricultural operations and providing manure to the fields and fuel for hearth. The livestock sector contributes 5.9 percent to country's Gross Domestic Product (GDP) and 30.3 percent to agricultural output at current prices. It is estimated that (1993-94) that almost 18 million people are employed in livestock sector in principal (9.8 million) or subsidiary (8.6 million) sectors (Planning Commission, 2001). During recent years a Livestock Revolution has been unfolding on Indian horizon which is demand driven unlike the Green Revolution which was supply driven. The population growth, urbanization and income growth has created a huge demand for food from animal origin. This is apart from the changing dietary preferences of rural people towards food from animal origin due to exposure of mass media. All this will place increasing pressure on livestock production system in which the traditional breeds and feeding systems are likely to give way to improved breeds and a greater reliance on cereal feeds. This paper attempts to analyze the changing livestock production systems, the factors driving the livestock revolution and the consequent demand for the cereal grains to fuel the revolution to continue.

Changing livestock production system

The livestock production in recent times has been undergoing a paradigm shift. From being a companion animal of the farmers in subsistence agriculture, they have come to occupy the center place as the main source of livelihood. The cows and buffaloes have moved from the interiors of villages to peri-urban areas to provide milk to urban consumers. Even in the interiors of the countryside, the dairy co-operatives have made their effective presence thereby giving a fillip to the business of keeping dairy cows and buffaloes. The traditional role of cattle as source of motive power to agricultural operations has greatly diminished which have left the oxen useless. We often come across with news reports of large-scale movements of zebu cows and bullocks to West Bengal and Bangladesh for slaughter. The economic considerations often overweighs the religious sentiments howsoever we may try to look otherwise. The farmers either simply drive away the non-productive cattle or even bargains for a little sum with the unscrupulous traders. This way he saves the precious feed resources to be put to more productive use through buffaloes or crossbred cows.

The traditional grazing lands have over the years shrunken due to encroachments not only by people but also by the government by giving away on pattas. The continued neglect of the village commons have resulted in decline in productivity and carrying capacity. They have just become the exercising grounds for livestock. A further increase in livestock production could be expected only from improved feeding in the stall and not from the grazing systems alone. Therefore, the role of compounded feed industry is vital in making available the quality feed at economic rates to livestock in peri-urban areas, commercial units and progressive farmers.

Similarly, the poultry industry has come of age from being in the backyard to factory style production adopting the latest technologies available globally. The country is now recognized as a major player in international market. There is however a regional skew ness with most of it being concentrated in south. The phenomenal growth in poultry industry has made available the products at rates, which the consumers used to pay a decade ago. Therefore, the changing livestock production system has a major implication on food and nutritional security for a large section of the society.

The driving force for livestock revolution

The livestock revolution unfolding on Indian horizon is being driven by factors, which include the huge human population base, rate of urbanization, growth in per capita income and change in consumption behaviour. A discussion on this aspect is relevant to the theme of the paper as both human as well as livestock both are the consumer of cereals.

Human population growth rate

The human population in India is 1033 million (2001) which is expected to reach 1312 million in 2020 (Table 1). The growth rate (Table 2) which was over 2 percent in 1980s has of late slowed down to under 2 percent in 1990s and will further fall down to 0.77 percent 2020s. Although the growth rate has been decreasing appreciably, still the huge population base provides market, which is very large.

Table 1: Human, urban and rural population in India (in million)

	2001	2010	2020	2030
Total population	1033	1174	1312	1417
Urban population	288	355	455	579
% urban pop	27.8	30.2	34.7	40.9
Rural population	745	819	857	838
% rural pop	72.2	69.8	65.3	59.1

Source: FAO (2004)

Rate of urbanization

The urban population which stands at 288 million (27.8 % of the total) is poised to increase by 58 percent by 2020 and double by 2030 when they will become 41 percent of the total population. Urbanization brings about a marked shift in the lifestyle of people including the change in dietary feeding habits. People tend to shed away the taboo towards meat and egg as prevalent in rural areas which results in increased demand for products of animal origin.

Table 2: Growth rate (% p.a.) in human, urban and rural population

	2000-10	2010-20	2020-30
Total population	1.44	1.12	0.77
Urban population	2.36	2.50	2.44
Rural population	1.07	0.46	-0.23

Source: FAO (2004)

Growth in per capita income and change in dietary habits

The per capita income in India is expected to grow at an average rate of 3.7 percent per year over 1993-2020 (Bhalla et al., 1999). The food consumption behaviour of people changes because of exposure to mass media, tempting to explore new tastes. It has been observed that expenditure elasticities for food of animal origin (Table 3) have a higher coefficient. The expenditure elasticity measures the percentage change in expenditure on a particular food group, given 1 percent increase in total expenditure. Therefore, any increase in per capita income will create more demand for livestock products. It is pertinent to note that the elasticity for meat and eggs is higher in rural areas than urban areas (Table 3) which indicates a huge insatiated demand for livestock products in rural areas.

Table 3: Estimates of expenditure elasticity for different commodities

Source		Year	Cereals	Meat and eggs	Milk and milk products
Kumar, 1998	Rural	1993-94	-0.007	0.848	0.458
	Urban	1993-94	-0.037	0.633	0.372
Bhalla et al., 1999					
	Rural	1993	0.29	1.01	1.53
		2020	0.10	1.25	1.53
	Urban	1993	0.18	0.71	0.94
		2020	0.10	0.74	1.05

Source: Kumar (1998); Bhalla et al., (1999)

Growth in livestock population

India is endowed with huge livestock population. They have been an integral part of the way of living of the rural people. But with changing times when economic considerations take paramount place affecting every sphere of activity, the livestock sector has not remained aloof. Trend in livestock numbers between 1961 and 2004 have been presented in Table 4 and their population projected up to 2025 taking into the growth rate of last ten years (1984-2004). A look at the growth rate (Table 5) of cattle reveals that its number increased up to 1990 after which a declining trend has set in which has become more pronounced during last five years, registering decrease of 1percent p.a. On the other hand buffaloes have shown a steady march since 1970 along with the Operation Flood Programme. In many quarters, the decline in cattle numbers have been a cause of concern, putting a question mark on the sustainability of the agricultural sector through diminished supply of manure to fields. But do we need to panic or just let the equilibrium find its way through interplay of economic factors. In fact, the combined population of cattle and buffalo (Table 4) have remained almost constant or exhibited a marginal decline (during last five years). The attrition in cattle numbers have spared the valuable feed resources to be put to more productive use through buffaloes and high yielding crossbred cows, providing income and employment to farmers. It is not known if the dung of cattle is superior to that of buffalo in supplying the organic matter to fields. Even otherwise, the government and the religious agencies together cannot possibly afford to arrest the decline howsoever it may try, when the farmers are not willing to retain the low productive cattle.

Table 4: Trend in livestock number 1961-2004, and their projection* 2005-2025 (number in million)

Item	1961	1971	1981	1991	2001	2004	2005	2010	2015	2020	2025
Cattle	176	178	189	204	191	186	184	176	168	161	154
Buffaloes	51	57	68	82	94	98	99	105	111	118	125
Sheep	40	40	46	50	60	63	64	69	75	81	88
Goats	61	67	91	114	121	120	120	122	123	124	126
Pigs	5	7	10	13	14	14	14	15	15	15	15
Chickens	108	132	197	300	377	425	441	529	635	762	915
Cattle+Buffalo	227	235	256	286	286	283	283	281	280	279	280

*projection based on growth rate of last ten years (1994-2004)

The population of goats has over the years remained stagnant in recent decades because the production system, which supports them, has come under threat. The public grazing land is getting reduced because of encroachment and their over use has caused a decline in the productivity and carrying capacity. Therefore, the demand for goat meat is not being met resulting in increase in its price, making it unaffordable to many. Hence, the traditional goat rearing practice has to undergo a change and supplementation under stall feeding condition may be promoted to get further increase in productivity. Pig in India is caught in its image as filthy animal surviving in drains and by-lanes, evoking strong aversion to the potential meat eaters. Its role in alleviating the food and nutritional security for the lower income groups and weaker sections of the society needs attention. Their excellent feed conversion efficiency need to be exploited as has been done in China and a facelift is required to make it more acceptable to consumers. The chickens have shown an impressive growth consistently over last three decades.

Table 5: Growth rate (%p.a.) in livestock no. during different periods

Item	1961-71	1971-81	1981-91	1991-2001	Last 20 years 1984-2004	Last 10 years 1994-2004	Last 5 years 1999-2004
Cattle	0.13	0.60	0.76	-0.62	-0.25	-0.88	-1.00
Buffaloes	1.06	1.73	1.98	1.40	1.44	1.20	1.18
Sheep	-0.03	1.47	0.69	1.96	1.38	1.66	1.19
Goats	0.97	3.11	2.30	0.57	0.94	0.22	-0.30
Pigs	2.36	3.92	2.67	1.07	1.65	0.37	1.01
Chickens	2.06	4.09	4.31	2.30	3.06	3.72	4.26
Cattle+Buffalo	0.34	0.88	1.09	0.00	0.27	-0.22	-0.28

Trend in milk production

The Operation Flood programme has revolutionized the dairy sector in India. The production now stands at 90 million tones (2004, Table 6) registering an average growth rate of 3.95 percent p.a. during last ten years. The share of buffalo milk is 55 percent, cattle 42 percent and goat 3 percent (Table 8). Based on the growth rate (Table 7) of last ten years the total milk production is expected to reach 170 million tones by 2020. Delgado et al., (1999) has projected it to reach 172 million tones by 2020 with a growth rate of 1.6 percent p.a. between 1993 and 2020.

Table 6: Milk production trend 1961-2004, and their projection* 2005-2025 (million metric tonne)

Item	1961	1971	1981	1991	2001	2004	Projected yield 2005	2010	2015	2020	2025
Buffalo Milk	11	12	19	29	47	50	52	65	80	99	123
Cow Milk, Whole, Fresh	9	9	14	23	36	38	39	47	57	68	82
Goat Milk	0.5	0.7	1.0	2.3	2.6	2.6	2.6	2.5	2.5	2.4	2.4
Milk,Total	20	23	34	54	85	90	94	114	139	170	208

*projection based on growth rate of last ten years (1994-2004)

Table 7: Growth rate (%p.a.) in milk production during different periods

Item	1961-71	1971-81	1981-91	1991-2001	Last 20 years 1984-2004	Last 10 years 1994-2004	Last 5 years 1999-2004
Buffalo Milk	1.11	4.31	4.28	4.98	3.80	4.39	3.06
Cow Milk	0.77	4.31	4.81	4.45	4.23	3.76	2.88
Goat Milk	2.35	4.31	8.60	1.02	3.79	-0.48	2.64
Total Milk	**1.00**	**4.31**	**4.65**	**4.60**	**3.97**	**3.95**	**2.97**

Table 8: Percent share of different component in milk production

Item	1961	1971	1981	1991	2001	2004
Buffalo Milk	54.4	55.0	55.0	53.0	55.0	55.3
Cow Milk	43.0	42.0	42.0	42.6	42.0	41.8
Goat Milk	2.6	3.0	3.0	4.3	3.1	2.9
Total Milk	**100.0**	**100.0**	**100.0**	**100.0**	**100.0**	**100.0**

Trend in meat production

The meat sector has shown impressive growth indicating the changing dietary habits of population. In 1987-88, only 43.7 and 31.5 percent of urban and rural households, respectively, consumed meat whereas more than half of both types of households consumed meat in 1993-94 (NSS 1990; 1996). The total meat production (Table 9) stands at 6.032 million tones (FAO, 2004). Delgado et al., (1999) projected the total production to reach to 8 million tones in 2020 with an average growth rate of 2.8 percent p.a. between 1993-2020. A look at the different components of the total meat production reveals that poultry contributes 28 percent, Buffalo and Beef &Veal each 24.6 percent and pig and goat each contributing 8 percent (Table 11). While the brolier is growing at the rate of 12 percent during last ten years, the growth rate in buffalo and sheep meat is slightly above 1 percent (Table 10). The growth rate in beef has declined in recent years and it is more so in goat meat production. It appears that the present production system of goat production has reached its zenith and therefore any increase in production may come through increased productivity in commercial manner for which supplementation through stall-feeding will be desirable.

Table 9: Meat production trend 1961-2004 (,000 metric tonne)

Item	1961	1971	1981	1991	2001	2004
Beef and Veal	506	640	863	1228	1452	1483
Buffalo Meat	551	683	847	1224	1433	1483
Goat Meat	235	244	313	434	469	475
Mutton and Lamb	122	138	159	185	230	239
Pig meat	154	194	279	434	483	497
Meat others	50	76	108	129	140	140
Poultry Meat	78	95	141	389	1307	1715
Meat, Total	1696	2070	2710	4023	5515	6032
Eggs Primary	170	308	598	1210	1870	1890

Table 10: Growth rate (%) in meat production during different periods

Item	1961-71	1971-81	1981-91	1991-2001	Last 20 years 1984-2004	Last 10 years 1994-2004	Last 5 years 1999-2004
Beef and Veal	2.38	3.04	3.58	1.70	2.17	0.87	0.85
Buffalo Meat	2.17	2.18	3.75	1.58	2.27	1.16	1.18
Goat Meat	0.38	2.51	3.34	0.78	1.59	0.63	0.38
Mutton and Lamb	1.21	1.41	1.53	2.23	1.46	1.35	0.93
Pig meat	2.36	3.68	4.52	1.08	2.48	0.41	1.02
Meat, others	4.28	3.58	1.79	0.82	0.99	0.59	0.43
Poultry Meat	2.02	4.03	10.67	12.88	12.05	12.07	14.42
Meat, Total	2.01	2.73	4.03	3.20	3.50	2.99	3.83
Eggs Primary	6.12	6.86	7.30	4.45	4.48	2.84	2.35

Table 11: Percent share of different component in meat production

Item	1961	1971	1981	1991	2001	2004
Beef and Veal	29.8	30.9	31.9	30.5	26.3	24.6
Buffalo Meat	32.5	33.0	31.3	30.4	26.0	24.6
Goat Meat	13.9	11.8	11.5	10.8	8.5	7.9
Mutton and Lamb	7.2	6.7	5.9	4.6	4.2	4.0
Pig meat	9.1	9.4	10.3	10.8	8.8	8.2
Meat, others	2.9	3.7	4.0	3.2	2.5	2.3
Poultry Meat	4.6	4.6	5.2	9.7	23.7	28.4
Meat, Total	**100.0**	**100.0**	**100.0**	**100.0**	**100.0**	**100.0**

Cereal demand for food and feed

The present production of cereals in India is 196.2 million metric tones (2001, Table 16), of which 158 million tones is used as food and 7.9 million tones as feed. It is also one of the important consumer and producer of coarse cereals in the world. However, in contrast to the developed countries where cereals are used for livestock feed, it is staple food for the people in India and a source of income and employment. Annual growth of total cereal in India during 1961 to 1999 was 2.82 percent. This growth kept pace with the population growth of about 2 percent and the increase in income. The growth was mainly contributed by wheat and rice while coarse cereal except maize had declined. Cultivated area under rice and wheat have increased while it declined for all coarse cereals except maize. With improvement in standard of living of the population, the demand for cereals has been shown to decline (Table 12; Ramesh Chand, 2003).

Table 12: Demand projection for cereals towards 2020, million tonne

Source	Year	Food	Feed	Sub total	Growth rate % p.a.	
					Food	Feed
Bhalla et al., 1993	1993	147.12	3.71	150.83		
	2020	246.08	50.11	296.19	1.92	10.12
Kumar, 1998	1995	150.6	6.54	156.60		
	2020	237.6	15.19	252.25	1.84	3.43
Delgado et al., 1999	1993		3			
	2020		14			5.87

Table 13: Changes in food consumption pattern in rural and urban India, 1977-1999 (kg/person/annum)

	1977	1987	1993	1999
Total cereals				
Rural area	192.6	179.5	163.0	152.6
Urban area	147.0	139.1	129.3	125.0
Milk/ milk product				
Rural area	24.6	58.0	51.4	50.5
Urban area	39.7	64.9	68.3	72.4
Meat, egg, fish				
Rural area	2.7	3.3	4.1	5.0
Urban area	4.8	4.9	6.3	6.8

There has been a sharp decline in both rural as well as urban areas in per capita consumption of rice, wheat and coarse cereals since 1987-88 (Table 13). On the other hand meat, egg and fish has shown appreciable increase (Ramesh Chand, 2003). This provides strong evidence that in India food consumption pattern is getting increasingly diversified towards non-cereal products.

How this increase in demand for livestock products will be realized? The surge in demand will place increasing pressure on livestock production systems. The traditional breeds and feeding practices are likely to give way to improved breeds and a greater reliance on high energy cereal feeds. Presently, the livestock production system depend heavily on crop by-products, household waste, and open grazing areas as sources of feed. Presently 7.9 million tones of cereals are being fed to livestock, which is 4 percent of the total cereal production. Further expansion of the traditional sources of feed to support a large increase in livestock production seems unlikely, particularly as available grazing areas are shrinking and are already seriously degraded (Repetto, 1994). The grazing systems are rapidly diminishing in importance and urbanization and crop production are encroaching on traditional grazing areas. Similarly, mixed farming systems also face limits. Innovations in crop production have reduced crop residues and nongrain biomass available for feeding (Delgado et al., 1999). Therefore, availability of feed grains for livestock production will determine if the demand for livestock products could be met in future. The annual growth rate in total cereal production during 1982-94 was 3.0 percent whereas it was 3.5 percent for total cereal use as feed. Delgado et al., (1999) have estimated that the annual growth rate of total cereal use as feed between 1993-2020 will be 5.0 percent taking it from 3 million tones (1993) to 14 million tones (2020). Kumar

(1998) has also reported a similar cereal feed requirement of 15.19 million tones in 2020. However, Bhalla et al., (1999) projected the cereal feed demand to be 50.11 million tones in 2020 during which time India could have cereal deficit of 36 to 64 million tones per year by 2020. The present level of requirement of animal feed is estimated at 114.35 million tonnes for all species of livestock including poultry and is increasing at the rate of 2.62 percent p.a. As per the Planning Commission (2001), the present level of production is 41.96 million tonnes, thus showing a deficit of 64.27 percent. This gap is likely to continue. Taneja (1999) has also shown a 47 percent shortage of concentrate. The increase in demand for quality feed for high producing animals, the concentrate feed use is likely to increase. Farmers in rural areas manage the deficit by the use of other grains like wheat and broken rice including kitchen waste for feeding the productive animals. Ramesh Chand (2003) has analysed the estimates for cereal demand growth and reported that estimate of Bhalla et al., (1993) was an overestimate whereas, that of Kumar (1999) underestimated the cereal demand. He opined that the growth in cereal demand in India could be 2.20 percent p.a. by 2020.

To meet the demands of huge livestock population and their increasing productivity, feed resources need to be matched accordingly. At present the country faces a net deficit of 61.1percent green fodder, 21.9% dry crop residues, and 64% in concentrate feed. In the concentrate feed, coarse cereals like maize, barley, sorghum and pearl millet has a role and the rest is constituted by various oil meals and cakes. In India, during 2000-01, the total availability of oil meal was 15.82 million tones, of which 2.35 million tones (2.18 soybean cake, 0.003 Groundnut cake and 0.167mt other meals) were exported. The balance 13.27 mt was left in the domestic market. This included 4.05 mt of cotton seed meal, 2.55 mt rice bran and 1.42 mt other minor meals, 1.32 mt soybean meal, 1.88 mt of GNC and 2.05 mt of rapeseed meal.

Among various oil meals and cakes used for livestock feeding, GNC, mustard cake and cotton seed cake are common. Mustard cake is substantially used in northern and eastern part of the country but the quality varies widely because of adulteration with rapeseed meal. Of the total 28.33 mt of oil seed (Table 14) produced during 2004, soybean, cotton seed and ground nut seed were 7.0, 4.8, and 7.5 mt respectively. substantial amount of rapeseed (6.8 mt) was also produced during the period. From 28.33 mt of oil seed produced, 10.55 mt of oil cake was produced for utilization as livestock feed. This supplied an equivalent of 4.0 mt of crude protein to animals. Soybean and ground nut cake which are exported in substantial quantity may be retained in the country to help bridge the deficit in concentrate feed.

Table 14: Production of oil seeds and meal in India, 2004 (,000 tonnes)

	Oil seed	Oil cake	Crude Protein yield
Soybeans	7000	2065	929
Cottonseed	4800	499	125
Groundnuts in Shell	7500	3368	1347
Sunflower Seed	1250	396	119
Rapeseed	6800	3788	1325
Sesame Seed	800	315	94
Linseed	179	120	34
Total	**28329**	**10551**	**3974**

The decrease in per capita cereal consumption (Table 13) and slow growth rate in use of cereal as food (Table 15) indicates a change in consumption basket. Increasing mechanization of agriculture in rural area has reduced physical exertion and access to transport facilities has reduced calorie intake and hence reduced the cereal demand as food. With increase in income people go for nutritious, balanced and healthy food rather than increasing calorie intake. Despite the observed growth in demand for livestock products, per capita consumption of meat, egg and fish in India remains very low (Ram Chand, 2003). This is largely due to socio-cultural factors of consumers. Even if it can be afforded, people in India do not take meat on a regular basis. For a vast majority of those who are non-vegetarian meat intake is preferred occasionally and not as a part of regular diet. Therefore, India is not likely to witness serious competition between food and feed uses of grain.

Table 15: Projected growth rates in demand for major food towards 2020 AD and recent growth in supply

Commodity	Demand growth rate 1995-2020	Output growth rate in last 10 years
Cereals	1.88	2.16
Milk	3.26	4.14
Egg	3.76	4.59
Fish	3.75	4.28
Pulses	2.98	0.63
Vegetable	2.91	4.79
Fruit	3.20	5.75

Ramesh Chand (1999)

Table 16: Domestic supply and utilization of cereals in India, 2001 (1000 Metric tons)

	Domestic supply					Domestic utilization					
	Prod	**Import**	**Stock**	**Exp**	**Total**	**Feed**	**Seed**	**F/Manu**	**Waste**	**Uses**	**Food**
Cereals	196267	44	-8056	5392	182863	7909	10402	74	6441	70	157980
Wheat	69681	10	1135	3016	67811	836	4742	0	2998	0	59235
Rice (Milled eq.)	93203	28	-9190	2220	81822	373	4269	0	934	32	76215
Barley	1431	0	0	1	1430	129	79	74	29		1119
Maize	13160	5	-2	124	13039	6300	733	0	1408	38	4560
Rye											
Oats											
Millet	11235	0		19	11216	180	304	0	552		10180
Sorghum	7557	0		0	7556	91	275	0	520		6670

Food Balance Sheet (FAO, 2004)

Central food grain stock and their disposal

For a vast country like India where occurrence of natural calamity is a regular phenomenon, creation of a buffer stock is vital to food security for its huge population. In recent years large quantity of cereals (rice and wheat) has piled up in government stock which has reached a level of about 60 million tone (Table 17). With food grain stock piling up in godowns, the government made an attempt to export wheat in 2001-02 at an implicit subsidy or loss of Rs.4000/- per tone of wheat (Ramesh Chand, 2003). The justification given for export of rice and wheat at a huge loss and a price below domestic market is that there is no alternative to dispose off the massive stock of wheat that has accumulated with government agencies. Releasing such stock in open market rather than its sale would put downward pressure on domestic prices and might force domestic prices to go below minimum support price. The more serious implication of such move would be its adverse impact on future output growth and supply.

Table 17: Central food grain stock: actual stock and the norm (million tonne)

Year	January	April	June	October
Actual stock				
1997	20.0	16.4	22.4	15.3
1998	18.3	18.2	28.5	24.2
1999	24.4	21.9	33.1	28.0
2000	31.4	21.7	42.2	40.0
2001	45.7	44.7	61.7	58.3
2002	58.0	62.4		
Norm	**16.8**	**15.8**	**24.3**	**18.1**

Source: Economic Survey 2001-02

The other alternate option to clear the massive stock by supplying them to livestock feed industry was not considered. Neither has the feed industry put forth its case to the government. It is better to divert the excess stock of cereals to feed manufacturing industry rather than exporting them at huge subsidy or keeping them in godowns. The industries in turn could make available the animal feed at lower rates thereby giving a boost to the livestock industry. This would start rolling a chain of events creating additional employment and income simultaneously strengthening the food and nutrition security in the country.

Role of feed manufacturing industry

The feed manufacturing industry will have to play an important role in coming years because the livestock production system in the country is changing its character. Livestock feed are manufactured by industries under the banner of 'Compounded Livestock Feed Manufacturers' Association of India' (CLFMA) and other co-operatives. The association was formed in 1967 with the objectives of helping the promotion of the concept of balanced feeding of animals in accordance with the nutritional requirements for deriving maximum output through productivity improvement. CLFMA, at present has an installed capacity of over 5 million tones/ yr and produces 2.585million tones of feed (Table 18) which include 1.105 million tones of cattle feed, 1.45 million tonnes poultry feed and 0.029 million tonnes other feed. Other small industries in the unorganized sector produces 2 million tones/yr, thus making a total of about 5 million tones per year against a total demand of 42 million tones/yr of concentrate feed (Pathak, 2003). Several state Agro-Industrial Co-op have also started manufacturing compounded feed and many poultry industries have established their own feed milling facilities but they require research and development to take care of the quality. The increasing crossbred cattle together with buffalo population and the phenomenal growth in poultry sector all look towards the feed manufacturing industry to meet their requirement to sustain the momentum in livestock sector to cater to the demands of human population in decades to come.

Table 18: State wise production (in tones) of cattle, poultry and other feeds by CLFMA during 2003-04.

	Cattle	Poultry	Other feeds	Total
Andhra Pradesh	7444	175378	5676	188499
Assam	1121	1207	-	2328
Bihar	23425	35405	-	58830
Chandigarh	2817	3587	-	6405
Delhi	230	9232	135	9597
Gujrat	289444	39520	-	328964
Haryana	17716	30455	-	48171
Karnataka	35007	209585	494	245087
Kerala	166702	-	7660	174362
Madhya Pradesh	12000	14592	9000	26592
Maharashtra	302708	267454	589	570752
Orissa	-	8436	-	836
Punjab	41074	113949	73	155097
Rajsthan	7870	10979	-	18849
Tamil Nadu	171169	329151	14471	514791
Uttar Pradesh	7597	2952	-	10549
West Bengal	18794	187183	212	206189
Grand Total	**1,105,120**	**1,451,067**	**29,312**	**2,585,500**

Source: CLFMA, 2004

The livestock production system in the country is galvanizing for change. The traditional livestock rearing practice in which they were considered more as a companion animal providing motive power to agriculture and manure to the fields is changing. They are now considered as an economic enterprise, which provides income and employment to people. Of late, the livestock rearing practices is changing with supplemental feeding and concentration of livestock activities in peri-urban areas to meet the surge in demand of food from animal origin. Increasing population, urbanization and income growth together with changing dietary habits have created huge demand for milk and meat and eggs not only in urban areas but also in rural areas. Analysis of the growth of livestock and poultry population has revealed that the total livestock population may witness little change in next two decades with the exception of poultry sector. The cattle will decline in numbers but simultaneously the buffaloes are increasing keeping the total large ruminant population almost constant. The proportion of crossbred is also increasing appreciably. The production system that supports goat production appears to have been stretched enough and hence any increase can be expected only through supplemental and/or stall-feeding. The growth rate in demand for milk and meat seen in conjunction with livestock numbers indicate that the productivity of livestock need to be increased in coming years to meet the demand of food from animal origin. This could be achieved through increased use of cereals/ energy sources as livestock feed and the feed manufacturing industries together with the conducive government policies will have to play an important role to meet the needs of small and medium sized dairy and livestock production units to help realize the livestock revolution unfolding on Indian horizon.

Bibliography

Bhalla, G.S., Peter Hazell and John Kerr. (1999). Prospects for India's Cereal supply and Demand to 2020. Food, Agriculture and Environment Discussion Paper 29, International Food Policy Research Institute, Washington.

Chand Ramesh. (2003). Government intervention in Foodgrain Markets in the New Context. National Centre for Agricultural Economics and Policy Research Policy Paper 19. NCAP, New Delhi.

Delgado, C., Rosegrant, M., Steinfeld, H., Ehui, S. and Courbois, C. (1999). Livestock to 2020: The Next Food Revolution. Food, Agriculture and Environment Discussion Paper 28, International Food Policy Research Institute, Washington.

FAO, (2004). FAO Statistical Database. http://www.fao.org. Accessed January, 2005.

Kumar Praduman (1998). Food Demand and Supply Projections for India. Agricultural Economics Policy Paper 98-01, Indian Agricultural Research Institute, New Delhi.

National Sample Survey Organization (NSS). (1990). Report on the fourth quinquennial survey on consumer expenditure: Patterns of consumption of cereals, pulses, tobacco and some other selected items. NSSO 43rd round (July 1987-June 1988). Report no., 374. New Delhi: Department of Statistics, Government of India.

National Sample Survey Organization (NSS). (1996). Consumption of some important commodities in India. NSS 50th round 1993-94. Department of Statistics, Government of India. Draft report no.404. New Delhi.

Pathak, P.S. (2003). Prospects of Feed crops in India: The role of CGPRT crops. Working Paper no. 64, CGPRT Centre, United Nations.

Planning Commmission (2001). Working Group Report for the 10th Five Year Plan. Planning Commission, Govt. of India.

Repetto, R. 1994. The "second India" revisited: Population , poverty and environmental stress over two decades. Washington, DC: World Resource Institute.

Taneja, V.K. (1999). Animal feed milling industry in India. Report of the 23rd Session of the Animal Production and Health Commission of Asia and Pacific. Kochi, India/FAO.

8
CEREAL PROCESSING

K.R..Yadav

Grain Processing Methods:

Grain processing methods are divided conveniently into dry and wet processes. The primary objective is to improve the availability and digestibility of starch which is present at about 70-80 per cent in grains. However, the method of accomplishing this is complicated because: (1) the type of starch varies among grains in its digestibility; and (2) availability of starch even varies from one grain variety to another, particularly in milo.

Grain processing

A. Dry Processing	B. Wet Processing
1. Grinding	1. Soaking
2. Dry rolling or cracking	2. Steam rolling
3. Popping	3. Steam flaking
4. Extruding	4. Pressure cooking
5. Micronising	5. Exploding
6. Roasting	6. Reconstitution
7. Pelleting	7. Ensiling at high moisture content
8. Dehulling	

A. DRY PROCESSING

Grinding

Grinding is that process by which a feedstuff is reduced to a particle size by impact, shearing or attrition. The process is common, economical and simple, other than soaking. A wide variety of equipment is available and all of it allows some control of particle size. Coarsely ground grains are preferred for ruminants while finer ground grains are more common for poultry and swine.

Dry rolling or cracking

The method refers to passing grain without steam between a closely fitted set of steel rollers which are usually grooved on the surface. It breaks the hull and/or seed coat and results in an end product of coarsely ground grain some times referred to as flaking. Cattle seem to prefer flaked grain to finely ground grain, and are usually better for it.

Popping

Most readers are familiar with popped rice (khai) and popped maize which is produced by action of the rapid application of dry heat, causing a sudden expansion of the grain which ruptures the endosperm. For increasing digestibility all grains may be processed by this method, but it appears that it is especially effective in processing sorghum or other milo grains. Popped milo requires more storage space due to its light density.

Extruding

Extruding usually involves grinding the grain, followed by heating with steam in order to soften it, then forcing the softened steamed ground grain through a machine with a spiral screw which expels the grain through a tapered head to produce a ribbon like product. Extruding animal feeds is generally confined to pet foods.

Micronising

Micronising is essentially the same as popping, except that heat is provided in the form of infra-red energy.

Roasting

Roasting is accomplished by passing the grain through a flame or heating it to the desired temperature in an oven for a period of time, resulting in some expansion of the grain, which produces a palatable product. The method may be used with whole soybeans to destroy heat labile inhibitors and thus improve nutritive value for poultry and swine.

Pelleting

Pelleting is accomplished by grinding the material and then forcing it through die openings by a mechanical process. Feedstuff usually is, but not always, steamed to some extent prior to pelleting. Pellets can be made into small chunks, or cylinders of different diameters, length and degrees of hardness. The advantages of pelleting feeds are as follows:

1. Feeds to be pelleted are usually ground first – the pellets so formed being appreciated by the consumers.
2. Pelleting feed to a free flowing form facilitates its handling and use in a self feeder.
3. Pelleted feeds are usually less dusty and more palatable.
4. The feed reduces storage space requirement.

The process involves about 10 per cent more cost than non-pelleted concentrates.

Dehulling (Corticated form)

Dehulling is the process of removing the outer coat of grain, nuts and some fruits as the hulls are high in fibers and low in digestibility in swine, poultry and other monogastric animals. The best known outer coverings of cereal grains are barely hulls, oat hulls and rice hulls. Presently hulls are combined with other residue from the milling of these cereal grains and are marketed as by-products.

The protein content of such unhulled (undecorticated) oilseeds as soybeans, cottonseeds, groundnuts, sunflowers, and safflowers is relatively low.

B. WET PROCESSING

Soaking

Hard grains soaked for 12 to 24 hours in water is a practice long in use by livestock feeders (which are not mechanically processed) for feeding of sore mouthed horses and mules. Benefits are also obtained by soaking oilseed by-products like mustard cake in water and thereby alleviating the toxicity factors like HCN.

Steam rolling

Rolling refers to a process by which grain is compressed into flat particles by passing it between rollers. Steam rolling is also called crimping, and steam crimping refers to exposing grain to steam for a short period of time, usually one to eight minutes, followed by rolling. The steam softens the kernel, producing a more intact, crimped-appearing product than that of produced by dry rolling. Steam rolling offers little or no advantage in feed efficiency over grinding or dry rolling. However, the product may be useful for very young animals before their teeth are fully developed or for very old animals with badly worn teeth.

Steam flaking

Steam flaking grains are prepared in a similar manner but with relatively rigid quality control. Grain is subjected to high moisture steam for a sufficient time to raise the water content to 18-20 per cent and the grain is then rolled to produce a rather flat flake. Thin flakes are better as they allow more efficient rupture of starch granules whereby a more desirable texture is produced.

Pressure cooking

The product is very similar to steam processed flaked grain. In the case of pressure flaking, the grain is subjected to steam under pressure for a short time, such as 50 psi (pounds per square inch) for one to two minutes. Steam is injected into the cooker till the grain in the chamber reaches a temperature approaching 300° F. the grain is then expelled from the cooker at a temperature below 200° F and with 20 per cent moisture these are flaked. In comparison with steam flaking, flakes produced by pressure are less brittle.

Exploding

Exploding is the swelling of grain, produced by steaming under pressure by releasing to the air. Stem is injected into high-tensile strength steel 'bottles' to raise pressure to 250 psi. after about 20 seconds, a valve opens to let the grain escape as expanded balls with the hulls removed. Under high pressure, moisture is forced into the kernels, which when released into the air swell to several times the original size.

Ensiling at high moisture content

High moisture grain refers to grain harvested at a moisture level of 20 to 35 per cent and stored without drying in a silo. It may be ground before ensiling or ground and rolled stored in either of the two ways.

1. It may be ensiled in a silo.
2. It may be preserved by the addition of 1-1.5 per cent propionic acid or a mixture of propionic acid with either acetic or formic acid to inhibit mould formation during storage.

This is a particularly useful procedure when weather conditions do not allow normal drying in the field and it obviates the need to dry the grain artificially.

It has been estimated that provision of an adequate quantity of balanced feed alone could increase production of livestock by at least 20% (Singh, 1989). Therefore, steps to improve nutrients utilization of existing feed resources by employing suitable technologies is the need of the hour. There are many processes by which the cereals are processed eg. 'reconstitution.'

Reconstitution

Reconstituted grain is the mature grain that is harvested at a normal moisture level (10-14 per cent), followed by addition of water to bring the moisture level to 25-30 per cent and the wet product is stored in an upright silo (for required compaction) for 15 to 21 days prior to feeding. The grains are rolled and ground at the time of removal. Properly reconstituted milo (sorghum) and steam processed flaked milo give similar results with fattening cattle. The similar type of definition has been given by Sullins et al., (1971) that Reconstitution is a conditioning of grain by adding enough water to air dried (10-13% moisture) grain to raise the moisture level to about 25-30% and the grain is then stored in air-limiting structures for a period, usually 21 days

Mechanism of action

The complete mechanism of action is not fully understood. Histological studies of sorghum grain which has been reconstituted reveal a complete disruption of the endosperm. The protein matrix become disrupted and freed the starch granules and protein bodies, which resembles with the process of germination. In germination, the embryo of the seed secretes gibberelins which then migrate to aleuronic layer of the seed and result in production of amylases and proteases (Luchsinger, 1966). The amylases stimulate starch solubility and the proteases increase the protein solubility. The in-vitro studies have shown that in reconstituted grain the utilization is improved to the extent of 40% (Newhaus and Tatusek, 1971).

Urea treatment of grains causes the seed coat to fissure and disrupt seed coat organization. The starch granules become less crystalline with a convex appearance and the organization among clusters of granules become more open in urea treated milo (Russel et al., 1988). Orskov et al. (1974, 79) observed minimal loss of nitrogen from urea treated grain of barley, corn, wheat and oat after 5-6 months of storage. During process of reconstitution the lactic acid increases from 0.01 in dry corn to 1.06 in reconstituted corn (Stock et al., 1991). Urea has the potential to preserve high moisture milo and sorghum grains.

Nitrogen solubility

Reconstitution increased the protein solubility in sorghum (Billing, 1972) and corn (Danley and Vetter, 1974). Laboratory evaluations have shown that reconstitution of sorghum grain increased 70% ethanol soluble protein

(Loynachan, 1970). Singh (1994) determined the nitrogen solubility of raw and reconstituted 1% urea treated Bajra grain in distilled water, bicarbonate phosphate butter and

McDougall's buffer. Nitrogen solubility in McDougall's buffer was highest and in distilled water was lowest.

Effect on feed intake and digestibility

The digestibilities of DM, OM and non-protein organic matter were significantly increased in reconstituted sorghum grain as compared to dry sorghum grain (McGinty et al., 1967). They have also reported that reconstitution of sorghum grain and then grinding prior to feeding increased protein digestibility by 16-22% and DM & OM digestibility by 17-29% in cattle. Ration containing reconstituted sorghum grain was consumed more rapidly than ration containing ground dried grain (Bush et al., 1979). The digestibility of starch increased in reconstituted sorghum grain than in ground grain (Hibberd et al., 1983).

Effect on growth and feed efficiency

Beeson and Perry (1956) reported that fattening beef cattle utilize high moisture ground ear corn from 10-15% more efficiently than regular ground ear corn. There has been apparent increase in body weight gain in beef cattle when were fed reconstituted sorghum grain (Riggs & McGinty, 1970). Feed efficiency improved significantly in steers fed reconstituted sorghum grain compared with dry rolled (Simpson et al., 1985).

Table 1. Effect of reconstitution and urea treatment on DM loss, pH, lactic acid, starch and total and reducing sugars of Bajra grain (21 days incubation)

Items	T_1 (Dry Bajra grain)	T_2 (Reconstituted)	T_3 (1% urea treated)
DM loss (%)	-	1.64^a	0.39^b
pH	6.04^b	4.33^c	7.53^a
Lactic acid	0.39^b	2.21^a	ND
Starch	66.36	65.77	64.65
Total sugars	2.34^c	2.97^b	3.98^a
Reducing sugars	0.46^c	0.60^b	0.72^a

Source : Kishore (1996)

Table 2: Effect of processing Bajra grain on nitrogen solubility (%) in solvents

Items	T_1	T_2	T_3
Distilled water	19.17^b	43.94^a	45.66^a
Bicarb phos. Buffer	32.01^b	58.70^a	61.20^a
McDougall's buffer	40.97^b	69.20^a	71.38^a

Source : Kishore (1996)

Table 3: Effect of processing bajra grain on in-vitro total gas, CH4, CO_2 and other per 200 gm DM/24 h.

Items	T_1	T_2	T_3
Total gas (ml)	53.36^b	60.77^a	60.04^a
CH_4 (%)	29.75^a	22.30^b	22.92^b
CO_2	70.25^b	77.70^a	77.08^c
Total-N (mg)	8.53^b	8.88^a	8.90^a
NH_3-N (mg)	2.60	2.50	2.74

Table 4: Effect of reconstitution of bajra gram on in-situ nitrogen and DM disappearance (%)

Hours	T_1	T_2	T_3
3 N-Degradability	24.28^b	47.10^a	49.73^a
DM-degradability	31.05^b	48.43^a	50.43^a
6 N-Degradability	35.87^b	48.34^a	50.87^a
DM-Degradability	43.91^b	56.90^a	57.75^a
12 N-Degradability	49.63^b	60.70^a	62.50^a
DM-Degradability	63.61^b	70.44^a	71.38^a
24 N-Degradability	62.48^b	73.23^a	75.64^a
DM-Degradability	78.62^b	89.88^a	90.97^a

Table 5: Effect of reconstitution and 4% urea treated reconstituted Bajra grain on DMI, digestibility and nutritive value in sheep.

Item	T_1 (Ground Bajra)	T_2 (Reconstituted bajra)	T_3 (4% treated reconstituted Bajra)
DMI (g/d)	705	703	704
CPI (g/d)	54.08^{b}	54.02^{b}	70.40^{a}
Digestibility (%)			
DM	50.55^{b}	54.78^{a}	55.17^{a}
CP	42.80^{b}	49.92^{a}	50.37^{a}
CF	51.64^{b}	53.94^{a}	54.78^{a}
Nutritive value (%)			
DCP	3.46^{c}	4.40^{b}	6.11^{a}
TDN	51.13^{b}	56.25^{a}	55.73^{a}

Table 6: DM intake, digestibility and nutritive value of experimental diets in buffalo calves

Item	T_1 (Barley based conc)	T_2 (Barley with Bajra in conc.)	T_3 (Reconstituted Bajra)	T_4 (4% treated reconstituted Bajra)
DMI (Kg/d)	4.15	4.13	4.14	4.16
CPI(g/d)	489	492	495	501
Digestibility (%)				
DM	60.7^{b}	54.1^{c}	61.6^{ab}	63.8^{a}
CP	68.1^{a}	61.7^{b}	68.6^{a}	70.5^{a}
CF	60.2^{a}			54.9^{b}
	59.9^{a}			61.5^{a}
Nutritive value (%)				
DCP	8.1	7.2^{b}	8.1^{a}	8.6^{a}
TDN	63.3^{a}	57.2^{b}	62.9^{a}	64.7^{a}

Table 7: Nitrogen balance, body weight gain and economics of feeding experimental diets in buffalo calves

Item	T_1	T_2	T_3	T_4
Nitrogen balance (g/d)	35.07	29.82	36.46	39.23
Body wt. gain (g/d)	508	443	515	530
Feed consumed/kg Gain (kg)	8.35[b]	9.40[a]	8.29[b]	7.93[b]
Cost/kg LW gain (Rs.)	23.51	25.80	22.38	22.21

Following conclusion are drawn from the above studies.

1. Reconstitution of Bajra grain did not alter its chemical composition or macro mineral content, decreased pH and increased lactic acid, total and reducing sugars. It leads to higher nitrogen solubility, higher total gas production and higher degradability of nitrogen and dry matter.
2. Urea treatment of Bajra grain increased its CP content, total and reducing sugars, nitrogen solubility and disappearance of nitrogen and DM.
3. It is effective in controlling fungal growth and rise in temperature in the process of reconstitution.
4. Constitution and 1% urea treatment of Bajra grain increased its nutritive value and nitrogen balance in sheep.
5. The digestibility co-efficient and nutritive value of reconstitution and 4% urea treated Bajra grain were at par to control concentrate and higher to raw grain in buffalo calves.
6. Buffalo calves fed reconstituted and urea treated Bajra grain gained faster and consumed less feed/unit gain.

Reconstitution and urea treatment of Bajra grain increased the feed utilization, feed efficiency and performance of animals and decreased the cost of production. However, urea treatment was superior to reconstitution as it increased the solubility of reconstituted Bajra grain. Hence, barley can be replaced with reconstituted Bajra grain and conventional concentrate mixture can be replaced with 4% urea treated Bajra grain successfully and economically in growing buffalo calves.

Bibliography

Beeson, W.M. and Perry, T.W. 1956. The comparative feeding value of high moisture corn with different feed additives for fattening beef cattle. Paper No. 1173. Purdue Univ. Lafayette, Indiana.

Billings, T.J. 1972. Biochemical changes in the proteins of sorghum grain during moisture reconstitution. M.Sc. Thesis. Texas. A. and M. Univ., College Station.

Bush, L.J. Netermayer, D.T. and Adams, G.D. 1979. Reconstituted sorghum grain for lactating dairy cows. J. Dairy Sci. 62: 1094.

Danley, M.M. and Vetter, R.L. 1974. Artificially altered corn grain harvested at three moisture levels. III. In-vitro utilization of carbohydrate and nitrogen fractions. J. Anim. Sci. 38: 430.

Hibberd, C.A., Wagner, D.G., Hintz, R.L. and Griffinm, D.D. 1983. Effect of sorghum grain variety and processing method on the site and extent of starch digestion. Oklahoma Agr. Exp. Sta. MP 114: 28.

Kishore, N. 1996. Effect of reconstitution and urea treatment of Bajra grain on nutrients digestibility and performance in ruminants. PhD Thesis submitted to CCSHAU Hisar.

Loynachan,T.M. 1970. The effect of temperature moisture and storage time on the utilization of reconstituted milo. Ph.D Dissertation, Univ. of Arizona, Tucson.

Luchsinger, W.W. 1966. Carbohydrates of barley and malt. Cereal Sci. Today, 11: 69.

McGinty,D.D., Breuer, L.H. and Riggs, J.K. 1967. Digestibility of dry and reconstituted sorghum grain by cattle. J. Anim. Sci. 27: 1163 (Abstr.)

Newhaus, V. and Totusek, R. 1971. Factors affecting the in-vitro digestibility of high moisture sorghum grain. J. anim. Sci. 33: 1321.

Orskov, E.R., Smart, R. and Mehrez, A.Z. 1974. A method of including urea in whole grains. J.Agric. Sci. 92: 185.

Orskov, E.R., Stewart, C.S. and Greenholgh, J.F.A. 1979. The effect of sodium hydroxide and urea on some storage properties of moist grains. J.Agric. Sci. 102:185.

Riggs, J.K. and Mc Ginty, D.D. 1970. Early harvested and reconstituted sorghum grain for cattle. J. anim. Sci. 31: 991.

Russel, R.W.; Lin, J.C.M.; Thomas, E.E. and Mora, E.C. 1988. Preservation of high moisture milo with urea: Grain properties and animal acceptability. J. Anim. Sci. 66: 2131.

Simpson, Jr., E.J., Schake, L.M. Pflugfelder, R.L. and Riggs, J.K. 1985. Evaluation of moisture uptake, aerobic and anaerobic phases of reconstitution upon sorghum grain digestibility and performance of steers. J. Anim. Sci. 60: 877.

Singh, J.D. 1994. Effect of reconstitution of Bajra grains on the performance of growing lambs. M.V.Sc. Thesis, CCS HAU, Hisar.

Singh, M. 1989. Proceedings of summer institute on "Animal feed technology in Livestock Production and Feed Industry". Department of Animal Feed Technology, CCSHAU Hisar.

Stock, R.A; Sondt, M.H. Cleale, R.M. and Britton, R.A. and Britton, R.A.1991. High moisture corn utilization in finishing cattle. J. Anim. Sci. 69: 1645.

Sullins, R.D., Rooney, L.W. and Riggs, J.K.1971. Physical changes in the kernel during reconstitution of sorghum grain. Cereal Chem. 48: 567.

9
STORAGE LOSSES IN FEEDS

Nand Kishore

If storage conditions are not optimum the feeds are damaged. These damaged feeds if induced in compound feeds may cause health and production problems. The factors that are responsible for storage losses can be divided into two groups:

1. Biotic factors: Includes insects, rodents, birds and microorganisms.
2. Abiotic factors: Includes temperature, moisture, breakdown of produce and type of storage.

Insects

Under Indian conditions the most important insects pests of stored grain are Sitophilus oryzae (Rice Weevil), Rizopertha dominica (Lesser grain borer), Trogoderma granarium (Khappra beetle), Callosobruchus maculates (Pulse beetle), Sitotroga cerealella (Grain moth), Tribolium castanium (Rust red flour beetle), Oryzaephilus surinamensis (Saw toothed grain beetle), Latheticus oryzae (Long headed flour beetle), Corcyra cephalonics (Rice moth), Cadra cautella (Almond moth) and Plodia interpunctella (Indian meal moth). Out of these 11 species of insects, first five are capable of damaging all kinds of stored material therefore, these are known as primary insects while last seven attack broken/ processed/milled food grain so called secondary pests.

After mating, the females begin to lay eggs; under favorable conditions a female lays about 200 eggs in one month. Moths lay their eggs within a few days and then die. Larva emerges from these eggs and it causes the greatest damage to the grain. Larva is converted to pupa and pupa into adult. Pupa is inactive and causes little damage. Pupa stage is 4 to 5 days. This type of development from egg to adult is called metamorphosis and the period is about 1 month under favorable conditions. The multiplication of insects is very fast due to laying large number of eggs and short development time. One pair of insects (male and female) could result in over 1 million individuals within about 5 months. The insect's growth is maximum at 12 to 14% moisture and 21 to 27°C temperature.

Rodents

During storage the rodents not only consume the stored material but also contaminat it with their excreta, hair and dead bodies. Each rat is known to void 10,000 droppings, 4 liters of urine and 5 lacs of hair annually. Each rat eats 8.5% of its body weight/day. The losses caused by rats are estimated to be 2.5% of the total stored products.

Microorganisms

The damage caused by microorganisms in stored products is excessive heat and discoloration. Fungi and bacteria are mostly seed born. Most of the storage fungi belong to Aspergillus and Penicillium groups and they are capable of producing mycotoxins.

Birds

The losses caused by birds are 0.85% of the stored material. They not only consume food grains, but also contaminate with their excreta and feathers. Each bird can consume on an average 25g grain/day.

Temperature

A produce can be stored safely even at high moisture content above the safe storage level provided the temperature is maintained low and uniform throughout the storage period e.g. cold storage. When temperature rises above 66°C the germination of grains is affected and the biochemical activities in the grain are increased that result into more breakdown of nutrients. Temperature ranging from 20-40°C accelerates the development of insects, but above 42°C and below 15°C the development of insects is retarded. A temperature below 10°C for longer period may cause death of insects. Temperature ranging from 2°C to a maximum of 63°C may influence the growth of storage fungi.

Grains being living matter respire to supply energy for biochemical processes i.e.

$$\text{Carbohydrates and fats} \quad \frac{\text{Respiration}}{O_2} = CO_2 + H_2O + \text{Heat}$$

In anaerobic conditions complete oxidation of food material does not take place so that incompletely oxidized substances such as alcohol and acetic acid are formed which deteriorate quality of food grains.

When grains are stored, the insect population is rapidly built up in a particular pocket and they respire at the rate of 20,000 to 1,00,000 times more than that of same weight of grains. Thus, heat is generated which raises the temperature of bulk grain from 38°C to 43°C and moisture content from 11% to 14%. Such heating is known as dry heating and the spot where temperature increased due to development of insect is known as hot spot. This hot spot forces the insects to migrate to cooler area or result in their death. This is known as sterilization heat. At the place of hot spot the moisture content is very high which invites the fungal infestation and increase the temperature from 43°C to 63°C and moisture content from 14% to 18%. This is known as wet heating. The same can be summarized in the Table given below:

Type of heating	Moisture content	Temperature range	Casual organisms
Dry heating	11-14%	38-43°C	Insects, mites
Wet heating	14-18%	43-63°C	Fungi

Some facts regarding temperature

1. Increasing temperature deep in bulk indicates the presence of insect or mould activity.
2. High temperature in all over storage structure indicates the biochemical deterioration.
3. Combination of high bulk temperature and cold weather indicates that the surface moisture will rapidly increase.

Moisture

In feed and feed ingredients, moisture is present in two main forms i.e. water of composition and water absorbed. The quantity of free water (water absorbed) held by the grain product is a critical factor, which plays a vital role in the safe storage of stored products. Free water may be defined as the loss in weight brought about by heating for 24 h at 102±3°C or the amount of water that can be removed without changing the chemical structure of the grain. The amount of water in dry feeds varies from about 5 to 30 percent. Cool and dried grain respired at normal rate, but grains containing moisture above critical level (Table below) respire fast, liberate more heat which can further increase respiration rate and moisture content. The metabolic activity of grain increases slowly from 11 to 14 percent but from 15-20 percent moisture content it increases rapidly. It is recommended that grain having a moisture content above a level in equilibrium with 70 percent RH should not be stored.

Table: Critical moisture content for safe storage of cereals at 70 percent RH and 27^{0}C temperature

Stored cereals	Moisture (%)
Wheat, Sorghum Barley and Corn	13.5
Oat	13.1
Soybean	12.2
Paddy	15.0

Moisture migration

In storage the moisture of the grain tend to move from the place having higher vapour pressure to lower vapour pressure to equalize the moisture content throughout the storage. This is known as moisture migration.

When environmental temperature falls below grain temperature, damage may take place at the top center, when ambient temperature rises above grain temperature, damage may take place at the bottom of storage structure.

When the environmental temperature is low, the air coming in contact with wall of the storage structure becomes cold and moves down and the air in grains being hot moves upwards. It carries moisture with it, which is absorbed by the grain at top center and hence the grains there are deteriorated. Reverse is the condition in hot environmental conditions.

Breakdown of produce

Improper storage conditions results in to break down of produce causing nutrient damage and decreases palatability. The loss is not merely in terms of quantity but also in quality of the feed ingredients. The qualitative loss is attributed to chemical changes in protein, carbohydrates, amino acids, fatty acids and vitamins, which affect the nutritive value of the feeds.

Type of storage

Bagged grains are stored in warehouses, which are also known as conventional godowns. The storage facility for bulk material is a flat or vertical bin also known as silo. The scientific requirement to minimize the storage losses; the storage facility should be:

i) Moisture proof
ii) Air tight
iii) Insects, birds and rodent proof
iv) Fire proof
v) Should have good aeration system to keep the grain dry and cool.

The losses due to rats, insects and moisture are considerably higher if the storage structures are not rodent, moisture and insects proof. If the storage structure is not airtight, then the stored material cannot be fumigated which results in higher storage losses.

Losses during storage

Storage is the most important post harvest operation. The losses during storage can be divided into two major categories:

i) Quantitative losses
ii) Qualitative losses

Quantitative changes are physical changes in weight and volume, which are easy to measure. While, qualitative changes refers to the biochemical changes which take place in the biochemical moieties of stored material.

Quantitative losses

Weight loss result from evaporation of moisture, from component parts of product being eaten by insects, rodents and birds; and from allowing quantities spill from the container in which the produce is stored. In some instances weight loss may be converted into a slight gain in weight due to reabsorption of moisture from the air. The weight losses in indigenous bulk storage are low than bag storage. The weight losses in the unsealed stacks are higher as compared to sealed stacks. It has been found that the percentage of grains holed by insects is 2 to 3 times the percentage loss in weight.

Weight loss during 12 months storage in different countries

Country	Commodity	% loss
Ghana	Legumes	9.3
Somalia	Grain	20-50
South Africa	Legumes	50
India	Wheat	8.3
	Food grain	9.3
U.S.A.	Maize	0.5
	Rice	1.5
	Sorghum	3.4
	Wheat	3.0
Thailand	Paddy	10
	Maize	10

According to an estimate the storage losses of food grain in India amounted to 6.6% of total production.

Estimates of food grain losses in storage in India.

Cause of loss	Wheat	Rice	Jowar	Bajra	Maize	Pulses	Total
Rodent	2.5	2.5	2.5	2.5	2.5	2.5	2.5
Birds	0.5	1.0	1.0	1.0	0.5	0.5	0.9
Insects	3.0	2.0	2.0	1.0	3.0	5.0	2.5
Moisture	0.5	0.5	2.0	0.5	0.5	0.5	0.7
Total	**6.5**	**6.0**	**7.5**	**5.0**	**6.5**	**8.5**	**6.6**

Assessment of storage losses

The reduction in weight registered over the storage period does not always provide an accurate record of the actual weight loss of produce. The tare allowance on bag and the variation in moisture or oil content of the bag fibres are made. The weight of dust, which may consist of powder from the product, insect and rodent frass plus the weight of any insects present, should be deducted from the weight of the product. Moreover, it may account for a 100 percent increase in weight loss; e.g. 3000 bags of maize infested with insects after two years in storage showed an apparent weight loss of 7 percent which increased to a 14 percent actual loss when the dust and insects were removed.

Shortage/Accounting for storage losses

Punjab and Haryana Govt. estimated the shortage in bag storage as follows: 0.2 percent per month of storage from September to May in case of wheat, 0.2 percent per month of storage in case of gram and barley; 2 percent during the first month, 2.5 percent during first 2 months, 3 percent during the first 3-4 months, 4 percent during he period of storage exceeding 4 months in case of maize, jowar and bajra. Rajasthan Govt. indicated that the maximum limit for writing off shortage in respect of wheat, stored with the state and central warehousing corporation was 1.5, 2.5 and 3 percent for storage of 2, 4 and 12 months. The Delhi Administration estimated a shortage of 0.5 to 1.0 percent of food grains during storage period in the fair price shops. Losses in various food grains due to insects in storage in Gujarat was recorded in wheat, rice, jowar, bajra, maize, gram, millets and pulses as 3.0, 2.0, 2.0, 1.0, 3.0, 5.0, 5.0 and 5.0 percent, respectively.

Methods for estimation of storage losses

Losses due to insects

Any of the following formula can be used for calculating the actual percentage loss:

i) The loss of grain in weight % = $\frac{(UKI-IK) \times 100}{UK}$

Where, UK = wt. Of 100 uninfested grain, IK = weight of infested grain, UKI = weight of equal number of uninfested grain.

ii) Loss (%) = $(W + G + M) \frac{100}{S} (W_1 + G_1 + M_1)$

Where,

W, G, M = Percent (by No.) of weevilled, germ eaten and mouldy grain

S = wt. Of 100 good grain in g

W_1, G_1, M_1 = Wt. Of W, G, M no. of weevilled, germ eaten & mouldy grain (g)

Losses due to fungi

The methods for estimating loss from insects are also applicable to fungal damage. However, when mould occurs a considerable proportion of the grain is rejected. The impact of fungal infestation on loss can be estimated by including the separation of mould damage from other types of damage during the analysis.

Losses caused by vertebrate pests and bird

Losses caused by such as rodents and birds are difficult to assess directly, since they result in the removal of grains from the store. It is difficult to obtain an accurate estimate without accurate weighing of the grain throughout the season. In captivity the Rattus rattus (roof rat) has been found to consume 8-12 g/day, the Mus musculus (house mouse) 3-5 g/day and the Bandicota spp (benedicoot rat) consume 25-30 g/day of food grains and feeds. While eating the rats also contaminates an estimated 10 times more food than they eat with urine, feces, hair and saliva.

2) Qualitative losses/Biochemical Changes

Biochemical changes are concerned with the major modifications which take place in the biochemical moieties of stored feed ingredients.

Carbohydrate changes

Alpha and beta amylases attack the starches of the grain and grain products during storage, converting them into dextrin and maltose. Amylase activity in wheat increases during the early stages of storage. Water is consumed in the starch hydrolysis reactions and thus, the dry weight of the products of starch hydrolysis is greater than that of the original. Although this hydrolytic action might be expected to result in significant increase in the reducing sugar content of grain, conditions that favor starch decomposition usually favor respiratory activity also so that the sugars are consumed and converted into carbon dioxide and water. Under these conditions that usually occur at moisture levels of 15 percent or more, the grain loses both starch and sugar and the dry weight decreases. At higher moisture levels, however, active carbohydrate fermentation may occur with the production of alcohol or acetic acid and resulting characteristic sour odors.

Soluble carbohydrates of grain germ stored for 8 days at moisture levels from 9 to 25 percent and temperatures from 29 to 50^{0}C produced characteristic increases of reducing sugars at the expenses of non-reducing sugars.

When damp grains were stored in air, extensive mould growth occurred, and the increase in reducing sugars was only about 1/4th as great as the decrease in non-reducing sugars, owing to the utilization of the former by the mould.

The changes in the di-and trisaccharide contents of grains and byproducts during storage under good and poor conditions indicated that under good conditions, concentrations of various sugars remained essentially unchanged, except for a slight decrease in sucrose content. When the wheat was stored at high moisture contents and temperatures, sucrose, glucose and fructose contents decreased, and the maltose content increased.

Changes in nitrogenous compounds

Total protein

In grains stored for 8 years under conditions, which might be used, for long-term commercial storage, crude protein remained unchanged.

Enzyme and free amino acids

Proteolytic enzymes in grain and in organisms associated with grain, hydrolyze the proteins into polypeptides and finally into amino acids. These reactions ordinarily proceed very slowly and are not readily measurable until the grain has reached an advanced stage of deterioration.

Lipids

Deteriorative changes in grain fats or oils may be either oxidative, resulting in typical rancid flavours and odour or hydrolytic, resulting in the production of free fatty acids. Grains contain fairly active antioxidants and the fats in unbroken kernels of grain are rather effectively protected against effects of oxygen in the air. For these reasons, the development of oxidative rancidity is rarely a problem in grain storage, although it is often a serious problem in the storage of grain oils and of milled products, particularly whole grain milled products.

Fats in grain are readily broken down by lipases into free fatty acids and glycerol during storage, particularly when the temperature and moisture content are high and thus favourable to general deterioration. Fat hydrolysis takes place much more rapidly than protein or carbohydrate hydrolysis in stored grain. For this reason, the free fatty acid content of grain has been proposed as a sensitive index of incipient grain deterioration.

Nutritive Change

Mineral changes

Although mineral matter is seldom gained or lost in storage the availability of phosphorus nutritionally important to animals and man, appears to increase in storage. Most phosphorus in grain is present in the form of phytin, a potassium magnesium salt of inositol phosphoric acid. During the storage of flour and more slowly in the storage of whole grain, phytin is acted upon by the enzyme phytase with the liberation of water-soluble readily available phosphorus compounds.

Carbohydrate changes

Freshly harvested rice is not digested as readily as rice that has been stored for a time. Fresh rice is said to contain an active alpha amylase that causes the rice to become sticky when cooked. This amylase presumably becomes partially inactivated during storage.

Protein changes

Although the total protein content of grain as calculated from its nitrogen content is generally assumed to remain unchanged during storage, a progressive though small increase was reported in the protein content of wheat during extended storage. This increase in protein on a percentage basis was the result of a loss in carbohydrates by respiration.

The proteins of wheat, corn and soybeans and their ground products were shown to decrease in solubility and in digestibility by pepsin and trypsin in vitro.

Simultaneously, there occurred an increase in amino nitrogen and a decrease in true protein nitrogen. Wheat containing approximately 11 percent of moisture showed a decrease in protein digestibility of 8 percent when stored in sealed jars at 24^{0}C for 2 years. Corn containing about 12 percent moisture similarly stored showed a decrease of 3.6 percent in protein digestibility in the same time. These changes, as well as changes in protein solubility occur much more rapidly in the milled products of grain than in whole grain.

Good feeding grain is characterized by high digestibility and biological value of the protein by the absence of toxin substances (mycotoxins, fungicides etc.) by the presence of lipids which have not been excessively hydrolyzed and/or oxidized and by relatively minor changes in water soluble and fat soluble (specially tocopherol) vitamins.

Vitamin changes

Cereal grains are generally good sources of thiamine, niacin, pyridoxine, inositol, biotin and vitamin E. they also contain significant quantities of pantothenic acid. Vitamin A activity occurs in yellow corn but is practically absent in all other cereal grains.

Wheat containing about 17 percent moisture lost approximately 30 percent of its thiamine in a 5-month storage period. This wheat deteriorated considerably during this period because of its high moisture content. At normal moisture level of about 12 percent the thiamine loss in 5-month period was in the neighborhood of 12 percent.

Studies on rice have also indicated that thiamine is quite stable during storage. Hulled rice stored in straw bags for 4 years retained most of its original thiamine content during the first 2 years but a significant drop occurred during the 3rd and 4th year of storage.

Very little information appears to be available concerning losses of the B vitamins, other than thiamine, found in grain (riboflavin, niacin, pyridoxine, pantothenic acid, para-amino benzoic acid and inositol). But it is generally believed that these vitamins with the possible exception of pantothenic acid are rather stable and are not readily destroyed in unbroken grain under normal conditions of storage. Riboflavin and pyridoxine are rather sensitive to light and may therefore, be unstable in milled products exposed to strong light.

Considerable losses of vitamin A have been shown to occur in yellow corn during storage. Corn stored in steel bins for 4 years contained less than half the crude carotene of fresh corn.

Precautions/measures for reduction of storage losses

1. The grain/feeds should be properly and reasonably dried before storage.
2. Temperature in the storage structure should be maintained below optimum by aeration to avoid moisture migration and reduce activities of microorganisms.
3. Insects should be kept under control to avoid dry and wet heating.
4. Storage structure should be rodent proof, leak proof and free from dampness.
5. Grain should be reasonably free from foreign matter, which enhances development of insects.

In short, the motto should be to keep the grains/feeds cool, clean and as dry as possible.

10
BIS SPECIFICATIONS FOR FEEDS

B. S. TEWATIA

Evaluation of the feed ingredients is important for achieving quality in the feed manufacturing process. Assessment of quality before unloading would save both trouble and money. Ingredients vary considerably in feeding value and wherever possible, they should be purchased on the basis of their nutritive value. To achieve uniformity in quality of feeds in the country, need of a single standard was ascertained. Thus Indian Standards Institution (ISI) started functioning in 1947. Agricultural and Food Products Division Council's subcommittee (Animal Feeds Sectional Committee) devises standards for animal feeds. Bureau of Indian Standards (BIS) certification is governed by the provisions of BIS Acts and the rules and regulations made there under. This mark conveys the assurance that they have been produced in compliance with the requirements of that standard.

SPECIFICATIOS FOR SOME AGRO-INDUSTRIAL BYPRODUCTS

Maize bran

It consists largely of the coarse and fine fibrous material obtained after separation of the germ in wet milling manufacturer of maize starch and other products. It is of two types:

Coarse bran: Consists mainly of the outer coating of the maize kernel, hence it is high in fibre and low in protein content.

Fine bran: Consists of fine fibrous material left as a residue after sieving the slurry subsequent to the removal of germ and coarse bran during wet milling. Its fibre content is lower as compared to coarse bran.

Rice polish

Also known as rice polishing and is the finely produced material obtained in polishing the rice (Oryza sativa) kernel after the hulls and bran have been removed.

Rice bran

It is the pericarp or bran layer, germ of rice, hull fragments and broken rice as is unavoidable in the regular milling of edible rice. Rice bran as obtained by milling rice by different techniques varies considerably in its composition, particularly in its fibre and acid insoluble ash content.

Solvent extracted rice bran

It is obtained by extraction of oil by means of a solvent from rice bran. Hexane of food grade is used for extracting oil from rice bran.

Wheat bran

It is the coarse outer covering of wheat (Triticum aestivum) kernel, as separated in the process of commercial milling.

Tur husk

It is a byproduct of Dal milling industry. It is obtained in the processing of clean arhar (Cajanus cajan) kernels for preparing tur dal. The husk is the outer covering of the seed.

Gram Husk

It shall be the outer covering of the gram seed obtained from cleaned gram (Cicer arietinum) kernels in the process of splitting the kernels for the preparation of gram DAL. It should not contain more than 10 percent by weight of fine powder.

Gram chuni

A byproduct obtained in the preparation of gram DAL. It consists of seed coat of green seeds with broken pieces of cotyledons including germ obtained as a by-product during the processing of gram pulse for human consumption.

Cane molasses

It is an important byproduct producing during the manufacturing of cane sugar both by vacuum pan process and the khandsari process. Molasses is used for production of ethyl alcohol, rum, yeast, acetone, butanol and certain organic acids.

Parameters	**Grade-I**	**Grade-II**	**Grade-III**
Density in degrees Brix Hydrometer at 25.5^{0}C Min.	85.0	80.0	80.0
Ash, sulphated percent by mass, Max.	14.0	17.5	17.5
Total reducing matter, Min.	**50.0**	**44.0**	**40.0**

Table 1. Specifications for some agro-industrial byproducts

Characteristics	Maize bran		Rice Polish	Rice bran		Solvent extracted bran rice bran		Wheat husk	Tur husk	Gram	Maize gluten feed	
	Coarse	Fine		G-I	G-II	G-I	G-II				Grade-I	Grade-II
Moisture, percent by mass, Max.	10.0	10.0	10.0	10.0	10.0	10.0	10.0	10.0	10.0	12.5	10.0	10.0
Crude protein (N×6.25) percent by mass, Min.	7.5	14.5	11.0	13.0	11.0	15.0	14.0	14.5	5.0	13.0	45.0	23.0
Crude fat, percent by mass, Min.	-	-	15.0	15.0	12.0	1.5	1.5	3.0	-	-	4.0	6.0
Crude fibre, percent by mass, Max.	18.0	9.5	4.0	10.0	12.0	14.0	16.0	11.0	44.0	12.0	3.5	8.0
Total ash, percent by mass, Max.	1.5	1.5	10.0	-	-	-	-	3.5	6.0	-	-	-
Acid insoluble ash, percent by mass, Max.	0.5	0.5	1.5	5.0	8.0	6.0	10.0	0.25	1.0	0.25	0.5	0.5

SPECIFICATIONS FOR SOME VEGETABLE PROTEIN SOURCES

Cottonseed oil cake

Decorticated oil cake: It is the product obtained from clean cottonseed composed principally of the kernel with such unavoidable portions of the hull and fibre which is be left during the extraction of oil.

Un-decorticated oil cake: The product obtained from whole, clean, de-linted cottonseed only after extraction of oil.

Table 2. Specifications for cottonseed oilcake

Characteristics	Decorticated		Un-decorticated	
	Type-I	Type-II	Type-I	Type-II
Moisture percent by mass Max.	8.0	8.0	10.0	10.0
Crude protein percent by mass Min.	41.0	37.0	24.0	20.0
Crude fat percent by mass Min.	5.0	5.0	7.0	7.0
Crude fibre percent by mass Max.	12.0	14.0	24.0	28.0
Acid insoluble ash percent by mass Max.	2.0	2.5	2.0	2.5
Castor husk or oil cake	Nil	Nil	Nil	Nil
Mahua oil cake	Nil	Nil	Nil	Nil

Guar meal

Guar meal is a byproduct obtained during manufacturing of guar gum. In the process, the hulls of the guar seeds are separated. After the separation of hulls, the seeds are subjected to grinding, milling and sifting to separate the germ and endosperm. Both the hulls and the germ together constitute guar meal.

Table 3. Specifications for Guar meal

Characteristics	Percent
Moisture percent by mass Max.	10.0
Crude protein percent by mass Min.	40.0
Crude fat percent by mass Min.	3.0
Crude fibre percent by mass Max.	12.0
Total ash percent by mass Max.	7.0
Acid insoluble ash percent by mass Max	0.5

Linseed cake

The oilcake derived from linseed (Linum usitatessimum Linn) is a feed of high nutritive value. It is the product obtained by expeller extraction of most of the oil from linseed. It is richly palatable and causes slightly laxative effect.

Table 4. Specifications for Linseed oilcake

Characteristics	**Expeller pressed**		**Ghani**
	oilcake Grade (HF)	**pressed Grade (LF)**	
Moisture percent by mass Max.	8.0	8.0	8.0
Crude protein percent by mass Min.	29.0	31.0	26.0
Crude fat percent by mass Min.	8.0	5.0	15.0
Crude fibre percent by mass Max.	10.0	10.0	9.0
Total ash percent by mass Max.	8.0	8.0	9.0
Acid insoluble ash percent by mass Max	1.5	1.2	2.5

Niger seed oilcake

The solvent extracted oilcake is obtained by extraction of oil by means of a solvent from Ghani or expeller pressed niger oilcake is obtained by pressing clean and sound niger seeds (Guizotia abyssinica). The meal is subjected to heat treatment under controlled conditions so as to remove traces of solvent.

Table 5. Specifications for Niger seed oilcake

Characteristics	**Grade-I**	**Grade-II**
Moisture percent by mass Max.	9.0	9.0
Crude protein percent by mass Min.	35.0	29.0
Crude fat percent by mass Min.	1.0	1.0
Crude fibre percent by mass Max.	18.0	20.0
Acid insoluble ash percent by mass Max	1.5	2.5

Table 6. Specifications for some vegetable protein sources

Characteristics	Decorticated safflower oil cake		Solvent extracted groundnut cake	Mustard oilcake		Sesamum oilcake	
	Expeller pressed	Ghani-pressed	Type-II	Expeller pressed	Ghani pressed	Expeller pressed	Ghani-pressed
Moisture, percent by mass, Max.	10.0	12.0	8.0	10.0	10.0	8.0	8.0
Crude protein (N×6.25) percent by mass, Min.	48.0	45.0	47.0	37.0	35.0	42.0	36.0
Crude fat, percent by mass, Min.	5.0	8.0	-	5.0	8.0	5.0	14.0
Crude fibre, percent by mass, Max.	15.0	15.0	10.0	8.0	8.0	7.0	7.0
Total ash, percent by mass, Max.	9.0	9.0	-	-	-	13.0	13.0
Acid insoluble ash, percent by mass, Max.	2.0	2.0	2.5	1.5	1.5	2.0	2.0

SPECIFICATIONS FOR ANIMAL PROTEIN SOURCES

Fish meal: Fish meal is obtained from fresh fish or fish wastes or from unsalted dried fish. It is prepared by cooking the raw material or by heat treating the dried fish, pressing the cooked mass, drying and pulverizing it to required mash size. It is in the form of powder that 99 % of material shall pass through 2.8 mm sieve.

Blood meal: An important animal product that is used as a protein supplement in animal feeds. For the preparation of blood meal, blood from slaughtered animals is processed within shortest possible time. Blood is subjected to an indirect slow heat and dried with constant agitation. Dried blood is then ground.

Meat meal: An important animal product that can be used as a protein supplement in animal feeds. Different methods employed for production of meat meal involving partial or complete removal of bones result in a highly variable product. On account of the presence of bones in varying percentage, the product is often termed as meat-cum-bone meal. The carcasses of dead animals, which may or may not have been de-boned are first boiled in open cauldrons or in closed vessels and then dried in steam-jacketed vessels. The dried material is then pulverized.

Table 7. Specifications for some animal protein sources

Characteristics	Fish meal I	Fish meal II	Blood meal	Meat meal	Meat-cum-bone meal
Moisture % by mass Max.	10.0	10.0	8.0	10.0	10.0
Crude protein % by mass Min.	60.0	50.0	80.0	70.0	45.0
Crude fat % by mass Max	12.0	12.0	2.0	6.0	10.0
Total ash % by mass Max	-	-	5.0	-	-
Acid insoluble ash % by mass Max	3.0	5.0	1.5	2.0	2.0
Phosphorus % by mass Max	-	-	-	1.0	5-7
Chlorine (as Nacl) % by mass Max	4.0	5.0	-	-	-

SPECIFICATIONS FOR COMPOUNDED FEEDS FOR CATTLE

There are two types of compounded cattle feeds differentiated on the basis of their crude protein and crude fibre content. Feed mixtures for cattle have been so compounded as to provide 14 to 16 percent DCP and 68 to 74 percent TDN. One kg of these feeds would be required per 2.5 kg milk in cattle and 2.0 kg in buffaloes.

Each bag has to be labeled to give the following information

Name and type of the material	Name of the manufacturer
Net mass in kg, when packed	Batch number
Crude protein percent	Crude fibre percent
ME Kcal/kg (Calculated)	Urea, if present

Compounded feeds for cattle should have the following characteristics

- Compounded cattle feed should in the form of a meal or cubes or pellets.
- It should free from harmful constituents, metallic pieces and adulterants.
- The feed should be free from fungal growth, insect infestation or any other objectionable odour.
- Urea when used should not exceed 1 percent.
- Availability of 10 percent by mass of easily digestible carbohydrates like molasses, cereal grains, potato starch etc. is mandatory with urea.

Table 8. Requirements for compounded feeds for cattle

Characteristics	Type-I	Type-II
Moisture, percent by mass, Max.	11.0	11.0
Crude protein (N×6.25), percent by mass, Min.	22.0	20.0
Crude fat, percent by mass, Min.	3.0	2.5
Crude fibre, percent by mass, Max.	7.0	12.0
Acid insoluble ash percent by mass, Max.	3.0	4.0
Common salt (as Nacl), percent by mass, Max.	2.0	2.0
Calcium, percent by mass, Min.	0.5	0.5
Phosphorus, percent by mass, Min	0.5	0.5
Vitamin A, IU/kg	5000	5000

SPECIFICATIONS FOR POULTRY FEEDS

Chicken feeds are of the following six types

1. **Broiler starter feed:** A ration to be fed to chicks up to the age of six weeks for meat production.
2. **Broiler finisher feed:** A ration fed to chickens from six weeks onwards for meat production.
3. **Chick feed:** A ration to be fed up to 8 weeks to chicks not intended for meat production.
4. **Growing chicken feed:** A ration fed to chickens from 8 weeks until laying commences.
5. **Laying chicken feed:** A ration fed to laying birds from 20 weeks onwards.
6. **Breeder layer feed:** A ration fed to breeding chicken.

Poultry feeds should have the following characteristics

- Feed should be in the form of pellets, crumbs or mash and it should be free from rancidity, toxic ingredients and adulterants.
- Antibiotics and coccidiostats may be added to the feed at a level recommended by the manufacturer.
- The aflatoxin B_1 content of the feed should not exceed 500 ppb
- The material shall be packed in clean, dry polyethylene-lined jute or laminated paper bags.

Each bag shall be suitably marked to give the following information

- Name of the material and brand name, if any
- Type of poultry feed
- Name and address of the manufacturer
- Net mass, when packed
- Batch No., month and year of manufacturing

Each bag shall have the following information

- Name and quantity of the antibiotic or coccidiostat added, if any
- Crude protein and crude fibre content
- Aflatoxin B_1 content
- ME (calculated) Kcal/kg
- Directions for use

Table 9. Specifications for chicken feeds

Characteristics	Broiler Starter feed	Broiler Finisher feed	Chick Feed	Growing Chicken feed	Laying Chicken feed	Breeder layer feed
Moisture, percent by mass, Max.	11.0	11.0	11.0	11.0	11.0	11.0
Crude protein, percent by mass, Min.	23.0	20.0	20.0	16.0	18.0	18.0
Crude fibre, percent by mass, Max.	6.0	6.0	7.0	8.0	8.0	8.0
Acid insoluble ash, percent by mass, Max.	3.0	3.0	4.0	4.0	4.0	4.0
Salt (as Nacl) percent By mass Max.	0.6	0.6	0.6	0.6	0.6	0.6
Calcium percent by mass Min.	1.2	1.2	1.0	1.0	3.0	3.0
Available phosphorus, percent by mass, Min.	0.5	0.5	0.5	0.5	0.5	0.5
Lysine, percent by mass, Min.	1.2	1.0	0.9	0.6	0.65	0.65
Methionine, percent by mass, Min.	0.50	0.35	0.30	0.25	0.30	0.30
ME (Kcal/kg) Min.	2800	2900	2600	2500	2600	2600

Table 10. Requirement for minerals, fatty acids, amino acids and vitamins in chicken feed

Characteristics	Broiler Starter feed	Broiler Finisher feed	Chick Feed	Growing Chicken feed	Laying Chicken feed	Breeder layer feed
Manganese (mg/kg)	90	90	90	50	55	90
Iodine (mg/kg)	1	1	1	1	1	1
Zinc (mg/kg)	60	60	60	50	75	100
Copper (mg/kg)	12	12	12	9	9	12
Vitamin A (IU/kg)	6000	6000	6000	6000	8000	8000
Vitamin D (IU/kg)	600	600	600	600	1200	1200
Vitamin E (mg/kg)	15	15	15	10	10	15
Vitamin K (mg/kg)	1	1	1	1	1	1
Thiamin (mg/kg)	5	5	5	3	3	3
Riboflavin (mg/kg)	6	6	6	5	5	8
Pantothenic acid(mg/kg)	15	15	15	15	15	15
Vitamin B_{12} (mg/kg)	0.015	0.015	0.015	0.01	0.01	0.01
Linoleic acid (g/100g)	1	1	1	1	1	1
Methionine + Cystine (g/kg)	0.9	0.7	0.6	0.5	0.55	0.55

MINERAL MIXTURES FOR CATTLE AND POULTRY FEEDS

Mineral mixtures for supplementing cattle feeds shall be of two types:

1. Mineral mixture containing salt
2. Mineral mixture without salt

All ingredients used should be of quality suitable for animal consumption. The mineral mixture shall be in the form of a free flowing powder, thoroughly mixed and completely homogeneous. It should be grounded to such fineness that in case of type-I material, not less than 70 % and in case of type-II, not less than 90 % by mass of the material should pass through 106 micron sieve. It should be free from adulterants, insects and undesirable odour. It should be free from spores of Bacillus anthracis and Clostridium sp. In case of type II mineral mixtures, salt should be added at the time of mixing the feed by the user, at the rate of 22 % by mass of the material. The percentage of chlorine as sodium chloride in the mixture after addition of salt shall be at least 22 percent by mass.

Each container shall be marked giving the following information

Name and type of material	Name of manufacturer	Net mass in kg
Date of manufacturing	Ingredients used	Guaranted composition

Table 11. Requirements for mineral mixture for cattle

Characteristics	With salt	Without salt
Moisture, % by mass, max	5	5
Calcium, % by mass, min	18	23
Phosphorus % by mass, min	9	12
Magnesium, % by mass, min	5	6.5
Salt, % by mass, min	22	-
Iron, % by mass, min	0.4	0.5
Iodine, % by mass, min	0.02	0.026
Copper, % by mass, min	0.06	0.077
Manganese, % by mass, min	0.1	0.12
Cobalt, % by mass, min	0.009	0.012
Flourine, % by mass, max	0.05	0.07
Zinc, % by mass, min	0.3	0.38
Sulphur, % by mass, max	0.4	0.5
Acid insoluble ash% by mass, max	3	2.5

Table 12. Requirements for mineral mixture for poultry

Characteristic	Requirements
Moisture, % by mass, max	3
Calcium, % by mass, min	30
Phosphorus % by mass, min	9
Iron ppm, Min	2000
Iodine, % by mass, min	0.01
Copper, ppm Min	500
Manganese, % by mass, min	0.40
Fluorine, % by mass, max	0.05
Zinc, % by mass, min	0.40
Acid insoluble ash % by mass, max	3

Bibliography

ISI (1958). Indian Standards Institution (IS: 1162) Specification for cane molasses.

ISI (1961). Indian Standards Institution (IS: 1942) Bone meal as livestock feed.

ISI (1962). Indian Standards Institution (IS: 2239) Specification for wheat bran

ISI (1965). Indian Standards Institution (IS: 3161) Specification for gram chuni

ISI (1966). Indian Standards Institution (IS: 3440) Specification for soloist extracted linseed oil cake as livestock feed.

ISI (1968). Indian Standards Institution (IS: 1664) Mineral mixtures for supplementing cattle feeds.

ISI (1968). Indian Standards Institution. Specifications for compounded feeds for cattle

ISI (1968). Indian Standards Institution (IS: 3593) Specification for solvent-extracted rice bran as livestock feed.

ISI (1975). Indian Standards Institution (IS: 3648) Specification for rice bran as livestock feed.

ISI (1992). Indian Standards Institution (IS: 1374) Poultry feed specification.

BIS (1992) Mineral mixtures for supplementing cattle feeds specification (IS : 1664).

11
GELATINIZATION

A.K.Tyagi and Nitin Tyagi

Starch is a homogeneous polymer (i.e. complex of simpler bits), a polysaccharide of thousands of simple sugars. "Simple" starch granules are very individual in structure and content and vary from 2-100 microns in size. A simple granule contains one nucleus. A "compound" starch granule has several nuclei and a rigid matrix structure. As the plant produces the starch molecules, it deposits them in successive layers around a central hilum to form a tightly packed granule. Wherever possible, adjacent amylose molecules and outer branches of amylopectin associate through hydrogen bonding in a parallel fashion to give radially oriented, crystalline bundles known as "micelles." These micelles hold the granule together to permit swelling in heated water without the complete disruption and solubilization of the individual starch molecules.

When a solid polymer contacts a solvent, the first stage of interaction is to form a GEL. With enough solvent it then forms a SOL. The gel/sol interaction is reversible, with increasing water and temperature and enzymic activity favoring the sol. The gel is a COLLOIDAL structure that is it has inter particle bonds (usually hydrogen bonds) of lower potential energy than starch in true SOLUTION. Thus enzymically unconverted mash starch extracted by later will form a gel haze by complexing when cooled and the lower thermodynamic condition is favoured. This is called "starch haze".

Gelatinization of Starch

Gelatinization of starch is a well-known process in the food and paper industries. This process is used to modify the rheology of various systems. When heat is applied to starch granules suspended in a liquid, the starch granules absorb water and swell. Starch molecules have many hydroxy groups which react with the water molecules, attracting and holding them. The smaller amylose molecules diffuse out of the swollen starch granule and form a 3-D network which traps additional water. The loss of free water and restricted flow of the water due to the enormously swollen granules occupying more space, contribute to the increased viscosity of the dispersion. This process is irreversible and it is termed as gelatinization of starch. Gelatinization temperatures are considered as ranges covering the temperatures at which loss of bi-refringence (characteristic of polarizing light) is first noticed and less than 10% remains. This temperature range is greatly influenced by the binding forces within the granule which vary with starch source. When the starch granule is heated in water, the weaker hydrogen bonds in the amorphous areas are ruptured and the granule swells with progressive hydration. The more tightly bound micelles remain intact, holding the granule together. Bi-refringence is lost.

When gelatinization is relatively complete, product expansion becomes possible. There are several successive and distinct phases of cereal conditions found during any process of gelatinization.

1) The first phase includes the slow absorption of water, with little if any swelling. During this period the starch granule maintains its characteristic of polarizing light, when light is passed through it.
2) The next phase includes an immense absorption of water, the loss of birefringence when light is passed through the starch granule and, in most cases, a very great increase in viscosity of the dough.
3) The final phase occurs at elevated temperatures: the starch loses its granular characteristic, with the starch becoming formless sacs, and the glucoside linkages between starch molecules breaking. During this period, the viscosity of the dough decreases.

Basically the gelatinization of starch has two results important to digestion:

i) Gelatinization enhances the ability of starches to absorb large quantities of water, and this leads to improved digestibility in almost all cases, and improved feed conversion in many cases.
ii) Gelatinization increases the speed at which enzymes (amylases) can break down the linkages of starch, thus converting starch into simpler and more soluble carbohydrates.

To make cereals or starches into expanded products, it is necessary to gelatinize the starchy portion of the ration, making the starch plastic and capable of intracellular expansion. Un-gelatinized starch particles will absorb only a small amount of water and will not adhere to one another.

KINETICS OF GELAINIZATION OF STARCH

Cooking of whole grains is the first step in the production of whole grain foods (Kent &Evers, 1994).The purpose of cooking is to convert the raw grain into a palatable, digestible, and workable form through gelatinization of starch in it. Gelatinization of starch has been recognized as a first-order irreversible reaction and described by the following scheme (Lund &Wirakartakusumah, 1984):

$$\text{Water + ungelatinized starch} \xrightarrow{\text{Heat}} \text{gelatinized starch}$$

$$\ln \beta = \ln \beta_0 - k_r t,$$

Where β is concentration of ungelatinized starch (%), β_0 is concentration of ungelatinized starch at the beginning of cooking (100%), k_r is reaction rate constant (s^{-1}), and t is cooking time (s).

Water molecules participating in the reaction are held by the gelatinized starch granules while the remaining travel forward (Bakshi & Singh,1980).The reaction rate constant from such a system is the apparent rate constant, which is a combined form of the true k_r and the grain resistance against the water transfer.

While the true k_r is affected by the characteristic attributes of the starch granules, the apparent k_r is additionally affected by the characteristic and geometrical attributes of the whole grain. In other words, the partition of water molecules between starch granules and cooking medium, and the gelatinization reaction are dominant in the course of the in vitro process. However during the in situ process, the partition of water molecules between whole grain and cooking medium, and water transfer within the grain in addition to the characteristic attributes of the immobilized starch granules are the dominant factors. The in situ system can also offer much more resistance to the heat transfer from the cooking medium than the in vitro system. Consequently, under the same cooking conditions it takes longer for the in situ gelatinization than the in vitro gelatinization.

Methods for Gelatinization

Several changes have occurred in the cattle feeding business which have focused attention on grain processing. The first of these was the arrival of big feedlots provided an opportunity to use larger and more sophisticated processing equipment at reasonable cost per ton of feed produced. Also, the need to minimize feed separation and digestive disturbances encouraged the use of more sophisticated methods of processing.

Steam flaking

This was the first "modern" technique which markedly increased feed efficiency and rate of gain in the case of milo. Grain is subjected to steam under atmospheric conditions for usually 15 to 30 minutes, before rolling. Large, heavy roller mills set at near zero tolerance produce a very thin, flat flake which usually weighs from 22 to 28 pounds per bushel and contains 16 to 20 percent moisture. As the flake density is decreased there is linear increase in both starch availability and flake durability (Sindt et al., 2003b). The flaking process causes gelatinization of the starch granules (hydration or rupturing of the starch molecule) rendering them more digestible. Steam flaking improves the value of sorghum grains for feedlot cattle (Theuer, 1986). The conversion efficiency by beef cattle is optimized when the grain is flaked to 0.283 to 0.361 kg/L due to improvement of starch utilization (Xiong et al., 1991) The flake quality is measured in terms of consistency of flake thickness, moisture level, durability and degree of gelatinization (Sindt et al., 2003 b) The degree of flaking and level of gelatinization appear to be influenced by such factors as steaming time, temperature, grain moisture, roller size and tolerance, processing rate, and type and variety of grain. Many feedlots equipped with steam-flaking mills apply moisture to corn prior to steaming to aid in the flake manufacturing process. Moisture is also an essential component of starch gelatinization. Without adequate moisture, starch gelatinization is incomplete. For complete gelatinization of starch to occur, moisture must accompany starch in a ratio of at least 2:1. Moisture concentration of corn prior to flaking generally ranges from 16 to 24%. Improving the gelatinization of starch by increasing the moisture content of corn prior to flaking may result in improvements in cattle performance. Extreme levels of moisture in flaked corn improve starch availability but do not appear to increase heifer performance or carcass value. As Sindt et al., (2003a) reported that feeding heifers high-moisture flakes decreased ($P<0.05$) dry matter intake and average daily gain compared to heifers fed conventional flakes. When grain is extensively flaked starch is made more available to ruminal degradation, resulting in a more rapid degradation and more rapid rate of fermentation. Variation in feed intake in response to altered feeding schedule, weather front and so on, predisposes feedlot cattle to subacute or acute acidosis. Flaking sorghum grain to 0.238 and 0.322 kg/L (Reinhardt et al., 1997) resulted in reduced intake and poor animal performance compared with 0.361 kg/L (58.7% starch gelatinization), a higher susceptibility to sub acute acidosis and higher costs of production was reported.

Pressure Flaking

The grain is subjected to steam under pressure for a short time, such as 50 pounds per square inch for one to two minutes. The continuous flow cooker is operated by air lock valves to inject and eject grain. Steam is injected into the cooker at the desired pressure. The grain in the chamber reaches a temperature approaching 300° F. When the grain is expelled from the cooker it is generally cooled (by use of a cooling and drying tower) to below 200°F and 20 percent moisture before flaking. Flakes produced from this method may be less brittle and less subject to fragmenting during the mixing and feeding operation than those from steam flaking.

Popping

Air-dry grain with a moisture content of 10 to 14 percent is popped by heating it with high temperature air at 700-800 °F for 15 to 30 seconds. Not all of the grain pops, but the resulting product very much resembles ordinary popcorn and has a moisture content of approximately 3 percent. Popping causes disruption of the starch granules by using natural moisture in the kernel to steam, gelatinize and expand the starch granules.

Roasting

Grain is passed through a gas or electrically heated roaster and is heated to about 300 degrees Fahrenheit and has a roasted odor with an oily, puffed and slightly caramelized appearance. This process appears to improve the performance of cattle, is less expensive than steam flaking and is found to be more suitable for small feeders. The Conglomeration process is also important to discuss at this juncture, it consists of grinding the grain, adding water, pelleting the mixture and roasting (Abdelgadir et al., 1996 a). It increases the starch gelatinization to five folds. Felsman et al. (1976) from the series of in vitro and in vivo studies concluded that temperature of roasting has important effect on quality of processed grain. Corn roasted at 127 or 137 °C had greater moisture absorbing capacity was more susceptible to enzymatic degradation and resulted in higher DM disappearance than raw corn or the corn roasted at 93, 104 or 116 °C. The Lysine content was reduced in corn roasted at 137, 148 and 176 °C whereas, arginine levels were reduced only at 176 °C. The performance of calves fed soybeans roasted at 146 °C plus raw corn was superior to that of calves fed soybean meal plus raw corn but was similar to the performance of calves fed soybean meal plus roasted corn (Abdelgadir et al., 1996 b), this means that performance was superior when calves consumed protein and corn sources with similar degree of ruminal ability. In other study (Yu et al., 1998) The pressure toasting of whole horse beans found to increase the bypass content of starch by decreasing rumen starch disappearance at all incubation time of 0,2,4,8,12 and 24 h with increasing time and temperature for both time and temperature. At the short time incubations, pressure toasting had strong effects on rumen disappearance but after the long rumen incubations, the effects tended to reduce.

Extruding

Extruded grain is produced by a machine which applies heat and pressure by means of friction as the grain passes through a tapered screw. Dry whole grain, with no moisture added, is crushed by an auger-like rotor and forced through an orifice, producing "ribbons" which break into flakes about 1/32 inch in thickness. Various factors, including moisture of the grain, influence the character of the final product. The pre-requisites to relatively complete gelatinization and expansion in an extrusion cooking system are:

a) Particle reduction to a reasonably fine condition (suggested maximum: 9% over U.S. Bureau of Standards screen No. 16).

b) Uniform blending of moisture (as water or steam or both) to elevate moisture content to approximately 18-27%. Gelatinization can be accomplished at lower moisture contents, but will usually require excessive power.

Increase of product temperature for required period of time.

Extrusion Cookers

There are many means of gelatinizing starch. When a grain or flour is boiled in water, it will be gelatinized. The pelleting cereal mixtures in a pellet mill equipped with adequate steam conditioning will result in a small percentage of gelatinization. Pressure steaming of grain, followed by rolling, will result in a moderate degree of gelatinization of starch. Drying of aqueous slurry of cereal flour on steam jacketed rolls will result in relatively complete gelatinization of starch. Handling and processing of materials for extrusion cookers depends on particle size and ingredients used. Extrusion cookers are capable of gelatinizing and uniformly expanding all ground cereal grains, mill feeds, degerminated wheat or corn meals, wet milled starches, flours of tubers and pulses

Basically, there are three types of extrusion cookers in use today, these being: (1) Short time, high temperature extrusion cookers, (2) Pressure cooking extruders and (3) Extrusion cookers which are not designed for preconditioning with steam, but which instead inject both steam and water directly into a long extruder barrel designed to build up product temperatures and moisture contents gradually.

Extrusion cooking in the feed industry

1. Expanded dry pet foods

The major application to date for extrusion cooking in the animal feed industry has been the production of expanded pet foods.

2. Expanded soft moist pet foods

Soft moist pet foods contain 25% to 30% moisture, and are basically mixtures of meat meal or meat slurries, soy, sugar and humectants.

3. Gelatinization of the cereals for animal feeds

There is considerable evidence (Burton, 1962) that the nutritive value of cereals and starches is enhanced for ruminants when the cereals or starches are gelatinized. In most reports, such feeding trials have shown substantial improvement in feed conversion when the starch portion of the total ration has been gelatinized.

Much work remains to be done on the optimum percentage of gelatinized cereals which will produce the greatest improvement in various rations, but it seems probable that gelatinization of some portion of the cereals used in ruminant rations will prove an economic process for tomorrow's feed industry. It does appear that one cannot economically justify the cooking (compete or partial gelatinization) of more than the cereal portion of ruminant rations at this time. The cereal portions of meal type dog foods mink foods, horse feed and fish foods are also gelatinized prior to mixing with other ingredients for maximum feed efficiency. Since cereals are generally gelatinized by themselves (no other products mixed prior to cooking), the whole grain is first ground in a hammermill. The ground material is conveyed to a bin or live bottom feeder above the extrusion cooker. After cooking, the product will be dried to the desired moisture level in a tunnel type dryer, will be cooled in a horizontal cooler, and many thereafter be reduced in particle size (crumble roll, hammermill, impact mill, or attrition mill) in those cases where small particle size of gelatinized cereal is desired. It should be added here that gelatinization of cereals does not invariably show improved feeding results, except for ruminants.

4. Textured soy protein

Textured soy proteins are made by extrusion cooking of defatted soy flours or grits (min 50% protein, max 1% fat, max 3% fiber, NSI 50-57%) to produce chewy, meat-like chunks. Such products are used in dry expanded pet foods and in canned pet foods because of their chewy nature and their meat-like appearance when they are rehydrated.

Certain grains, notably barley and milo, have not achieved maximum utility in ruminant rations when simply cracked or ground before feeding. Cardon (1966) determined by chemical analysis that as much as 40% of the starch remained in fecal matter when ground rations high in milo content were fed to cattle. Some means of improving digestibility of barley and milo were clearly needed. The rolling of flaking of milo and barley has been adopted by many qualified cattle feeders.

Theoretically, the complete gelatinization of milo or barley should fill these objectives. But the preponderance of evidence available indicates that complete gelatinization of milo or barley may not be required for maximum economic utility of these cereals by ruminants. Partially gelatinized milo (steam rolled) was reported by Cardon (1966) to produce virtually the same daily rate of gain as completely gelatinized (autoclaved) milo, and to provide somewhat better rates of feed conversion.

Two method of steam rolling of barley and of milo are in use today:

a) Steam preconditioning at atmospheric pressure for 8 to 20 minutes in a vertical steaming chamber positioned immediately above the roller mill. This method usually results in grain temperatures of 210° to 215°F and in moisture contents of 18 to 20% prior to rolling. This method usually results in approximately 5 to 19% gelatinization after steaming, and 20 to 30% gelatinization after rolling.

b) Pressure preconditioning in a horizontal pressure processing unit for 50 seconds to 2 minutes at steam pressures of from 20 to 60 psi (250° to 300°F). Grain is discharged from this pressure cooker with 20 to 25% gelatinization and moisture content from 18 to 25% dependent on moisture content of incoming grain, and retention period selected for the pressure cooker. The grain is thereafter rolled in large diameter rolling mills, and will normally be 45% to 60% gelatinized after the rolling mills. A cooler is sometimes used as a tempering device and at times, as a method of reducing moisture content of the steamed grain between cooker and roller mill. Where incoming milo is very low in moisture content, a few percentage points of moisture is sometimes applied as water to the milo in a screw conveyor feeding the pressure cooker from a holding bin.

Bibliography

Abdelgadir, I.E.O., Morril, J.L. and Higgins, J.J (1996 a) Effect of roasted

Soyabean and corn on performance and ruminal and blood metabolites of dairy calves. J. Dairy Sci. 79: 465-474

Abdelgadir, I.E.O., Morril, J.L. and Higgins, J.J (1996 b) Ruminal availabilities of protein and starch: Effects on growth and ruminal and plasma metabolites of dairy calves. J. Dairy Sci. 79: 283 -290

Bakshi, A.S and Singh, R.P (1980) Kinetics of water diffusion and starch gelatinization during rice parboiling. J of Food Sci., 45, 1387-1392.

Burton, D.W. (1962) "Expanded concentrates vs. Ground concentrates vs. pellets for dairy heifers" Feedstuffs, Dec 1, 1962.

Cardon, B.P. Feedstuffs. May 14, 1966.

Felsman, R.J., Harvey, R.W., Linnerud, A.C. and Smith, F.H. (1976) Effect of roasting temperature on corn grain characteristics. J. of Anim. Sci. 42 (2) 476 – 480.

Kent, N.L. and Evers, A.D. (1994) Technology of cereals (4th Ed., pp. 233-258).

Oxford, UK : Pergamon.

Lund, D.B. and Wirakartakusumah, M. (1984). A model for starch gelatinization

phenomena in : B.M. McKenna (Ed.), Engineering and food, Vol 1. Engineering sciences in the food industry (pp. 425 -432). London UK : Elsivier

Reinhardt, C.D, Brandt, R.T, Jr., Behnke, K.C., Freeman, A.S and Eck, T.P (1997)

Effect of steam flaked sorghum grain density on performance, mill production rate and subacute ketosis in feedlot steers. J. Anim. Sci. 75: 2852 – 2857.

Sindt, J.J., Drouillard, J.S., Kessen, T.J., Sulpizio, M.J., Loe, E.R and Montgomery,

S.P (2003 a) Effect of feeding conventional or high-moisture, steam-flaked corn to finishing heifers. Cattlemen's Day 156 – 159.

Sindt, J.J., Drouillard, J.S., Montgomery, S.P and Loe, E.R (2003 b) Effect of processing variables on characteristics of steam- flaked corn. Cattlemen's Day 160 – 165.

Theuer, C.B. (1986) Grain processing effects on starch utilization by ruminants. J. Anim. Sci. 63. 1649.

Turham, M., Gunasekaran, S. (2002) Kinetics of in situ and in vitro gelatinization of hard and soft wheat starches during cooking in water. J. of Food engineering 52, 1-7.

Xiong, Y., Bartle, S.J. and Preston, R.L. (1991) Density of steam-flaked sorghum grain, Roughage level and feeding regime for feedlot steers. J.Anim.Sci. 69. 1707.

Yu, P., Goelema, J.O. and Tamminga, S. (1998) Influence of pressure toasting onstarch ruminal degradative kinetics and fermentation characterstics and gelatinization of whole horse beans (Vicia faba) in lactating dairy cows. Asian-aus. J. Anim. Sci. 12 (4) 537 – 543.

12
FEED MICROSCOPY

Ram Singh and S. S. Kundu

Good quality feed ingredient should mean the ingredient which possesses the excellence of its nutritive value in terms of both chemical composition and nutrient utilization. The demand for quality products is universal, and animal feed and feed industry are no exception to this. The quality of the feed ingredients which come from the same origin may exhibit a variation. The factors which affect the quality of the feed ingredients as well as complete feed are adulteration, damage and deterioration due to weather or storage conditions, natural variation and processing. Fine particle feed ingredients are prone to adulteration with one or more cheaper fine materials which may or may not have required/optimum nutritive values. Fish meal may be adulterated with common salt. Rice bran may be adulterated with rice hulls. Feed ingredients may lose their quality through damage and deterioration during inappropriate handling and storage. Feed grain is commonly damaged by insects under improper storage conditions. The chemical composition of plant products may be varied due to the fertility of the soil as well as the variety of the plant itself. Differences in the agro-industrial processing techniques will produce products or by-products with different quality. The feed quality can be determined by chemical analysis, feed microscopy, and spot and quick chemical tests.

Chemical analysis

The chemical analysis includes the estimation of moisture, crude protein, ether extract (fat), fibre, ash and mineral content and the quality is evaluated by comparing with the standard check. In general, feed ingredient free from adulteration and contamination will exhibit chemical composition very close to a standard or mean value recommended or reported in the region. The chemical analysis shows the total nutrient content of the feed ingredient and the data can be used directly for feed formulation. The chemical analyses are the traditional quality control tests. These methods require a well equipped laboratory and trained chemists. The total expenses per sample analysis are rather high. Also, chemical analyses do not tell us the source of nutrients in a given feed. For example, protein is one of the most important nutrients as for as quality assurance and feed formulations are concerned, which is determined by Kjeldahl method and expressed as crude protein. The results thus obtained do not reveal the sources of nitrogen whether it comes from protein in the ingredient or protein in adulterants or non-protein nitrogen contaminated or adulterated in the sample. Crude fat is still extracted primarily with petroleum ether using Soxhlet apparatus. There is a constant risk of fire and explosion with these solvents. The chemical analysis requires lot of time, therefore, there will be a significant time delay from receipt of sample to final quality determination. This delay in quality determination causes practical hindrance for unloading the supply and can be critical for larger feed mills that need to maintain the flow of incoming ingredients in unloading areas. Thus, routine chemical analysis fails to identify the purity, soundness, infestation, adulteration and contaminants which have significant bearing on quality. Feed microscopy can be the suitable additional tool and provide solution to such type of problems.

Spot and quick chemical tests

Many spot and quick chemical tests have been developed for testing the presence or absence of certain chemical substances which influence the quality of feed. Say, contamination of urea in feed ingredients such as fish meal is easily detected by using urea test. Many of the methods are very simple and can be practiced by the farmers. However, some of the techniques require expensive chemical reagents. Hence, its application is also limited to commercial feed production.

Feed Microscopy

What is Feed Microscopy ? Determining and evaluating the quality of feed ingredients and finished feeds and the extent of adulteration and contamination with the help of microscope is called as feed microscopy.

Importance of feed microscopy

Due to shortage and high prices of feed ingredients, adulteration is one of the main problems for feed manufacturers and cattle breeders. (Singh, 1994; Ahuja et al., 1995) Identification of adulterants and contaminants in feed ingredients is the most important application of feed microscopy. It is a simple, rapid technique that can tell more about the quality of an ingredient or finished feed, in a shorter time, as compared to chemical analysis. A feed microscopist, can often give more information about the quality of an incoming ingredient in ten minutes than several chemists can determine in the lab in several hours. And because the concepts and equipment are relatively simple, some level of feed microscopy is affordable to every feed manufacturers and organized farm without the cost of an elaborate laboratory. Feed microscopy involves the identification and evaluation of feed ingredients and foreign materials alone or in mixture, via either surface features or cellular characteristics. If ingredients and adulterants or contaminants are separated and proportional measured, then feed microscopy can be used for quantitative evaluation of feed ingredients. Thus, feed microscopy can satisfactorily tell the purity of the feed ingredient and the acceptance and rejection decisions are made just after comparisons with standard photomicrograph catalogue. Similarly, the presence of certain moulds and mould spores identified microscopically, assists in the determination of mould metabolites and feed refusal factors. Thus, weathering effects, moulds, heat and insect damage, filth, adulterants and contaminants can be observed readily under the microscope and compared to acceptable standards. Feed microscopy is the complement to precise chemical analysis by novel techniques in quality control laboratory. For example, feed microscopy reveals the source of nutrients in a given feed, whereas, chemical analysis gives the total amount of nutrients in a given feed. Therefore, for complete quality assurance programme, feed microscopy and chemical analysis should be taken up together.

Microscopy of feed ingredients

There are two types of microscope for identifying the structures or features of feedstuffs. One is the compound microscope and other is the stereomicroscope. The first one is used to identify the components of internal structure of feed and the second one is used to identify the external structure. The identification of feedstuffs by stereomicroscope involves arrangement of equipment/ materials of stereomicroscope, sample preparation and finally the inspection under stereomicroscope.

Materials required for stereomicroscopy

Stereomicroscope with light

A set of sieves and pan

Sharp pointed forceps and needle

Petri dishes

Beakers (100-150 ml)

Stainless spoons

Reagent bottles

Mortar and pestle

Sample preparation

There are several forms of feed like mash, pellet, crumble or cake etc. If they are brought for examination under stereomicroscope, it is very difficult to observe the structure of feed particles. Therefore, for accurate and dependable results, it is necessary to prepare the sample before examination as follows:

About 10g of the ground sample is placed on 40 mesh sieve to separate the particles by using RO-Tap shaker. Sieving removes the fine starchy dust and other fine particles in the feed for more positive identification. In case of expeller pressed cakes, it is necessary to treat them with chloroform before sieving. A floatation technique is used where the sample is soaked in the solvent (chloroform) then stirred and allowed to settle until the two fractions are clearly separated. The top layer is of organic and the bottom layer is of inorganic material. The top layer is removed in petri dish and allowed to dry at room temperature. The use of chloroform not only causes separation of organic and inorganic material but also removes fat from the sample, which does help for a more clear identification. This organic material is sieved as above.

Stereomicroscopic inspection: Samples of feedstuffs and mixed feed have the same process for inspection. First, colour and texture must be determined for primary information. Additional information can often be obtained from smell (burned, musty, rancid, ferment) and taste (soapy, bitter, sour) of feedstuffs. Next the sample is prepared by screening or floatation for microscopic examination.

- Set the stereomicroscope at lower magnification and adjust the focus.
- A fraction from the prepared sample should be spread separately on petri dish and examined under the stereomicroscope. Searching is facilitated by starting with coarse particles and working from one end of petri dish to the other.
- Searching the fraction (coarse and fine particles) under stereomicroscope, extra ingredients and similar ingredients should be raked aside, then restudied to confirm identification of certain ingredients.
- Adjust the proper magnification to examine characteristics of ingredients for accurate identification.
- Identification of feedstuffs structure is performed by looking for physical characteristics such as colour, hardness, softness, transparency, translucency, opacity and surface texture. Therefore, the investigator has to practice, observe and remember the physical characteristics of feedstuffs.

- Extra ingredients that are not components of feedstuffs, are called contaminants if found in small amount and adulterants if in large amount.

Stereoscopic features of commonly used feed ingredients: The feed ingredient samples are ground and passed through 1mm sieve. For the preparation of photomicrographs, the ground material is sifted through 40 mesh sieve using a pan. The material retained on 40 mesh sieve is used for the preparation of photomicrographs, as these particles give the clear picture. Thus, the particle size for the preparation of photomicrographs may range from 425 μm to 1mm and the photomicrographs are taken at 25X magnification. The microstructures of various feed ingredients are described below:

Microstructure of energy feed ingredients

(1) Avena sativa seeds *(Oat seeds)*

Under stereomicroscope, oat hull fragments and starch particles are visible. Hull fragments are elongated and range from light grey to tannish grey in colour and are semi-glossy. Starch particles are opaque and white in colour. In some of the fragments, starch particles are attached which represent the inner portion of the hulls. The texture of ground oats is fine and gives sweet odour of ground grain with no mustiness.

(2) Cicer arietinum by products *(Gram pericarp / bran / chuni)*

Gram chuni consists mostly of seed coat of gram seeds with broken pieces of cotyledons including germ obtained as a by-product during the processing of gram pulse for human consumption. The by-product has no other value except for animal feeding. The seed coat particles are hard, having sharp edges and give flake-like appearance. The outer portion of the seed coat is black, whereas, the inner portion is yellow in colour but still possessing blackish appearance. The cotyledonous material is semi-glossy, opaque, floury and white in colour. To the surface of the seed coat particles, cotyledonous material remains attached. The germ portion appears light yellow in colour.

(3) Hordeum vulgare seeds *(Barley seeds)*

In case of barley, the kernel is surrounded by a hull. Under stereomicroscope, the hull fragments and starch particles are seen. The hull fragments are light grey to tannish grey in colour. They are elongated and possess a dull luster on the surface. The starchy material is lustrous, opaque and white in colour and irregularly shaped. The white coloured elongated fragments represent the inner portion of the barley hull to which starchy material is attached. Ground barley resembles ground oats in overall appearance, whereas, ground barley fragments are slighty bigger in size than that of ground oats. Also, the starchy material, in case of ground oats, gives a cloudy appearance. The ground barley gives a fresh and sweet odour of ground grain (Pfost, 1976).

(4) Oryza sativa by-product *(Rice bran)*

Rice bran consists of the pericarp or bran layer, germ of the rice and some grain fragments remained during milling rice for human food, and it should contain only such quantities of hull fragments as are unavoidable in the regular milling process. From this type of rice bran, oil is removed and a product of better keeping quality, known as solvent extracted or deoiled rice bran, is obtained. In rice bran, the hull fragments are always present. On the outer surface of the hull fragments, longitudinal striations which run parallel to each other are clearly visible as they are shiny and form a cross-hatching pattern on the outer surface. The hull fragments are irregular in shape and yellow to brown in colour. They have a smooth surface and exhibit translucency.

(5) Pennisetum typhoides seeds *(Pearl-millet or bajra seeds)*

Under stereomicroscope, different coloured particles are visible. The outer portion of the seed coat exhibits slightly dark appearance, whereas the inner portion is pale yellow in colour. The starch is lustrous and white in colour. The particles are irregularly shaped but often globular to triangular in shape. The seed coat is hard and may not break by applying pressure with a needle. The texture of ground bajra is fine and gives a pleasant sweet odour of ground grain.

(6) Sorghum bicolor seeds *(Red sorghum seeds)*

The outer portion of the bran coat is black or dark red, whereas, the inner portion is red brown or pale yellow in colour. The sorghum grain has two types of starch, hard which is from the outer endosperm and soft which is from the inner portion of endosperm. The hard starch is corneous, opaque and has rough surface, whereas, the soft starch is shiny, white and exhibit floury appearance. The bran coat remains closely attached to the hard and corneous starch. The ground sorghum has sweet odour of ground grain and free from mustiness. The taste of the ground grain is slightly bitter. The stereoscopic features of white sorghum are same as in case of red sorghum except colour of seed bran coat. In case of white sorghum, the colour of bran coat is light yellow and that of micropyle is dark red.

(7) Triticum aestivum by-product *(Wheat bran)*

Wheat bran is the coarse outer covering of the wheat kernel as separated in the usual process of commercial milling. The wheat bran particles are thin, different in size and exhibit flake-like appearance. They are yellowish brown in colour. The germ appear pale yellow in colour and oval in shape. Starch particles are white, semi-translucent to opaque and semi-glossy. On inner surface of the bran particles, a floury coating is visible which is due to the presence of starch particles, adhered to the inner surface of the bran coat.

(8) Zea mays seeds *(Yellow maize seeds)*

Under stereomicroscope, the bran coat and endosperm particles are visible. The bran particles are thin, irregular in shape, semi-transparent and glossy. They range from light yellow to golden yellow in colour. The endosperm starch particles are of two types: white which are soft, lustrous, opaque and have floury appearance; and light yellow that are somewhat hard and exhibit translucent characteristic. The white coloured particles dominate the light yellow particles. To the inner portion of the seed coat starch particles are attached.

Microstructure of protein feed ingredients

(9) Arachis hypogaea cake *(Groundnut cake)*

Groundnut cake particles range from light brown to dark brown in colour. Some have white cotyledonous material attached which is lustrous, white, soft and fluffy. On critical examination of the photomicrograph, the dark coloured material as groundnut husk fragments could be identified. Cake resembles coconut meal in many of the stereoscopic features, and smells like that of roasted groundnut kernels.

(10) Brassica spp. cake *(Mustard cake)*

The seed coat and kernel fragments are fused together and cannot be separated but are friable. The seed coat is thin, somewhat hard and varies from dark or red brown to black in colour. Under stereomicroscope, the red brown and black colour represents the outer surface of the seed coat. The kernel fragments are irregularly shaped and yellow to brown in colour. The mustard cake has the characteristic odour of mustard oil. The stereoscopic features of solvent extracted mustard cake are similar, except that the particles are crumbly and more friable in case of solvent extracted mustard cake.

(11) Cicer arietinum seeds *(Bengal gram seeds, black)*

Under stereomicroscope, seed coat fragments and cotyledons are visible. The outer surface of seed coat fragments is light black in colour, whereas, the inner surface is dark brown. To the inner surface of seed coat fragments cotyledon is attached which is white in colour and forming a network pattern. The whitish yellow particles are that of cotyledons. They are different in shape and size. Some of the particles are globular amd some are triangular in shape. They possess odour like that of ground seeds.

(12) Cicer arietinum seeds *(Bengal gram seeds, white)*

Under stereomicroscope, seed coat fragments and cotyledons are visible. All the particles are whitish-yellow in colour, opaque, semi-glossy, and exhibit dull and somewhat uniform appearance. The seed coat fragments are flat and possess flake-like appearance. The cotyledon particles are different in shape and size. Most of them are either globular or triangular in shape as in case of black bengal gram. The odour is like that of ground seeds.

(13) Cocos nucifera cake *(Coconut cake)*

The coconut cake particles are brown to reddish brown in colour. The reddish brown colour represents the testa portion. Some has white endosperm attached. The endosperm is white, soft, lustrous and fluffy. The stereoscopic features in terms of shape, size and colour resembles very much to that of groundnut cake, but there are slight colour differences, on the basis of which, they can be differentiated. In addition, they possess different odours and tastes. Coconut cake has a pleasant nut-like odour, resembling roasted coconut.

(14) Cyamopsis tetragonoloba by-product *(Guar corma)*

Guar corma is a by-product obtained during the production of gum from guar seeds. In stereoscopic features, the particles are of different shape and size. The seed coat particles are dark brown and pale yellow in colour, which represent the outer and inner portion of the seed coat, respectively. They are hard, thick, greasy and semi-glossy. The cotyledons are comparatively soft. They are glossy and cream white in colour.

(15) Glycine max meal *(Soybean meal, solvent extracted)*

In soybean meal hull particles are often seen. The hull particles have rough, porous and blackish brown inner surface whereas the outer surface is smooth and shiny. The kernel particles are cream to yellowish brown in colour, opaque and exhibit dull appearance. The particles of soybean meal are hard, brittle, irregular and flat in shape. The dark brown colour of some of the particles indicates over-heating of the soybean meal. It possesses a sweet and pleasant odour but the taste is somewhat bland.

(16) Gossypium spp. cake *(Cottonseed cake expeller)*

Under the stereomicroscope, the hairs or fibres in cottonseed cake are seen in bundles and overlapping each other. These are yellow and white in colour, long, flattened in shape, (Voughan, 1970) semi-transparent and lustrous. In cake the hulls are usually present, which are dark brown and black in colour, thick, tough, hard and opaque. The hull fragments look like pieces of stones under stereomicroscope. Cottonseed cake has a sweet and pleasant odour but the taste is somewhat bland.

(17) Helianthus annuus cake *(Sunflower cake)*

Under stereomicro-scope, the sunflower cake particles exhibit a woody appearance and are hard and brittle. The particles of hull fragments are white and black in colour, whereas, that of kernel are yellowish brown or dark brown. The hull fragments differ in size, shape and length and possess white or white and black stripes on the surface. Due to mechanical actions, the hull fragments may lose white and black stripes, and appear cream coloured and exhibit smooth and lustrous appearance. The particles of kernel are irregularly shaped, small in size and have dull appearance. The particles resemble that of castor husk closely.

(18) Juglans regia cake *(Walnut cake mechanically extracted)*

The shell of walnut cake is extremely hard and covers the two-lobed, wrinkled kernel. Under the stereomicroscope, two types of particles are visible: brownish yellow and brownish black. The latter particles are that of shell portion and brownish yellow particles represent the fragments of kernel portion. The shell particles are very hard, irregular in shape and possess rough surface. The kernel fragments tend to be rectangular in shape. They are hard and possess smooth surface. Walnut cake has a pleasant odour but somewhat bland taste.

(19) Lathyrus sativus seeds *(Khesari, chickling vetch or grass pea seeds)*

Under stereomicroscope, the dark brown and black coloured particles are seed coat fragments. The fragments are hard, thin, opaque and dull and flake-like in appearance. The cotyledons are semi-glossy and whitish yellow in colour. They are different in shape and size. Most of the cotyledon particles are either globular or corneous in shape.

(20) Linum usitatissimum cake *(Linseed cake)*

The linseed cake particles are different in shape and size but uniform in appearance, and grey brown to dark brown in colour. The particles are semi-glossy, somewhat hard and opaque. The white coloured tiny particles are that of cotyledon which exhibit bright and shiny appearance. The odour of the cake is like that of ground linseed or somewhat characteristic odour of linseed oil.

(21) Madhuca indica cake *(Mahua seed cake)*

The particles are somewhat globular in shape and brown to reddish brown in colour, but a few pale yellow coloured particles may also be seen. The particles are opaque, semi-glossy and uniform in appearance. The cotyledon is white and yellow in colour, glossy and fluffy. The mahua seed cake has a characteristic pungent odour.

(22) Pisum sativum seeds *(Pea seeds)*

Under stereomicroscope, different coloured particles are visible. They are brown, whitish-brown, whitish-yellow and light green in colour. The seed coat particles have thin, flake-like appearance and sharp edges. The cotyledon particles are thick and possess reticulation like spongy appearance. The light green colour is the characteristic colour of pea seed coat. Pea seeds possess odour of ground pea seeds and bland taste.

(23) Zea mays by-product *(Maize gluten feed)*

Maize gluten feed is a by-product obtained after the removal of most of the starch and germ from maize in wet milling manufacture of maize starch. Maize gluten feed consists of maize gluten meal and maize bran. It may also include part of the maize germ oil meal. Thus, the three products gluten, bran and germ are mixed together and sold as maize gluten feed (McDonald et al., 1995). Under stereomicroscope, different coloured particles are visible. Most of the particles range from yellow to dark brown in colour, but light yellow and whitish coloured particles are also seen, the white colour may be due to the presence of starch particles. Dark brown coloured material indicates heat damage during the manufacturing process. The particles are irregular in shape and size. Maize gluten feed has a sweet odour of toasted maize. The odour characteristic of desirable maize gluten feed is one of the most distinctive odours among grain products (Pfost, 1976). It is slightly acidic in taste and has coarse texture.

(24) Fish meal

The muscle fibres are seen as different sized fragments and are yellow or yellow brown in colour. The muscle fibre fragments have dull surface and are slightly transparent. The muscle fibres can be easily separated by applying little pressure with needle and tweezers. Bones are thick, hard, opaque, and different in shape and size and range from white to yellowish-white in colour. Fish scales are shiny, flat and creamy white in colour. Fish meal possesses a sharp fishy odour of cooked fish.

(25) Meat meal

Meat meal is the finely ground, dry residue from animal tissues exclusive of hide, hoof, horn, hair, and blood and stomach contents except in such traces as are unavoidable during processing operations. Under stereomicroscope, the red brown particles are the blood particles. These are hard and semi-lustrous. The other particles are that of meat scrap. They are hard, opaque, and brown and black in colour. The meat scrap particles possess uniform appearance but a coarse texture. Meat meal possesses odour like that of cooked meat.

Microstructure of adulterants

Quality assurance aims to produce a least-cost and balanced feed which is palatable, digestible, free from adulterants, contaminants and infestants and meets the nutritional requirements of the animal. Compound feeds could be mixed with various adulterants such as rice husk, groundnut husk, castor husk, wheat straw and saw dust. Therefore, photomicrographs of commonly used adulterants in animal feeds have been prepared and their microstructures have been defined as follows:

(1) Acacia nilotica *(saw dust)*

The particles are different in shape and size, whitish brown to dark brown in colour and woody in appearance. They are thick, hard, opaque, somewhat lustrous and do not break even after applying pressure with needle and tweezers. They possess wood-like odour.

(2) Arachis hypogaea husk *(groundnut husk)*

The husk fragments are pale yellow in outer portion and white opaque and glossy in inner portion. The husk fragments possess longitudinal ridges forming a reticulate pattern. The thin, papery, red coloured particles are that of pericarp of groundnut kernel that enclose the kernel loosely.

(3) Oryza sativa husk *(rice husk)*

The rice husk particles are yellow in colour and irregular in shape and size. They are somewhat hard and possess sharp edges. They exhibit flake-like appearance with longitudinal striations forming a cross-hatching pattern on the outer surface of the particles.

(4) Ricinus communis husk *(castor husk)*

The particles are dark brown and black in the outer layer and whitish yellow in the inner layer. They are hard and exhibit a woody appearance. The castor husk particles closely resemble that of sunflower cake. The most striking difference between the two is that the former does not bear stripes on the surface of their particles, only the fibrous strands are visible.

(5) Triticum aestivum straw *(wheat straw)*

The particles are elongated in shape and dull white to brownish yellow in colour. They are thin, semi-glossy and semi-transparent. In some of the particles, the fibrous strands are clearly visible.

Identification of feed ingredients and adulterants in compounded cattle feeds:

The microstructure of feed ingredients and adulterants were applied for their identification in compounded cattle feeds. Twenty five samples of compounded feeds were collected from the farmers' houses in the villages of Chamba district of Himachal Pradesh and examined for their chemical and physical constituents. The physical constituents were determined by feed microscopy in which the microstructures of various feed ingredients and adulterants were compared with their respective standards. The analysis of proximate principles and physical constituents of compounded cattle feed is given in Table 1. The proximate composition was compared with BIS specifications and it was found that none of the twenty five samples fulfilled the BIS requirements for cattle feed type1 in terms of crude protein and ether extract. Of the twenty five samples one (4%), fulfilled the BIS requirements for cattle feed type 2. Twenty four (96%) samples failed to fulfill BIS requirements due to lack of BIS specifications in these samples in terms of crude protein. The perusal of the data showed a high percentage of CF and acid insoluble ash in these samples. This might be due to the presence of adulterants in these samples.

Table 1: Proximate composition (%DM basis) and physical constituents of compounded cattle feeds:

Cattle feed	Proximate composition				*Physical constituents			
	CP min.	CF max.	EE min.	AIA max.				
BIS type 1	22.00	7.00	3.0	3.0	-	-	-	
BIS type 2	20.00	12.00	2.5	4.0	-	-	-	
CF-I	18.03	13.01	2.03	5.26	BA	GN	WB	CS
CF-II	15.15	15.21	2.39	5.02	MZ	MC	GN	RH
CF-III	14.21	15.38	2.56	6.22	MZ	GN	WB	RH
CF-IV	15.81	14.78	2.60	6.42	GN	WB	MZ	RH
CF-V	20.23	12.60	2.89	3.98	BA	RB	CS	GN
CF-VI	13.12	15.89	2.86	8.29	RB	BA	CS	RH
CF-VII	12.80	16.29	2.02	7.56	MZ	GN	WB	RH
CF-VIII	15.75	14.28	2.35	6.66	BA	SB	RB	
CF-IX	16.01	14.99	2.18	5.49	MZ	RB	CS	RH
CF-X	16.92	14.98	2.09	6.46	MC	BA	WB	RH
CF-XI	18.68	13.58	2.35	3.23	MC	BA	RB	RH
CF-XII	15.35	13.85	3.02	6.92	MZ	FM	RB	RH
CF-XIII	16.21	13.92	2.05	5.82	SC	WB	BA	RH
CF-XIV	17.81	14.05	2.55	5.51	BR	SB	BJ	RH
CF-XV	18.29	13.28	2.30	4.25	GN	BA	PA	RB
CF-XVI	19.12	11.55	2.19	3.15	WB	BA	CS	
CF-XVII	18.25	14.23	2.11	5.25	RB	WA	GN	MZ
CF-VIII	16.02	14.25	2.24	6.51	BA	WB	SB	RH
CF-XIX	16.82	13.90	2.35	6.12	CS	GN	MZ	WB
CF-XX	15.12	14.75	2.40	8.12	GN	CS	BA	RH
CF-XXI	17.21	13.92	2.35	6.70	MZ	GN	WB	CS
CF-XXII	18.21	13.55	2.98	5.85	BA	SB	MC	WB
CF-XXIII	19.05	13.25	2.76	2.08	OT	CS	MZ	GN
CF-XXIV	18.85	15.25	2.26	2.65	MC	WB	CS	RH
CF-XXV	18.98	14.92	2.78	3.02	CS	WB	MZ	GN

• SB, Soybean meal; PA, Peas; BA, Barley; WB, Wheat bran; GN, Groundnut cake; MZ, Maize ; CS, Cottonseed cake; GNH, Groundnut husk; BJ, Bajra; OT, Oat; RH, Rice husk; RB, Rice bran; MC, Mustard cake; SC, Sunflower cake; BR, Broken rice; FM, Fish meal; GC, Gram chunni; MG, Maize gluten; MM, Meat meal;.

The microscopic studies of these samples revealed their physical constituents as shown on Table 1. On microscopic examination, it was found that many of the samples were adulterated with rice husk as a result of which higher percentage of cattle feeds samples failed to meet the BIS specifications. Thus, rice husk is the most commonly used adulterant in compounded cattle feeds in the region and wherever, adulterant is detected the protein content in the sample is relatively low. Therefore, for complete quality evaluation of feeds, chemical analysis and feed microscopy should be considered together. The study further concludes that the colour and shape of the particles of feed ingredients and adulterants are the most important criteria for their identification singly or in mixture, though other criteria like opacity, translucency, transparency, hardness and softness, texture, odour and taste are also helpful in this regard. Although, quality evaluation by microscopic inspection is based on the ability of feed microscopist to recognize the normal constituents of the various feedstuffs as compared with contaminants or undesirable ingredients. Hence, it is imperative for the feed microscopist to be familiar with microstructures of different feed ingredients and adulterants.

Bibliography

Ahuja, A.K., Gupta, B.K. and Ichhponani (1995). Nutrient content and availability of different compounded cattle feeds. Indian J. Dairy Sci. 48: 6, 390-394.

McDonald, P., Edwards, R.A. and Greenhalgh, J.F.D. (1995). Chemical composition of foods. In: Animal Nutrition, ELBS, edition of fifth edition. pp. 546-563.

Pfost, H.B. (19876). Product control. In; Feed manufacturing technology. American Feed Manufacturing Association Inc., Virginia. pp. 249-298.

Singh, B. (1994). An analysis of the marketing of cattle feeds in Punjab. Indian J. Dairy Sci. 47: 569-573.

Voughan, J. G. (1970). The structure and utilization of oilseeds: Champman and Hall. London. Pp.145-192.

13
LIQUID FEEDS HANDLING

Nityanand Pathak

The most important food of any mammalian life is the milk (preferably the mother's milk). Milk is one of the most valuable gifts of the Almighty. Immediately after borth the life of mammalian infant is supported by the milk suckled direct from the mammary glands. Besides milk there are other types of liquid feeds that need handling right from the stage of production to feeding and the intermediary stages of storage and transportation etc. During the process of development of feed technology different kinds of liquid feeds have been developed in different countries. The composition and method of preparation of liquid feeds depends on the sources of food items and concept of the livestock owners, e.g. the composition of slurry or gruel fed to cows and buffaloes during the first fortnight of calving is more or less similar to that prepared for the feeding of ladies during the first 10-15 days immediately following the delivery. These gruels or slurries are prepared preferably from the high protein and high energy ingredients along with other herbal ingredients considered useful for the cleaning of womb and involution of uterus. Feeding of liquid diets to livestock is an age old practice in India and it starts from the birth. Different kinds of liquid feeds used for the feeding of livestock may be listed as follows :

1. Milk and milk products

Whole milk, skim milk, reconstituted milk, whey, butter milk and mattha etc.

2. Slurry and gruel

These are made of cereal flour, leguminous flour or mixture of cereal and leguminoud flour. These also contain jaggary or rob (crude thick syrup prepared by boiling sugarcane juice in large pans). These may also contain some medicinal ingredients like dried ginger powder, cumin,chiraita and some dried herbal products for feeding during the first week of calving.

3. Milk replacer

The composition of milk replacer varies greatly in different regions of the country where it is used. It invariably contains milk products which may be mattha, curd or skim milk.

4. By products of sugar (khand) and jaggary industries

These include scum screened during boiling of the sugarcane juice, washings of the pan, molasses and press mud etc.

• Former Director, CIRB(ICAR)-113 B, Vatika, Sun City Vistar Bareilly - 243122, U.P.

5. Molasses based liquid feeds

These are mostly urea containing products and may be fortified with minerals and vitamins. The common molasses based feeds are urea-molasses liquid diet (UMLD) standardized by author during 1970-72 at the Indian Veterinary Research Institute, Izatnagar for the utilization of unutilized surplus molasses for the feeding of livestock as the main source of energy. During seventies of previous century about one-third of total molasses produced in the country was declared surplus and storage became a serious problem with the sugar factories. At that stage taking clue from the Cuban system of beef fattening, the preparation and feeding of UMLD was standardized and used for the feeding of growing cattle and buffaloes and lactating crossbred cows. Ad libitum feeding of UMLD supplied 50 to 65 % dry matter intake and the rest 35 to 50 % constituted fodders and protein supplements. The other important molasses based product is the urea-molasses-minerals supplement (UMMS).

6. Therapeutic liquid feeds

These include normal saline, glucose saline, calcium-borogluconate, etc.

Handling of liquid feeds

Most of the handling processes for the use of liquid feeds are common and require different size of utensils and pots for preparation, storage, packaging, transportation and feeding. Arrangements for protection from flies, reptiles, rodents and birds commonly present at the place of preparation and feeding is required. This is more important for the molasses based products because these are used for longer duration from the day of preparation. Wire net, wooden plank or covers made of light weight galvanized iron sheets are used.

1. Milk and milk products

Depending on the quantity to be handled earthen pots and metallic cans are used. For longer storage chilling arrangements are done and bulk is transported in refrigerated tankers mounted on trucks and trains. For short duration and short distance indigenous low cost method of wrapping cans with wet gunny bags is quite common.

2. Slurry and gruel

These are prepared daily and used as supplement for the supply of concentrates and increasing the voluntary intake of coarse roughages. Common utensils available in the house are used for the handling of these feeds. This is also used for the handling of milk substitutes.

3. Byproducts of jaggary and khand industry

Large quantity of scum is separated during the processing of sugarcane juice by boiling. The scum contains sugar, minerals and nitrogenous fraction. During the season most of the pig farmers camp with their pigs at a suitable place near the processing plants. The scum is fed ad libitum to pigs alongwith deoiled rice bran or ghuta (rice bran available from small rice milling plants. It contains polish, bran, kanaki and fine hull particles). The pigs are also allowed scavenging for few hours daily. Small quantity od scum and sugar rich can washing is also fed to bovines.

4.Molasses and molasses based liquid feeds

The molasses is sored in kuccha or pucca tanks or overhead tanks depending on the amount produced. Molasses is transported in tankers mounted on truck or train. UMLD is prepared by hot method to destroy the urease activity, if any in the molasses but for feeding in less than a week cold process may be used. UMMS is prepared by hot process and dispensed in polipacks of 500g to 10 kg capacity. Bulk supply is made in molasses tankers, but supply of UMMS in tankers must contain clear written instructions for feeding the UMMS only after thorough mixing for uniform dispersal of minerals in the feed.

5.Therapeutic feeds

These are proprietary products and handled as per the industrial standards.

At the end it would be appropriate to conclude that so far no serious attempt has been made to collect information on the types of liquid feeds used for the feeding of livestock. Similarly no information is available about the handling, storage, transportation and feeding of different types of liquid feeds fed in different regions of the country. Animal Nutrition and feeding literatures of India are dominated by the indigenous practices of northern region and these are highly deficient for the practices of southern and eastern regions including the north-east states. There is need of serious efforts of the collection and compilation of information on the indigenous methods used for the preparation, handling and feeding of different kinds of feeds, and also the purpose and merits associated with the systems.

14
FEED PLANTS AND THEIR MANAGEMENT

Jai Singh

India is the richest in livestock wealth and is the largest milk producing country in the world. But milk produced by individual lactating animal is just at the bottom. The productivity of the animal is a function of both the genetic and phenotypic environment. Under the various phenotypic environmental factors, feeding is of utmost importance as feed account for 60 – 70 % of total cost of livestock production. Feeding animals with optimum quantities of nutrients is instrumental in exploiting their full capabilities. The concept of scientific feeding requires that the animals are fed the right quantity and quality of feed and fodder. But there is acute shortage of feeds and fodders which is the major constraints in livestock productivity. While there is some debate on the exact size of the current deficit, there is shortage of 40.4 % dry fodder, 24.7 % green fodder and 47.1 % concentrate feed.

The compounded feeds are concentrated sources of energy and protein. The main energy sources in it are the cereals and cereal by products. However, to reduce cost and to earn more profit, the incorporation of grains is minimal. The bulk of the feeds have been found containing poor energy sources like deoiled rice polish. The feed ingredients used in compounded feeds are adulterated with cardboard, rice husk, poor quality grains. Such feeds reduce the feed intake and milk yield.

The feed manufacturing strategy should be based on physiological state of the animals and their production potential; livestock rearing system in different techno-socio-economic conditions; availability of raw material and ingredients; frequency and intensity of the natural disasters such as droughts and floods, etc.

The design criterion for a suitable feed plant, selection of feed plant and its capacity, management of the feed plant, conventional and potential feed ingredients, types of feeds, feed standard, status of the present feeds, etc have been appropriately described and discussed in this chapter.

2.0 Present Status in Cattle Feed Production

During the last decade, the production of compounded feed for cattle has increased from 3 million tones to 10 million tones. It is far less than the requirement. The feed is manufactured by the organized sector who are the members of Compound Livestock Feed Manufacturers Association (CLFMA) of India, by the small scale feed producers, by Government Institutional Farms and small private dairy units. The present total production is just sufficient to meet the 25% of the total feed requirement. Apart from feed produced by the industry, the dairy farmers offer to their animals small quantity of grains, oil cake, bran, kitchen wastes and agro industrial byproducts available locally.

The supplementary feed industrial units are also coming up in the country to assist the feed manufacturers. They produce and supply vitamin pre-mix, mineral mixture, protected protein, protected amino acids, protected fat, toxin binders, pellet binders, herbal complex, flavors, etc. The research institutions have developed several feed formulations for better animal performance. Improved feed processing technologies have also been developed to increase quality and quantity of feed at effective costs.

3.0 Bureau of Indian Standards specifications

Many feed manufacturers have registered with Bureau of Indian Standard (BIS) and adopted BIS specifications. There are many lacunas in adopting the BIS specifications such as non availability of quality feed ingredients, lack of experience and technical man power, cost of ingredients , non availability of quality control facilities, etc.

3.1 BIS Specifications for Animal Feed

BIS have laid down specifications and guide lines for the feed manufacturing so that uniform quality standard feed could be manufactured. There are two types of BIS specifications Type – I, IS : 2052, 1979 (Table 1) and Type – II, IS : 2052, 1979 (Table 2). The type –I contain higher protein and fat contents but lower level of fibre. This feed is of concentrate type. It is suitable to cover the requirements of high yielding animals and also during the early lactation period. The specifications Type-II have been proposed by the Compound Livestock Feed Manufacturers (CLFMA) Association of India.

Another Type-III feed is the Specialty Feeds (Table 3) which are nutritionally equal or superior to BIS specifications, particularly high protein concentrate having high quality protein ingredients with high by-pass protein, high energy concentrate with higher level of oil and or with high by-pass fat. Levels of structural and non-structural carbohydrates have also been maintained in such formulations. Some of the manufacturers and members of CLFMA are producing Specialty Feeds.

Recently the protected feed nutrients are taking its entry in to feed formulations. Energy is the first limiting nutrient affecting the productivity of animals. Higher levels of grains in the ruminant diet have been found to reduce fibre digestion. Concurrent to this, the energy utilization from cereal grains is improved when it is digested post-ruminally. Supplementation of ruminally protected methionine and lysine to higher yielders also increase milk production (Sharma, 2004), fibre digestibility as well as acetate level and acetate : propionate ratio improved. Milk production increased on increasing the of un degraded protein (UDP) in ration (Table 5)

Table 1: Bureau of Indian Standard Specifications for Cattle Feeds (Except moisture, all are on dry matter basis)

Ingredients	**Type-I IS: 2052, 1979**	**Type-II IS: 2052, 1979**
Moisture, % maximum	11	11
Crude protein, % minimum	22	20
Crude fibre, % maximum	7	12
Crude fat,% minimum	3	2.5
Acid insoluble ash, %, Maximum	3	4

Table 2. CLFMA Specifications for Cattle Feeds

Ingredients	**Dairy Special**	**Type-I**	**Type-II**	**Type-III**
Moisture, %, Maximum	12	12	12	12
Crude protein, %, minimum	22	20	18	18
Fat, %, minimum	3.0	2.5	2.5	2.0
Crude fibre, %, Maximum	7	7	12	14
sand silica, %, Maximum	3.5	4.0	4.5	5.0

Fat % recommended by BIS = 2.5 to 3.0
Fat % recommended for total mixed ration = 5
Protected or prilled fat % recommended = up to 9

Fat source recommended 1/3rd from natural feed, 1/3rd from oil seed and 1/3rd from by-pass source

Table 3. Ingredients in Kilogram for Concentrate Feed Formulations Adopted by Various Feed Industries

Ingredients	Type-I	Type-II	Type-III	Type-IV
FFS	5	-	-	-
Soymeal	7	8	-	-
Cotton seed cake	4	-	-	-
mustard oil cake	18	14	20	12
Groundnut oil cake	-	12	13	-
Sunflower cake	-	4	5	3
Maize gluten	-	-	-	-
Guar korma	7	-	-	-
Maize	10	8	8	10
Barley	10	8	-	-
Wheat	5	7	6	-
Rice kani	5	7	7	-
Rice polish	-	5	7	16
Deoiled rice bran	20	18	24	18
Phak	-	-	-	28
Urea	1	1	1	1
Mineral mixture	2	2	1	0.5
Common salt	1	1	1	2
Calcite powder	-	-	1	1.5
Molasses	5	5	6	8
CP, %	22	22	22	15
TDN, %	74	74	72	69

Table 4. Rumen Undegadability of Protein in Selected Feeds

Feed/ Feed ingredient	Crude protein, %	Undegra-dability	RDP (g/kg DM)	UPD (g/kg DM)
Babul seed meal	15.9	0.42	92	67
Coconut cake	25.4	0.44	142	112
Formaldehyde treated	-	0.62	97	157
Cotton seed cake	38.2	0.47	202	180
Cotton seed extraction	41.0	0.60	164	246
Gingely oil cake	36.9	0.45	203	166
Formaldehyde treated	-	0.52	206	223
Guar meal	43.4	0.17	360	74
Karanja cake	33.4	0.45	184	150
Mustard seed cake	34.1	0.12	300	41
Formaldehyde treated	-	0.69	106	235
Niger seed cake	32.0	0.39	195	125
Rape seed meal	36.6	0.21	289	77
Formaldehyde treated	-	0.79	77	289
Safflower cake	32.3	0.29	229	94
Soybean meal	50.7	0.46	274	233
Formaldehyde treated	-	0.69	157	350
Heat	-	0.64	183	324
Extrusion	-	0.59	208	299
Sunflower cake	30.1	0.46	163	138
HCH)	-	0.63	111	190
Soybean full fat	38.0	0.26	281	99

Table 5. RDP : UDP Ratio on Milk Production

Parameter	70 : 30	52 : 48	37 : 63
DMI (% live weight)	3.1	3.4	3.7
milk yield (kg/day)	6.3	7.2	10.1
Milk protein (%)	3.4	3.5	3.6

RDP – Rumen degraded protein
UDP – Undegraded protein

4.0 Protected Feed Nutrients

The protected feed nutrients are taking entry into feed formulations, though at slow rate. The energy utilization from cereal grains is improved when it is digested post-ruminally. Several methods have recommended from time to time to bring a shift in the site of digestion of such feeds without altering the rumen function. Some success in this direction have been achieved by treatment of grains with formaldehyde. The formaldehyde forms cross linkages with starch which prevent swelling of starch granules or there may be a formation of protein matrix which become resistant to microbial action. Thus protecting the underlying starch granules. Formaldehyde treatment at 1 per cent level increased fibre digestion in the rumen and also availability of glucose in the intestine which favoured higher production.

5.0 Quality of Commercially Manufactured Feeds

The scientists of Punjab agricultural University collected samples of compounded feeds and feed ingredients from farmers, Govt and semi- Govt organizations and analyzed for quality parameters during 1996-97 to 2003-2004. During the year 1998 and 1999 (Table 6) more than 70 % cattle feed samples failed BIS specifications. The deoiled groundnut cake showed no sign of improvement in spite of quality monitoring but samples of mustard cake, soybean meal and deoiled rice polish were improved as not more than 30 % of these samples failed BIS standard specifications. During 2002 – 2003 (Table 7) some improvement in cattle feed sample was noted with respect to crude protein as only 27 % samples failed BIS specifications. The groundnut cake, however, continued to be of poor quality. The crude fibre content was very high in almost all the ingredients like rice polish, rice bran, wheat bran, mustard cake, etc. The rice polish samples were suspected to have been adulterated with rice husk. The feed samples received from Govt. organizations generally met the CP specifications but the urea content was much above the recommended level (Table 8). The feeds with high urea content can be more harmful to the animals as excessive urea can change the pH of the blood and affect the reproductive performance of the animals. A comparison of the quality of cattle feed received from the industry and Govt. farms is presented in Table 8.

Table 6: Summarized Analytical Data of Feed and Feed Ingredients during 1997-2001

Samples	1997		1998		1999		2000		2001	
	No. received	% failing	No. received	% failing	No. received	% failing	No. received	% failing	No. received	% failing
Cattle feed	35	45.7	42	69	91	73.6	224	25	167	35.3
DGNC	15	66.7	27	88.9	12	58.3	7	71.4	67	76.1
Mustard cake	29	27.6	12	-	12	-	23	-	117	28.2
Soybean meal	2	50	5	-	12	38.5	9	-	44	29.5
DO Rice bran	13	38.5	23	8.7	24	29.2	18	-	108	29.6

Source: S Saizpaul and S.S.Sikka, Department of Animal Nutrition, PAU, Ludhiana, DOS Workshop, NDRI, October-2004

Table 7. Summarized Analytical Data of Feed and Feed Ingredients during 2002-2003

Feed Ingredient	No.	CP% Range	BIS	% failing	CF % Range	BIS	% failing	EE% Range	BIS	% failing
Cattle feed	221	12-32	20-22	27	5-32	7-12	76	1-10	2.5-3.0	9
Maize	9	8-12	9	11	2-5	2.4	25	4-5	4	-
Rice kani	4	8-10	7.9	-	3	1.4	90	2	1.7	-
Barley	5	11-12	12	50	9	6.5	100	1	2.8	100
Bajra	3	12-24	12.5	67	3-4	2.2	100	6	4.9	-
Mustard cake	57	6-42	35-38	9	3-28	8	92	6-15	5.8	-
Soybean meal	14	46-54	42	-	7-12	6	100	1	1	-
Guar meal	7	39-52	40	14	12-23	12	43	4-5	3	-
Groundnut cake	9	33-51	43-48	55	17-29	8-12	100	1-7	6-7	-
Maize guletin	4	55-65	23-45	-	2	3-8	-	5-9	3-4	-
Rice bran	40	7-12	11	43	13-31	11	100	5-24	12	48
Wheat bran	52	8-17	13	42	8-35	12	88	3-7	-	-

Source: S Saizpaul and S.S.Sikka, Department of Animal Nutrition, PAU, Ludhiana, DOS Workshop, NDRI, October-2004

Table 8. Comparative Results of Cattle Feed Collected from Industry and Govt. Farms 9 2003 – 2004)

Parameters	Industry Range	% Feed Type I	% Feed Type II	% Failing Totally	Govt. Farms Range	% Feed Type I	% Feed Type II	% Railing Failing
Moisture, %	5.22-12.19	80	-	20	8.97-12.49	94	-	6
CP	16.3-25.07	30	35	35	17.88-30.18	74	13	13
Ash	8.1-16.2	-	-	-	8.86-17.49	-	-	-
CF	6.5-14.5	5	59	39	7.9-16.68	-	93	7
EE	1.36-10.64	85	-	16	1.67-5.23	53	20	27
AIA	0.6-7.2	50	13	37	2.03-3.36	74	26	-
Urea	0-1.2	-	-	-	0-3.09	20	-	80

5.1 Quality of Commercial Compounded Feeds

The compounded feeds should conform to BIS Type II specifications. The survey conducted by S.N. Rai of NDRI, Karnal, revealed that CP (12-16 %) and fat (0.5 – 1.0 %) contents were invariably lower and CF (20 – 22 %) and sand silica (6 – 8 %) contents were very high. This implies that the energy content of these feeds is quite low which does not seem to be a healthy sign to the growth of feed industry in the country. There is need to establish effective mechanisms for ensuring quality standards and quality assurance.

6.0 Codex on Animal Feed

During 1990's, after the outbreak of food born diseases from Salmonella and E.coli in the United States and subsequently Bovine Spongiform Encephalopathy (BSE) and dioxin crisis in Europe, food safety became a subject of inceased importance internationally. Thus a way to secure food safety was to have surveillance of animal feed stuffs to trace back the feeds that pose a risk to human or animal health or to the environment. As a consequence, in the year 1997, FAO convened the Expert Consultation on Animal Feeding and food safety. The cosultation developed the draft Code of practice for Good Animal Feeding, which was discussed in various meetings and finally, during the 26th Session of the Codex Alimentarius commission, held in Rome in June 2003, the Draft Code of Practice on Good Animal Feeding was developed by the Commission.

Purpose and Scope of the Codex : The objective of this code is to ensure the safety of food for human consumption through the adherence of good animal feeding practice at the farm level and good manufacturing practices (GMP's) during the procurement, handling, storage, processing and distribution of animal feed and feed ingredients for food producing animals. This Code of Practice applies to the production and use of all materials destined to animal feed and feed ingredients at all levels whether produced industrially or on farm.

7.0 TYPES OF MANUFACTURED FEEDS

7.1 Based on Physical Shape

a. Pellets

Pellet is high density cylindrical form of hammer mill processed mixture of concentrate based feed ingredients. Diameter of pellet is varied from 3 mm for prawn, 4 - 6 mm for fish and 6 – 8 millimeter for cattle. Pellet size for sheep and angora rabbits can be decided in consultation with the concerned scientists. Dry mixture of feed module is prepared and hand mixed. Thereafter the mixer is further mixed in a mechanical mixer. The mixer is processed in hammer mill to specific fineness and graded through gyro screen. It is further mixed and cooked in dynamic stage. Molasses and other feed improving ingredients are also added here. Finally, the powder form of feed is steam treated and fed into pellet mill. Here the feed is pressed out through the die with the help of revolving hammer. The feed comes out of the die in the form of smooth cylinder of pre - set diameter and length. In some machines the die revolves while the rollers remain stationery. The true and bulk densities of palletized feed are 900 and 500 kg per cubic meter, respectively. The advantage of pellet form of feed is ease and economy in storage, handling and transportation. Pelleting also reduces dusty condition and selectivity of feeds.

b. Briquetts

Briquett is also high density cylindrical form of the feed module. Diameter of briquetts varies from 22 – 24 mm and length varies from 50 to 75mm. Normally briquetts are produced from herbage based feed module such as chaffed grass mixed with subabool leaves and berseem / lucerene hay. True density and bulk density of briquetts is around 750 and 360 kg per cubic meter.

c. Wafer

Wafer is a thin circular slice of 80 - 100 mm diameter and 15 – 25 mm thickness. It is produced by compressing the chaffed grass/ straw / wheat bhusa with leguminous material in 1: 1 proportion.

d. Complete Ration Block

The complete ration feed block is a mixture of hammer mill processed fodder (wheat straw or any other roughage material) grains and cakes along with minerals and salt, etc. Size of such block is 28 * 25 * 5 inches. The weight of one block is 14 kg which is sufficient for a normal milch animal. Protein content of this feed is kept at 6, 10 and 14 per cent level for different categories of producing animals. This block is wrapped in thin woven plastic cover for marketing. These are produced using hydraulic operated compressing machines.

e. Complete Feed Brick

The complete feed brick is a mixture of fine straw, grains, cakes, mineral mixer, salt, etc. Size of the brick is 200 * 100 * 100 mm. The bricks are wrapped in plastic cover. These are produced using hydraulic operated compressing machines.

f. High Density Feed Bales

High density bales are produced from chaffed dry grasses or chaffed rice straw or stovers or wheat bhusa with or without mixing the cultivated legumes / fodder tree leaves. Ammonia / urea treated straw can also be used. Molasses and salt can also be added to the feed materials while producing high density bales. These bales are tied with single or two wires. The bales are of 300 * 300 mm cross section. The length of the bale is kept according to the weight of the bale which varies from 15 – 25 kg . The density of bale ranges between 350 – 400 Kg per cubic meter. Such bales are cheaper and are recommended for the drought / flood affected areas.

g. Powdery Coarse Grained Feed

This type of feed is prepared by crumbling the feed pellets produced for prawn and fish. Such small granuled feed is consumed in fish hatchery. Fish feed module having protein value of 18 – 35 per cent is used. The grain size varies from 1.5 mm to 3 mm in the same lot.

h. Crumb Feed

Crumb feed is produced by further processing the palletized feed of poultry feed module. Such feed is suitable for the poultry. It contains crumbs of varying sizes from 1.5 – 3 mm.

7.2 Based on Feed Modules / Formulations

a. Commercial Concentrate Feeds

Feed formulations of conventional feeds are given in Table 3 and 4.

b. Non - Commercial Feeds

Module – 1

Non - Cereal Complete Feed

Low cost non-cereal based complete feeds was developed utilizing poultry droppings, urea and molasses with cheaper by products from cereals like 85 % deoiled rice bran, 10 % molasses, 2 % urea, 2 % mineral and 1 % salt.

Module –2

Non - Cereal Complete Feed

Low cost non-cereal based complete feeds were developed utilizing poultry droppings, urea and molasses with cheaper by products from cereals like 85 % deoiled rice bran, 10 % molasses, 2 % urea, 2 % mineral and 1 % salt. Urea can be incorporated at 2, 3 and 4 % along with 10, 15 and 20 % molasses. In these feeds deoiled rice bran, mineral mixture (2 parts) and salt (1 part) can be added. Such non-conventional concentrate feed can produce a body weight gain up to 500g/ day when sorghum silage is offered ad lib (Rai, 2004).

Module – 3

Herbal Fortified Grasses, Crop Residues and Byproducts Based Feed:

Conventional concentrate feeds are costlier source of nutrients especially in rural areas where sufficient fodders are produced. The feeding cost is about 70 % of the total cost of animal production. This can be reduced by 40 % by replacing costly concentrate mixture with highly digestible dried legume forage. A growth rate of 0.5 to 0.6 kg per day is desirable under normal feeding of concentrate mixture along with good quality hay and green fodder. Similar growth rate was obtained when each kg concentrate was replaced by 1.0 to 1.3 kg by dried cowpea, berseem and Lucerne (Rai,, 2004).

Module – 4

The feed explained in formulation 1 above will be fortified with tree leaves, berseem, alfalfa or other leguminous fodder in certain proportion to suit to the condition of the animal.

Module – 5

Herbal Energy and Nutrition Feed

This is a leaf meal prepared using tree leaves such as leucaena, siris, khejri, berseem, alfalfa and other legumes. The leaves are dried, ground and pelletized.

The dry leaf production will be about 12 tonnes per ha. In case of trees 47.6 tonnes wood mass will be additional. This wood mass if converted in to charcoal and briquetted will fetch Rs 1.08 lakh / ha / year. The leaf biomass can be either pelletized (12 – 15 mm diameter and 20 – 25 mm length) or briquetted (20 mm Daimeter, 25 – 35 mm length). Average density of finished product will be 800 – 1000 Kg / cubic meter.

Module –6

Roughage Based Complete Feed Block

These feed blocks are prepared using crop residues, tree leaves, leguminous material, concentrate constituents, urea, molasses, salt, mineral mixer and lime in appropriate proportion for different category and productivity of animal. Such blocks can have brick, rectangular / cubical blocks or briquettes.

Module –7

Straw Based pellets

Wheat straw based pellets containing wheat straw (40 %), deoiled rice bran (36 – 50 %), calcite powder (1.5 %), common salt (1 %), rice polish (5 %), urea (1 %) and molasses (15 %) can be produced. The straw based pellets / briquettes can be used in deficit areas caused by drought or floods.

Module –8

Similarly rice straw based feed comprising rice straw (50 %), deoiled rice bran (32 %), mineral mixture (2 %), urea (1 %) and molasses (!% %) can be produced. This feed will provide 10 % crude protein and 45 – 50 % TDN. Production of this feed can be recommended in rice grown areas

Module –9

Leaf Meal Based Complete Feed Block / Briquette

These feed blocks are prepared using tree leaves, leguminous material, concentrate constituents, urea, molasses, salt, mineral mixer and lime in appropriate proportion for different category and productivity of animal. Such blocks will be in the form of a brick wrapped with thin plastic.

c. Low Cost Concentrate Feed Formulations

Module –10

This was found suitable in Santhal Parganas, hazaribagh, Giridhi, Dhanbad, Ranchi, Darbhanga, Samastipur, Madhubani, Begusarai, Purnea and Kathar.

The feed comprised rice bran 25 %, wheat bran 5 %, maize 18 %, mustard cake 20 %, linseed cake 10 %, gram chuni 20 %, salt 1 %, and lime 1 %.

Module –11

This was found suitable in Assam plains. The feed comprised: Mustard cake 30 %, rice bran 30 %, maize 18 %, Kalai churi 20 %, salt 1 % and lime 1%.

Module –12

Low cost goat feed comprised of dried tree leaves (ber, pipal and siris) 68 %, barley grain 30 %, mineral mixer 1 %, and salt 1 %.

Module –13

The complete feed formation hydraulic press type machine costs about Rs 4.0 lakh. It produces rectangular polythene covered feed blocks of 0.5 cubic feet. The cost of such feed is about Rs350 per 100 Kg. The blocks are made of wheat bran, rice bran, mustard and groundnut cake, urea, molasses, mineral mixer and salt.

Module –14

Using local feeds low cost concentrate mixer was formulated. It was found suitable for sustainable milk production in north Bihar. The feed comprised: Rice bran 15 %, wheat bran 15 %, maize 18 %, mustard cake 15 %, linseed cake 15 %, gram chuni 10 %, masur chuni 10 %, salt 1%, and lime 1 %.

Module –15

Fish Feed

Fish feed is manufactured using fish meal – 20 %, Deoiled cake Soybean – 25 %, rice bran – 20 %, GOC / mustard cake – 20 %, molasses – 8 %, soy oil – 2 % , vitamin mixture and salt, etc. Total protein content of this feed is about 31 %.

8. MAJOR CONSTITUENTS OF THE FEED PLANT

8.1 Machinery

The mechanical constituents of the feed plant include: weighing machine, hand mixing platform, primary dry mixer, grinding mill, gyro shifter, jacketed paddle – mixer – cooker – conveyor, molasses storage and applicator unit, steam generator, steam conditioner, pellet mill, pellet crumbler, pellet sieve, pellet grader, aspirator and dust control system, water softener, electric control panel, safety control switches, main switch gear, bucket elevators, structures and walkways, water and steam supply system, transit holding bins, bag filler and bag closer, wheel barrow and tools, etc.

8.2 Building

Asbestos Cement Corrugated sheet covered shed of 24 m length, 16 m width, partly 5.7 m and partly 10 m height to install and operationalize the feed plant in vertical design for gravity flow of the material from one unit to another unit, side ways stores for the raw and finished product, plant engineer room, record room, visitors room, security and lorry ways, sanitary fittings, etc.

8.3 Water and Power Requirement

The plant needs connected electrical load of 33 KW. The running load will be around 25 KW. Two taps water supply will be needed for the plant and tree taps for other uses.

8.4. Equipment and Machinery for Non Conventional Feed Manufacturing

The following plants and machinery will be required to manufacture herbage based feed pellets, wafers, feed blocks, densified feed blocks and leaf meal processing.

8.4.1: IGFRI Reciprocating ram type forage densifying machine

The machine consists of a frame work, a gear drive, a crank and ram mechanism, a receiving chamber, compression chamber and a split extension chamber. The drive consists of two fly wheels and a pair of cylindrical gear wheels. For densification, the fodder or formulated module of feed is pressed in to the compression chamber. The reciprocating ram / piston cuts the upper edge of the fodder and presses it to the compression chamber. Here the fodder is compressed and pushed in to the split extension compression chamber for controlling density and stabilizing the bale shape. The pressed bale / block is tied wit two / three wires of 14 gauge. This machine reduces the stack volume of grasses, tree leaves and paddy straw from 15.4 cubic meter / tonne to 2.8 cubic meter / tonne and that of manually pressed wheat bhusa and chaffed stovers from 5.9 to 2.6 cubic meter / tonne. Urea, molasses, tree leaves, leguminous fodder, grains, salt, lime, etc can be mixed according to the feed module for different category of animals. The machine produces rectangular bales / blocks of 15 – 25 kg of 350 – 400 kg per cubic meter density. These blocks can be stored safely for a period of 3 years . they are easy and economical in handling and long distance transportation.

8.4.2: IGFRI Feed Pelletizer

The machine mainly consists of an auger, auger housing, main shaft to drive the auger, set of multi – hole pressure plates, feeding hopper and flat belt power transmission system with 7.5 kw 3 – phase electric motor.

A mixture of poultry droppings / cattle dung / other textured cellulosic materials in suitable combination with cake, wheat bran, mineral mixture, molasses, salt, etc or the ingredients specific to the selected feed module. The mixture is fed into the machine through the feeding hopper which is carried in by the revolving augor and pressed against the pressure plate. Finally the material comes out through the holes of the pressure plate in the form of cylindrical pellets. The pellet diameter is adjustable between 6 to 8 mm for goats, sheep, rabbits and 8 to 16 mm for cattle 25 mm and length between 20 – 40 mm.

8.4.3: Feed Pelleting for Cattle

The IGFRI feed pelletizer has been found satisfactory in pelleting wheat bhusa and chaffed grasses mixed with concentrate in 1 : 3 proportion (w / w) and 1 : 1 proportion with subabool leaves or berseem or the selected feed module.

8.4.4: Feed Brquetting

The IGFRI feed pelletizer has been found satisfactory in briquetting wheat bhusa and chaffed grasses mixed with concentrate in 1 : 3 proportion (w / w) and 1 : 1 proportion with subabool leaves or berseem or the selected feed module. The brequetts were 22 – 24 mm in diameter and 20 – 40 mm in length.

8.4.5: IGFRI Feed Wafering Machine

The machine mainly consists of frame, crank and piston mechanism, compression chamber, split extension stabilizing chamber, feed hopper with agitator and V – belt transmission with 14 kw electric motor. The piston covers 80 strokes per minute with a stroke length of 25 cm.

Chaffed grass / straw / wheat bhusa with leguminous material in the proportion of 1 : 1 is fed in to the compression chamber through the hopper and is pressed during the forward stroke of the piston.

8.4.6 Compound Feed Brick Making Machine

It works on the principle of IGFRI forage densifying machine. The difference is that compression takes place by the application of hydraulic force. The mixed ingredients of feed are fed in to the hydraulic cylinder where it is pressed and stabilized in brick shape. The brick is wrapped in plastic cover.

8.4.7 Commercial Complete Feed Block Manufacturing Plant

The concept to prepare complete feed blocks emerged from National dairy Research Institute, Karnal. M/s Anmol Feeds pvt. Ltd., Bulandshahr, M/s Poshak Feeds (India) Pvt. Ltd., Karnal and M/s Godrej Agrovet, Khanna, Punjab have established plants to undertake manufacturing of compound complete feed and total mixed ration.

9.0 Animal Feed Manufacturing Technology Identification

The following points need to be considered

a. With Respect to Interested Group

- People / consumer or business with needs and or wants
- Range of needs / wants
- Plan , develop and produce the item in demand
- Price it, promote it and deliver to consumer / interested group
- Profit level and range

b. With Respect to Market Search

- Search and study the relevant facts
- Domain / target area - local and or export
- Effectiveness of advertising
- Economy of the group

c. With Respect to Product Manufacturing

- Finding quality raw material at good price
- How many products, quantity, quality can be made
- Continuous improvement in quality and quantity
- Packaging, size, quality and face attraction
- Storage of raw material and finished product
- Delivery and transport
- Manufacturing processes
- Plants and machinery
- SWOT analysis
- Cash flow, break even point, return on investment
- Proofing for fluctuating demands

d. With Respect to Feasibility Study

- Choose a product manufacturing or service
- Kinds of product, quantity, quality
- Alternates available in the market
- New or part of the ongoing business
- Plant and machinery and material
- Internal management, finance, personnel, production, selling, marketing and Promotion
- Government policies taxation, subsidy - assistance, license,
- Routines, work process, implementation, operation for the business
- Case - Study on relevant business

10. ANALYSIS OF NEEDS

a. General

- Dairying is an integral part of agriculture in India
- Milk is contributing 9 % to India's GNP
- Feeds and fodders are of crucial importance
- In the post – GATT / WTO scenario, the standard of milk hygiene are going to be enforced most strictly
- Animal feed demand is increasing @ 0.7 % per annum
- Milk and animal products demand is ever increasing
- Per capita / day availability of milk is 178g against the recommendation of 250 g
- Feed cost is 50 – 70 % of the production cost
- Present feed production is just 25 % of the demand
- Physical form and chemical composition of feed varies with species, growth stage and production environment
- Feed manufacturing units set up in foreign collaboration import feed ingredients
- Large capacity units of 5 – 7 t / hr capacity cost Rs 10 – 12 crores and are mostly under utilized

b. Plant and machinery specific

- The plant should be of smaller capacity and cost so that number of plants can be located in different raw material production catchment and governmental policy friendly

- The plant should be able to improve and or modify the manufacturing processes with the scientific developments.
- The plant should be able to utilize different location specific raw materials as per seasonal availability
- The plant should be able to switch over to other product in the event of market fluctuation and government policies.
- The plant should be of indigenous design to lower the cost on commissioning, operation and maintenance
- State the reasons for your choice

c. Feed Specific

- Animals raised on the low quality hay or grazed on poor quality pastures often are energy deficient.
- Protein deficiency in lactating animals may increase the incidence of silent heat and lower conception rate
- The forage to concentrate regulates the metabolic activity of the animal
- When diet excess 60 % grain on DM basis, rumen pH is depressed and metabolic activity shifts from milk production to fattening. The effects of low quality forage can not be overcome by increasing grain feeding.
- Total Mixed Ration (TMR) is getting encouragement as it ensures forage to grain ratio. TMR avoids own unique diet based on preference of ingredients.
- Feed production is increasing @ 1 % per annum.
- The present feed production is just 25 % of the demand. Feed provide densified energy.
- Feed regulates particle length more than 10 – 20 mm can maintain
- There is high promise to utilize local produce and local agro industrial by products.

11.0 MANAGEMENT OF FEED MANUFACTURING PLANT

In this section some ideas about your place in the world of feed manufacturers and identify the mind, money and muscle resources of your business venture have been listed in brief.

10.1 Successful Traits of a Feed Manufacturing Manager

- Problem Solver: He should like the challenge of problem solving.
- High Energy: He should have good health and high energy levels
- A Sense of Urgency: They are restless unless they work

- Self Confidence: They have abilities and believe in their ideas.
- Organization: They organize work in logical system.
- Vision: He keeps track of the whole business and visualize how diverse parts fit.
- Flexibility: They continue to find ways to do the job.
- Persistence: They do not quit when the going gets through.
- Optimism: They are optimists and think that work going to be great.
- Independence: They think they can do the job better than others.
- Emotionally Stable: They are not given emotional highs and lows as moods change.
- Commitment: They ensure the success of their ideas.
- Risk Taking: They like pitting abilities against adversity, not afraid of failure.

10.2 Chances of Survival and Failure

The business survives with good sale, adequate funding, good economic funding, good economic cycle, loss less debts and cometition. On the basis of this analysis he needs to decide as to whether he wants to go for production or service or sales. He has also to decide the type of business he wants to go for , such as – Sole proprietorship, Partnership, Inventer, Duplicator, Developer, Scalper, Company innovator, Corporator, Cooperative.

10.3 Planning for Business

The following considerations are essential for business planning.

- Preparation of business plan to serve as a road map
- Decision for product or service
- Assessment of competitions to be faced
- Assessment of resources - technology, technical personnel and finance.
- Gaining knowledge about regulations
- Delineation of market area
- Location of the unit
- Employment of the personnel
- Unit organization
- Unit financial aspects
- Goal setting – immediate, short term, long term
- Assessment of road blocks or obstacles
- Evaluation of potential conflicts.

10.4 Operational Management of Feed Plant

The following points need to be considered

- Development of market niche – potential customers, their habits, opinions, and preferences.
- How much where and when is the demand
- Research to expand product or service or both.
- Location of the plant – city or town, area within city or town, traffic pattern , building facilities and space , service facilities, local ordinances and regulations.

10.5 Financial Management for a Feed Plant

The following points need to be considered

- Hidden costs
- Starting cost
- Decoration and remodeling
- Starting inventory
- Deposits with public utilities
- Legal and professional fees
- Licenses and permits
- Funds for unexpected expanses
- Estimated monthly expanses
- Fixed and variable cost

10.6 Product Price Management

The following points need to be considered

- Pricing types – Odd ending price, multiple price, wholesale price, competitive price, market price, mark – down or reduction price, discount prices
- Brake – even analysis
- Rate of turn – over
- Installation expanses
- Establishing prices by cost (direct labor, direct material, overhead, profit).
- Price sensitivity – supply, demand, available substitutes, frequencies of purchases, buyer's budget.
- Pricing regulations if any

10.7 Production Schedule Management

The following points need to be considered

- Goal – to turn raw material in to products and cash flow
- Production lay out - organize machinery step – by – step operation to avoid idleness and un necessary movements.
- Factory work load
- Work and time standards
- Variable factors – delayed supply or shipping delay
- Tools for scheduling – check list operation process
- Sequence check list
- Quality of out put
- Effect on profit

10.8 Management of Production Risk

The following points need to be considered

- There is no tried and true path for risk management. One can introduce small risks and watch and gain experience
- Know the reasons of risk – such as poor market evaluation, poor planning, underestimating the cost, failure to specify concrete terms of supply, lack of support , dishonesty in dealing
- Risk management – by risk avoidance, risk reduction, risk retention, risk transfer, setting losses techniques.

10.9 Product Standard Management

To establish the product standard, the following points need to be considered.

- Product Policy Manual – it will state working hours, overtime hours, salary schedule, benefits and customer relations.
- Personnel training program to asquint with recent developments in technology, product and market.
- In house communications should be elaborate, accurate and quick.
- Record keeping must be perfect
- Personnel records
- Delegation of work and responsibilities
- Maintaining control
- Customer management
- Product advertisement

Now you can call yourself a suitable and successful feed and feed plant manager

Bibliography

Singh, Jai. (1988). Hay making and densification. Proc. International Grass land Congress, New Delhi. Pp 393 – 413

Singh, Jai. (2000). Aqua feed pilot plant. Technical Report. Central Institute of Agricultural Engineering, Bhopal

Singh, Jai. (1995). Technical Bulletin. Technology for grass and fodder harvesting and processing. Central Institute of Post Harvest Engineering and Technology, Ludhiana.

Singh Jai. (2004). Livestock feed security systems under natural disastrous conditions. All India DHO Workshop compendium, National dairy Research Institute, Karnal.

Rai, S. N. (2004). Feeding strategies for sustainable livestock production. All India DHO Workshop compendium, National dairy Research Institute, Karnal.

Sharma, D.D. (2004). Deviation of feed industry towards quality feed production. All India DHO Workshop compendium, National dairy Research Institute, Karnal.

Saijpaul, S. and Sikka, S. S. (2004) Quality of dairy feeds available in Punjab. All India DHO Workshop compendium, National dairy Research Institute, Karnal.

15
AGRO-INDUSTRIAL BY PRODUCTS

S.K.Tomar and S.K.Sirohi

Millions of small holders in India are rearing animals under diverse and risk prone environments. A wide range of feeding systems have evolved, each adapted to local ecological conditions and intimately linked with the local culture. These traditional animal farming systems are not static, they have changed over the generations particularly over the last few decades in response to economic pressure. In South Asian countries more and more grains are utilized by human and most of the cultivated land is used for grain production resulting in acute shortage of both roughages and concentrates. The gap between availability and demands of feeds is very wide, there is a deficit of about 48% for concentrate, 31% for green fodder and 17% for dry fodder (*Aneja et al.* 2002).To mitigate this shortage a large number of agro-industrial byproducts have been tested for their nutritional value. Some of these byproducts were found to be very promising. But majority of these agro-industrial byproducts adversly affected the performance of animals when fed as such, particularly at higher levels of inclusion for longer periods. These adverse effects were due to one or the other indiscriminating or toxic factor (s) present in them. The present paper deals in brief the availability, toxic factor(s) present and safe level of inclusion of the important agro-industrial byproducts available in India in complete feeds.

Agro-industrial byproducts as feeds

Before considering the different groups of byproducts it is necessary to examine the contrasting types from the feed value point of view. This is particularly important in relation to least cost ration formulation when different ingredients are evaluated as source of energy, protein, minerals, vitamins in relation to their cost and then included in complete feed subject to constraints in relation to specific nutrients or anti-nutrient properties.

Ørskov (1980) proposed that byproducts should be considered in four main categories viz. a.) byproducts low in digestible and low N content, b.) by products low in digestibility and high N content, c.) byproducts high in energy and low in N content in relation to their contents of metabolizable energy and nitrogen. This is particularly relevant in relation to ruminants, where there is a degree of interdependence between these two major nutrients. The microbial population of the rumen thus has a requirement for nitrogen, which varies according to the proportion of the organic matter digested in the rumen.

Byproducts of low digestibility and low content of nitrogen (A)

By products of this category include straws, husks, pods and haulms. Very often the nitrogen content in these by-products is so low that supplementary degradable nitrogen (e.g urea) is required to speed up both rate and extent of digestion in the rumen. If given as a high proportion of diet, these byproducts have slow rates of digestion and long retention times in the rumen consequently levels of voluntary intake are low.

Rice hulls : Rice hulls or husk is the largest byproducts of rice milling industry and most of it is either burnt or used as bedding for poultry and animals. It contains 3.2% CP, 1.4% EE, 32.7% CF, 38.7% NFE, 23.6% ash, 16.0% silica, 69.4% NDF and 38.0% ADF (Ranjhan,1990). Ground rice husk is often mixed to adulterate the rice polishing /bran (Singh and Kundu,2003). Husk when substituted at 0, 33, 66 and 100 percent of rice straw in growing crossbred calves ration, the growth rate was depressed with the increase of rice hulls, however at 33% level the depression was not significant as compared to that in the control. The DCP and TDN of rice hulls were 0.16 and 11.7 per cent, respectively.

Maize husk : It is superior to even gram husk in its nutritive value. It has about 8% CP. Fifty per cent of the dry roughage portion in complete feed of adult non-producing cattle and buffaloes can be replaced by this byproduct.

Sugarcane bagasse: Bagasse is one of the most important byproduct of sugar industry. It is a source of cellulose but poor in protein and high in lignin. Cattle and buffaloes can consume about 80% of their expected dry matter intake through bagasse impregnated with 1 - 2 per cent urea. About 60 kg compelete feed consisting of 20 kg bagasse, 6 kg molasses, 0.34 kg comman salt, o.34 kg mineral mixture and 65 litres of water forms a maintenance ration along with 800 g of groundnut cake for adult animals weighing 400 kg. Sengar et al. (1993) reported that sodium chloraite treatment of bagasse had decreased the lignin content and increased in situ dry matter digestibility.

Babul pods : Babul (Acacia spp.) pods contain aout 13% CP and 50% TDN (Punj,1988). The use of babul pods as animal feed is limited due to its high tannin content (Barman and Rai, 2003b). The main degraded product of Acacia nilotica tannin in ruminants are phloroglucinol and resorcinol. The concentrations of these products decreased noticeably from 18 to 42 h in buffalo rumen and 4 and 6% tannin levels (Siddhuraju et al. 1996).

Cocoa pod husk : The dried cocoa (Theobroma cacao) pods are brittle and the husk contain 6% CP, 31% CF, 3 % EE, 12% ash. It can be used upto 10-15% in the complete feed of ruminants.

Cotton straw : Cotton straw in ground form could be used as roughage source upto 30% in complete diets for lactating cattle and buffaloes. The palatability and nutrients utilization of cotton straw was improved by expandor method without enhancing the cost of feed on production basis (Nagalakshmi et al., 2004).

Cassava (Tapoica) waste: Cassava (Manihot esculenta) feeds and roots are poor in CP (2%) but rich in NFE (85%) where as tapoica starch waste has 2% DCP and 64% TDN. It has been recommended that tapoica waste can be safely included in the complete feed with a considerable economy for maintaining body weight, milk yield and butter fat production in cattle and buffaloes.

Byproducts of low digestibility but relatively high in nitrogen (B)

By products of the food industry, such as coffee residues, fruit pulp and cocoa meal are of low energy value, but are relatively high in nitrogen. In addition, animal excreta tend to have an excess of nitrogen in relation to available energy.

Coffee waste : Coffee (Coffea arabica and C. robusta) is cultivated commercially in coastal regions of India and is availiable about 70,000 tonnes which yield about 45,000 tonnes of coffee husk. It has about 9% CP, 40% CF, 10% EE and 5% ash. It has 3.4% DCP and 42.2% TDN and can be incorporated in the compelete diet of large ruminants (Ranjhan,1990)

Leguminous pulse straws: The residues of pulses are composed of husk of pod with leaves and tender stems which are more nutritious than the cereal straws and stovers. They contain 8.0-12.5% CP and 40-50% NFE. The voluntary intake varies from1.8-2.5 per cent of body weight in cattle and buffaloes. Groundnut straw along with wheat straw (35%) and wheat bran (1.0 kg) can meet the nutritional requirement of a buffalo weighing 450 kg producing 5 kg milk.

Pineapple waste : Pineapple (Ananas camosus) caunery waste consists of outer peels (shells), the crown and bud ends of fruit, fruit trimmings, the inner core and the pomace of the fruit from which the juice has been extracted. The pineapple waste contains 80-90% moisture and 5% CP. Two per cent of dry matter through this waste can be consumed in complete feeds by cattle and buffaloes.

Jackfruit waste : It contains 13.3% CP, 5.09 % EE, 12.4% CF, 0.21 % Ca and 0.35% P. It can be incorporated in ruminants compelete diet upto 10-15%. Banana peels, orange peels, mango peels, lemon peels have about

6-13% CP and 55-74% NFE and can be included in the compelete feed of cattle and buffaloes. Cauliflower leaves, papaya leaves, cabbage leaves and pea pods have 12-27% CP, 38-55% NFE, 1.0 - 4.5% Ca, 0.05-0.60% P and can be included in the complete diets of ruminants.

Citrus waste : In complete feeds citrus waste can be fed to large ruminants upto 40 kg/head/day without any harmful effects (Umoh,1982). After processing oranges, lemons or grapes for juice, the left over which comprises the pod seeds and rag etc. amounts to 40-60% by weight of the fruit could be very palatable to cattle and buffaloes. Citrus pulp contains a relatively high amount of pectin and soluble carbohydrates and for this reason dried citrus pulp has been used to replace cereals in ruminants diet (Bhattacharya and Harb,1973).

Sea-weed : Historical records show that the use of sea weeds in agriculture is very old and some species are used as feed and fodder for pig, horse, chicken, cattle and buffaloes. Vitamin content is higher as compared o wheat and milk. There is possibility of using these seaweeds either after drying or preserved with chemicals before using as ruminant feed. Agar agar is being extracted from Sargussam seaweed and its byproducts can be used in complete feeds for livestock feeding. This byproduct contain about 10% CP and 67% organic matter (Tomar,2004).

Byproducts of high energy value but low in nitrogen (C)

The byproducts of the sugar industry (molasses, sugar beet pulp), the byproducts of fruit horticultural industry and products such as stock feed potatoes are come in this category. Because of the rapid rate of their digestion, there is usually a substantial requirement for supplementary sources of readily available nitrogen to be given to balance the excess of energy. With monogastric animals this may take the form of skim milk, blood meal, fish meal, soy bean meal or dried yeast. In ruminants where the need in for a highly degradable source of nitrogen in the rumen, heat-treated proteins are unsuitable.

Fats and oils are the best examples of byproducts in this category. Animal fat can be included in the diet of pigs and poultry but at levels, which are usually less than 5% of complete diet (Cooke and Pugh, 1980). At higher levels of use, there may be problems of physical structure and adverse effects on carcass composition. In the case of pigs, the use of vegetable oils containing linoleic acid may lead to soft fat, particularly if the linoleic acid content of the diet exceeds 16 g per kg (Wood et al., 1984). With ruminants, there may be problems of maintaining cell wall digestion in the rumen if the proportion of fat in complete diet exceeds 5%.

Sugarcane molasses : Molasses is about 3% of the sugarcane or about 1/3rd of the quantity of sugar produced. It contains about 61% sugar and 3% protein and has been used in complete feeds of ruminants at 5-10% levels. Molasses is mainly used as (a) carrier for urea impregnation of poor quality roughages (b) as binder for commercial pelleted feeds and (c) as sweetener for increasing the voluntary intake of unpalatable feeds.

Mango seed kernels : The annual availability of mango seed kernels is about 5,00,000 tonnes (SEA, 2000). It has a high content of starch i.e.92% of its total carbohydrate content. It contains about 68-70% natural lipids of the total lipids (Dhingra and Kapoor, 1985). Stearic and oleic acids are the main components and saturated and unsaturated fatty acids which were 40 and 60%, respectively. Histidine and cystine were in greater amount as compared to other amino acids in the mango seed kernel (Barman and Rai, 2003a). Growth rate was found to be 440 g/d/ animal when used 20% mango seed kernel in the concentrate mixture of calves.

Potato waste : Potato waste is the byproducts remaining after extraction of starch with cold water. 16-20% of starch is produced and 3-3.5% dried potato waste is obtained for feeding in complete diets to cattle and buffaloes ((Boucque and Fiems, 1988).

Tomato pomace : Dried and ground pomace contained 22.36% CP and 28.11 % CF with a nutritive value of 13.7-15.8% DCP and 60.8-73.3% TDN. Tomato waste can be incorporated upto 35-40% of the concentrate mixture in the compelet diet of cattle and buffaloes.

Byproducts of category (B) are therefore well suited to being used in mixture with those of category (C). They are also suitable for use with other feeds of high energy content but which are low in N, such as cereal grains.

Byproducts high in energy and nitrogen (D)

Byproducts in this category include products such as blood meal and poultry offal meal, fish meal, extracted oil seed meals/cakes and waste vegetables such as carrots. Care is needed to ensure that potentially toxic compounds are recognised and that the inclusion of the byproduct in the complete diet will not adversely affect flavour and acceptability. Thus it is not recommended to use blood meal in calf complete diets (Cooke and Pugh,1980). There is also a need to ensure that the byproducts do not deteriorate during storage. Those based on leaves,(e.g cauliflowers, cabbages, pea pods) may have a short shelf life and in consequence are better suited for use near the place of their production.

Blood meal : Blood meal is a major slaughter house byproduct but much of it is wasted. It is usually made by coagulating the blood by steaming or by boiling, then drying and milling. Blood can also be soaked on wheat bran/rice bran and then dried .This can be an ingredient in the poultry complete feeds. Blood meal contains over 80% protein but poor is in Ca and P. As such it is unpalatable to animals. However, supplementation of basal cereal free complete diet with 3,6, and 9 per cent of blood meal gave performance similar as the control ration containing 10% fish meal.

Poultry offal meal : Offal meal, a byproduct of poultry dressing plant is available for use as a meal. It consists of head, feet, lungs, wind pipe, oil glands and intestines. After processing it in a valuable protein source which contains about 58% protein and 2910 kcal ME/kg. Offal meal is poor in methionine and lysine. Its inclusion in poultry complete feed beyond 2.5% lowers the overall performance of birds.

Fish meal : Fish meal is the most valuable by product and has been accepted as balanced source of protein for poultry, swine, newborn growing calves, lambs and kids.

Frog meal : Frog meal is a left over of the frog leg industry. About 1000 tonnes of this byproduct is available annually alone in Kerala. It contains about 60% protein and can replace fish meal twice by weight in the poultry complete diets both for growth and egg production.

Oil seed meals/cakes : Groundnut, soybean, mustard, lineseed, til, cotton seed and coconut cakes /meals are conventional protein supplements and costly items for animal production. All these cakes had 30-45% CP and high energy value. In addition to annually cultivated crops, there are many oil bearing perenial trees, for example sal, rubber, neem., mahua, castor, kosun, niger, karanj etc. All these fall into the category of unconventional oil seed cakes /meals. In India, the potential of unconventional oilseeds available from these trees is estimated to be 6.7 million tonnes to yield about 1.0 million tonnes of oil and remaining available as cakes (Ranjhan,1990). However, due to lack of facilities and awareness only about 3.5% of total potential is collected and utilized.

Waste vegetables : Vegetable wastes like carrots,cabbage, cauliflower, lady's finger, empty pea pods can be included in the compelete diets of cattle and buffaloes (Rai and Barman, 2004).

Matching byproducts to system of animal production

It is important to assess the feed value of byproducts in relation to the type of animal and the system of production in which the material is to be used. Thus low quality byproducts in categories A and B are best suited to use with animals which have relatively low nutrients requirements such as dry dairy cows, and goats. Such feeds may aso be used tactically at times of feed shortage to reduce the cost of the diet. By products in categories C and D are most appropriately used in more intensive systems such as pig and poultry production. They also have wide application in ruminant livestock operations. Thus oilseed cakes and animal byproducts are regularly part of compounded feeds for high yielding dairy cows. The fact that many are heat treated means that the protein is less readily degraded in the rumen and more likely to enhance the total supply of amino acids to the animal.

There are clear limitations to the extent to which certain byproducts may be recycled directly into the complete feeds of livestock. Apart from a low feed value, there may also be logistical problems of matching their availability to the supply of animals for their consumption. This problem may be exacerbated by a short life of the byproduct and restrictions on use imposed by compositional factors such as toxins or physical factors which might be associated with rapid deterioration. Strategic supplementation is justified because of regular feed shortages that occur and the fact that ruminants subsist for most of their life on agro-industrial byproducts on small farms. Added costs of detoxification and supplements often discourage byproducts use. There is a need for future systematic research on the optimization of the use of agro-industrial byproducts in complete feeds and develop strategies for their optimum supplementation in different animal species.

Table : Important agro-industrial byproducts, their recommended levels of inclusion in complete feeds and antinutritional factors.

S.No.	Particulars	Recommended level of inclusion in complete feed			Antinutritional factor (s)
		Calves	Milch cattle/ buffalo	Poultry	
1.	Rice bran		30 %	20 %	
2.	Wheat bran	15 %	30 %	15 %	
3.	Deoiled Groundnut cake	10 %	15 %		Aflatoxin
4.	Deoiled Mustard cake		20 %		Sinalbin
5.	Linseed cake	10 %	20 %		Linamarin & NCN
6.	Cotton seed cake		20 %		Gossypol
7.	Mahua seed cake	15 %	25 %		Mowrin
8.	Rubber seed cake	20 %			HCN
9.	Kosum cake	35 %		17 %	Cyanogens
10.	Babool seeds	30 %	15 %		Tannins
11.	Water hyacinth		15 %		
12.	Acacia seed chuni	30 %	45 % (bullock)		Tannins
13.	Mango seed kernel		10 %		
14.	Tea spent waste	20 %		10 % (broilers)	Tannins
15.	Panewar seed (Cassia tora)		15 %		Crysophonic acid
16.	Safflower cake		10-15 %		
17.	Niger seed cake		20-25 %		
18.	Karanj cake	10 %	15 %		
19.	Guar meal	5 %	10 %		Gum, Trypsin
20.	Bone meal	2.5 %	5 %	2.5 %	
21.	Blood meal		2 %	2 %	
22.	Poultry offal meal	1.0 %	2.5 %	2.5 %	

Bibliography

Aneja, R.P., Mathur, B.N., Chandan, R.C. and Banerjee, A.K. 2002. Technology of Indian Milk Products. A Dairy India Publ., Delhi, India, pp- 34.

Barman, K. and Rai, S.N. 2003a. Potential of mango seed kernel (Mangifera indica) as an animal feed. Indian Dairyman, 55 (8) : 59-62.

Barman, K. and Rai, S.N. 2003b. Utilization of tenniferous feed in animal ration : Chemical composition, amino acid profile and tannin fractionation of certain Indian agro-industrial byproducts. Anim. Feed Sci. Technol. (Accepted)

Bhattacharya, A.N. and Harb, M. 1973. Dried citrus pulp as a grain replacement for Awassi lambs. J. Anim. Sci. 36 : 1175-1180.

Boucque, C.H.V. and Fiems, L.O. 1988. Vegetable byproducts of agro-industrial origin. Livestock product Sci. 19 : 97-135.

Cooke, B.C. and Pugh, M.L. 1980. Slaughter waste in animal feeding. In : E.R. Ørskov (Editor), By-products and Wastes in Animal Feeding. Occasional Publication No. 3, BSAP, pp. 79-83.

Dhingra, S. and Kapoor, A.C. 1985. Nutritive value of mango seed kernel. J. Sci. Food Agric. 36 : 752-756.

Nagalakshmi, D., Reddy, D.N. and Kumar, M.K. 2004. Performance of Murrah buffaloes fed expander pelleted cotton straw based diets. Anim. Nutr. Feed Sci. 4 : 23-32.

Ørskov, E.R. 1980. Nutritional principles in utilization of wastes and by-products. In : E.R. Ørskov (Editor), By-products and Wastes in Animal Feeding. Occasional Publication No. 3, BSAP, pp. 13-17.

Punj, M.L. 1988. Availability and utilization of non-conventional feed resources and their utilization by in South Asia. In : Non-conventional Feed Resources and Fibrous Agricultural Residues, Strategies for Expanded utilization, Hisar, India, March 21-29, 1988, pp. 50-81.

Rai, S.N. and Barman, K. 2004. New animal feed resources : problems and potential. Proc. XI Animal Nutrition Conference on Nutritional Technologies for Commercialization of Animal Production System, held at J.N.K.V.V. Jabalpur (M.P.) from January, 5 – 7, 2004.

Ranjhan, S.K. 1990. Agro-industrial Byproducts and Nonconventional Feeds for Livestock Feeding. ICAR, New Delhi, pp. 7-91.

SEA (Solvent Extraction Association of India) 2000. Millennium Hand Book on Indian Vegetable Oil Industry and Trade (7th ed.) SEA Publication.

Sengar, S.S., Tomar, S.K., Lall, D. and Mehra, U.R. 1993. Effect of sodium chlorite treatment of straws on their cell wall constituents and in situ dry matter disappearance. Indian J. Dairy Sci. 46 ; 130-132.

Sidduraju, P., Vijaykumari, K. and Janardan, K. 1996. Chemical composition and nutrition evaluation of an under exploited legume, Acacia nitolica (L), Food Chem. 57 : 385-391.

Singh, R. and Kundu, S.S. 2003. Quality evaluation of some animal feedstuffs available in Haryana. Anim. Nutr. Feed Technol., 3 : 143-150.

Tomar, S.K. 2004. Unconventional feed resources for buffaloes in various agro-climatic regions. In : Kundu, S.S., Mishra, A.K. and Pathak, P.S. (Editors), Buffalo Production Under Different Climatic Regions. International Book Distributing Co., Charbagh, Lucknow, India, pp. 299-320.

Umoh, J.E. 1982. The use of concentrate and byproducts in beef cattle production : Emphasis on use of concentrate on pasture. Proc. National Conf. on Beef Production, July 27-30, Kaduna.

Wood, J.D., Brown, A.J., Enser, M. and Jones, R.C.D. 1984. Tissue quality in lean pigs. In : A. Cuthbertson and R. E. Gunn (Editors), Matching Production to the Markets for Meat. Occasional Symposium, BSAP, pp. 97.

16
HERBAL FEED ADDITIVES

K.K. Singhal and S.S. Thakur

The cow has been held in high esteem since ancient in India and played a prominent role in ancient economy. The inscriptions and stone edicts of king Ashoka (270-329 BC) reveal that there were hospitals for both men and animals and there were books exclusively devoted to treatment of animal diseases. Susruta Chakradata (200-500 AD) and similar treatises deal with metabolism, circulation, total development and heredity, which is very close to modern day science of nutrients (panch tatva) and their metabolism. With this background knowledge of nutrients, some herbs or their mixtures are used traditionally in India to promote feed intake and to cure ailments in human beings as well as in animals. India is rich in such herbs and the knowledge to utilize them for the welfare of mankind. Some regional variations have been recorded for the preference of herbs in human food. Such herbs are having some flavoring and medicinal agents, which stimulate the digestive system and the performance of human as well as livestock including poultry. Herbs, which include the whole plant or its specific part including roots, contain numerous active principles and that have not been identified and characterized clearly so far. These active principles are dependent on the parts of plant, region of its availability, maturity stage etc. Many a times effectiveness of a herb depends on the cocktail of herbs used simultaneously. Chemistry of herbs, particularly from their beneficial angle, is still not fully investigated scientifically, in spite of the fact that vast literature is available in Ayurveda. Invariably following chemicals are responsible for their beneficial/ pharmological effects.

1. Alkaloids
2. Saponins
3. Tannins
4. Glycosides
5. Essential fatty acids
6. Proteins and/ or amino acids

Generally, it is observed that use of herbs for a short period is sufficient for toning the body due to their medicinal values but their essential oil content and other unidentified chemicals also play a role in enhancing the animal performance. Besides, these are less expensive and safe than the chemical additives as side effects are rarely observed. Usually, mixture of several herbs is used rather than a single one to obtain the desired effect.

Alkaloids: Many plants such as comofrey (Symphytum officinate), borage (Borago officinalis), crotalaria (Crotalaria sagittalis), senecio (Senecio jacobea), rall fescue (Festuca arundinacea), datura (Datura stramonium), lupines (Lupinus spp.) etc contains various types of alkaloids depending upon their chemical structure. Alkaloids are generally known for their toxic effects in humans and in livestock.. Toxic effects of plant alkaloids are due to their bioactivation in the liver to toxic metabolites called pyrroles. .Type and extent of toxicity varies with the species of livestock. Sheep are more resistant than cattle and goats to the alkaloids. It was demonstrated that plant alkaloids are transferred from feed to milk, however, in a study it was reported that milk of lactating goats fed on S. jacobaea was offered to the rats for a prolonged period without significant affect on liver pathology (Goeger et al., 1982). However, small amounts of the herbs containing alkaloid are being used as medicine for humans and animals.

Saponins: Saponins are steroids or triterpenoid glycosides, commonly present in a large number of plants and plant products, which are used as herbs or for their health promoting properties (Fenwick et al., 1991). These components are present in soybeans, alliums, tea, spinach, sugar beet, quinoa, sunflower, ginseng, peppers, asparagus, yam, fenugreek, yucca, Sesbania sesban leaves, etc. A number of factors such as physiological age, environmental and agronomic factors have been shown to affect the saponin content of plants. Shikakai and Reetha are some important saponin rich herbal products, which are used for the washing of hairs and woolen clothes in India. Immature plants have higher saponin contents than more mature plants of some species. Yucca schidigera is the most common commercial source of steroid saponins.

Extensive research has been carried out into the membrane permeabilisting, immunostimulant, hypochloestrolaemic and anti-carcinogenic properties of saponins and they have been reported to have profound affect on growth, feed intake (Mader and Brumm, 1987) and reproduction in animals (Francis et al., 2002). Makkar and Becker (1996) reported that Quillaja saponins increased the efficacy of in vitro rumen microbial protein synthesis and decreased degradability of feed protein. Recently, it has been reported that dietary supplementation of saponins reduced the methane emission from ruminants and thus reduces the loss of dietary energy and keep the environment free from pollution from methane, which is considered a major green house gas that destroys the protective ozone layer. These structurally diverse compounds have also been observed to kill protozoans (Lu and Jorgensen, 1987) and molluses, to be anti-oxidants, to impair the digestion of protein and the uptake of vitamins and minerals to the gut, to cause hyperglycaemia and to act as antifungal and antiviral agents. Yucca extract, a rich source of saponins, has been reported to improve the ammonia – N utilization by binding with saponins when ammonia is in excessive quantity and release it later when ammonia concentration goes down (Hussain and Cheeke, 1985), which may prove a great advantage while feeding urea supplemented diets (Makkar et al., 1999). Excessive intake of saponins may be detrimental for livestock. These compounds can thus affect animals in different ways.

The positive effects of saponins were more pronounced when they were directly administered into the rumen rather than added to the feed (Odenyo et al., 1997) due to their surfactant action on the feed constituents that alters the rate of digestion (Killeen et al., 1998). Dietary saponins were often suspected of having a role in causing ruminant bloat, but evidence of this kind are lacking in the literature. Saponins such as those present in mahuwa (Bassia latifolia) oil cake are toxic to fish because of their damaging effect on the respiratory epithelia (Roy et al., 1990). Y. schidigera has been found to improve growth, feed efficiency and health in poultry and pigs, however, the mechanism of the action is not clear so far (Anthony et al., 1994).

Some of physical and chemical properties of saponins (e.g. surface active properties, methane reduction and N binding capacity) have sparked research into their use in livestock production applications. Decreased ruminal ammonia concentration (Hussain and Cheeke, 1995), increased propionate (Valdez et al., 1986) and improved animal performance (Ki. et al.,1994) has been reported with Yucca saponins.

Tannins: Plant tannins are phenolic compounds that are water soluble compounds containing one or more phenol groups. Many herbal feed ingredients such as sal seed (Shorea robusta), mango seed (Mangifera indica), tamrind seed, babool pods (A. nilotica), tree leaves namely robina, papal, oak etc. and forages viz sorghum are rich source of tannins. Barman and Rai (2004 a) reported that Babool pods contain highest level of total tannins (18.71±0.68 %) followed by mango seed kernel (8.39±0.59%) and sal seed meal (7.98±0.45%). The compounds having more phenolic hydroxyls are called polyphenolics and tannins are such compounds, which have the property to bind with proteins such as salivary proteins, dietary proteins, intestinal mucosa. Due to this property, tannins are generally considered anti-nutritional factor as they affect nutrient absorption.

Barman and Rai (2004b) reported that on increasing dietary level of tannins (from A. nilitica) in cattle, buffaloes and goats, CP digestibility the decreased significantly in all species and decrease was in the order of goat > cattle > buffalo, which showed that tannins at low level are beneficial for aiding the digestion. It is also evident from ancient Indian tradition of offering the guests with tannin rich herbs such as betel leaf (pan) with a layer of catechu and lime along with araci nut (supari) after the meal, which give an astringent taste as tannins interact with salivary protein and glycoprotein in the mouth. It seems that the metabolites of the tannins are having some benefical effects. Phloroglucinol, gallic acid, resorcinol and (+) catechin are the metabolites in all species, however, phloroglucinol and resorcinol were the major and gallate and catechin were minor end products of tannin degradation in in cattle and buffalo rumen fluid. Work conducted at NDRI, Karnal indicated that metabolites of tannins (phloroglucinol, gallic acid, + catechin and epicatechin with one other unidentified compound) get secreted in to the milk following the feeding of tanniferous plant material. Besides these metabolites, resorcinol was detected in urine of cows fed on babool pods containing diet (Barman and Rai, unpublished report). There are reports to indicate that cow's milk and urine possess medicinal value for human beings. It appears that cows grazing on different herbs secrete the metabolites in to their milk and urine, which are responsible for their therapeutic value, if any.

Although tannins are generally regarded as anti-nutritional, certain type/ kind of tannins at low concentration are known to alter rumen fermentation of carbohydrates and proteins (Barry and Duncan,1984) and microbial protein synthesis (Makkar et al., 1995) Since tannins are widely distributed in tropical feedstuffs, identification of tanniferrous feedstuffs having beneficial effects on ruminant digestion would help to exploit the use of such feedstuffs to improve the efficiency of ruminant digestion. It has been reported that Tamarind seed husk, an tannin rich feedstuff, incorporation at 7.5% level in the concentrate mixture alters the rumen fermentation beneficially resulting in improved performance (Bhatta et al., 2000).

Herbal liver stimulants have been extensively used in farm animals including poultry. Such stimulants improve the metabolism of nutrients to increase the body cell mass in pre-ruminant and ruminant stage of farm animals without additional requirement of nutrients (Arora and Madhu Mohini, 1984). Mahanta et al. (1983) showed the efficacy of such stimulants in recovery of damaged liver due to the consumption of dietary antinutritive factors in buffaloes. Herbal medicines were reported to decrease the aflatoxin toxicity in farm animals.

Glucosinolates: Gucosinolates are thioglucosides present in the plants of Brassica spp. such as mustard/ rapeseed, raddish, kale etc. These are present in stem, leaves and seeds of these plants. These are water soluble compounds. As such these are harmless compounds, but due the action of endogenous enzyme known as myrosinase, these are metabolized into thiocyanate, isothiocyante, nitriles, which may cause the pungency as well as goiter in human and livestock. Though these compounds are not being consumed in large quantities except that in ruminants, which consume mustard cake as a sole protein supplement. Goiter has not been recorded in livestock even after prolonged feeding of mustard cake in crossbred calves. Recently, metabolites of glucosinolates have been reported to be anti-carcinogenic and anti-fungal. It is evident from our traditional practice that massage of mustard oil is recommended for human beings as isothiocyantes are reported to be antifungal in nature. Metabolites especially thiocyanates get secreted in milk following the feeding of glucosinolate containing diets, which may stimulate milk preservation through lactose peroxidase (LP) system..

Galactogogue: Certain herbs like Smrita, Kambojinin and Jivanti (Leptadenia reticulate Wight and Avn) contain galactogogue ,which improve milk production if given in a suitable mixture for few days to lactating animals. Medicinally, these are restorative and are known as early as from the time of 'Atharveda Cherak Sanhita' for their lactogenic property termed 'stanya garbphprada' and thus have been shown to increase milk yield without affecting milk composition. These are claimed to be effective therapeutic agents for treating cases of hypogalactia. A commercial preparation containing these herbs improved the milk yield during the whole lactation of crossbred cattle following the supplementation of their diets with this mixture (50g/day) for 30 days (Arora et al., 1983) which was attributed to the efficient utilization of absorbed nutrients (Table 1). Buffaloes showing agalactis also responded positively (Kulkarni, 1976) and improved milk production (Gahlot 1982) following the supplewmentation of this feed additive for few days. Fenugreek (Trigonella foenum) seeds, known as methi seeds are aromatic, carminative tonic and galactogogue.

Table 1: Average milk yield of cows fed on galactogouge preparation

Attributes	Control	Experimental
Body weight (kg)	313.7	308.7
Lactation yield (kg)	3480.6	3689.7
Milk yield/day (kg)	12.89	13.66
Fat %	4.4	4.4
DM intake/kg milk (kg)	0.92	0.93

Flavoring agents: Some herbs like Jeera, dhania, ajwain, ginger, pepper have essential oils which can be used as flavoring agents in broiler diets to promote feed intake and feed efficacy (Gunther, 1991). Besides providing the flavour to mask the unpalatable feed ingredients they act as emollient for inflammation of the intestinal tract. Therefore, these seeds form the constituent of conditioning powder for cattle, horses and sheep and also used to render musky hay and compressed fodder palatable (Anon,1976). Garlic (Allium sativum) contains strong smelling agent known as allcin which has anti-parasitic, antifungal and anti bacterial properties. Though garlic is known to improve feed efficiency in broilers but it imparts off flavour to milk when supplemented in the diet of lactating animals.

In a recent review, Wenk (2002) concluded that herbs can replace antibiotics for raising young animals. Herbs contain many antioxidants having a high potential for the protection of nutrients against oxidation in the digestive tract, in metabolism as well as in the products.

Thirteen plant extracts, selected for their high falvonioid content, were screened by Broudisco et al. (2000) for their action on fermentation and protozoal numbers in 1 lit dual out flow fermenters supplied with 50:50 orchard grass hay + barley diet and reported enhanced acetate, butyrate and propionate, increased gas production and decreased methanogens etc. with some plant extracts selected for their high falvonoid content. Based on these results few extracts have been elected for further study.

Orgegano, which is use to treat gastro-intestinal disorders and retarding food spoilages, is another feed additive of interest. Oil of Oregano has two very active phenols, carvarcrol and thymol that work in synergy. The mode of action of these phenols against organisms such as bacteria is through its toxic effect on the bacterial cell wall, by denaturing and coagulating the protein within the cell wall structure (Basset, 2000) Orego-stin R has been studied in swine and poultry. More Research is needed in ruminants.

Two hydroxymethylglutarly-SCOA (HMG-COA) reductase inhibitors, mevasatin and locastatin inhibited the in vitro growth and production of methane by strains of Methanobrevil bacter isolated from the rumen. Mevastatin or lovastatin did not inhibit growth of species of rumen bacteria that are essential for fermenting cellulose, starch and other plant polysaccharides to acetate, propionate and butyrate. In vitro studies suggests that supplementation of ruminant feeds with HMG –COA inhibitors could decrease ruminant methane production and increase the efficiency of feed utilization (Miller and Wolin, 2001).

Phytoestrogens: The role of plant estrogens in human food has attracted the attention of scientists world over (Price and Fenwick, 1985) since these and other substances have been suggested to act as anti-carcinogens for estrogen-induced tumors. The estrogenic isoflavones are the most common group of estrogenic substances in plants and occur mainly as water soluble glycoside conjugates. Estrogenic activity has been ascribed to pastures or forages all over the world. Leguminosae family of the plants is the most important sources for phytoestrogens in animal feed. Phytoestrogens have very low potency as compared to estradiol 17 â but they can produce significant biological effects due to their large consumption. Such effects include temporary infertility, dystokia, and permanent infertility. Mohsin and Pal (1975) reported the phytoestogenic content in some Indian fodders. However, Kaur et al. (1999) used sophisticated analytical technique (HPLC) and reported that total phytoestrogen content of leguminous fodders such as berseem, lucerne, shaftal, subabool and senji was 1079.11, 460.62, 216.84, and 60.58 ppm, respectively. Non-leguminous fodders such as maize, guinea grass, mustard, oats, hybrid napier, and blue panic grass contained less than 100 ppm phytoestrogens. Daidzein and genistein constituted a minor fraction of total estrogenic activity in all the plants. Major phytoestrogenic substance in all the plants was coumestrol.

The presence of phytoestrogens in soybeans has been recognized for some time and it was reported that because of estrogenicity of these compounds, soybean meal was beneficial as diethylstilbestrol as a growth promoter in farm animals.

Urease Inhibitors: The rapid hydrolysis of urea results in nearly instantaneous ammonia release in the rumen following consumption of a diet containing urea, often exceeding the capacity of microbial population to utilize it. Such excessive release of ammonia can result in a asynchronous ruminal fermentation and subsequent inefficient utilization of NPN products such as urea. One possible method for increasing the utilization is through the regulation of microbial urease via the controlled use of urease inhibitors. (N- butyl) thiophosphoric triamide (NPBT) is capable of short term inhibition of microbial uresae activity in the rumen (Ludden et al., 2000a). However, the ruminal micro flora is capable of adopting a chronic NBPT administration (Ludeen et al., 2000b). Supplementation of NBPT at a level sufficient to cause a 77% reduction in ruminal urease activity was incapable of producing a sustained release of NH from Urea. Further, more ruminal metabolism of NBPT may produce metabolites of NBPT molecule that have a negative post absorption effect on N metabolism in the animal thereby limiting its practical use in improving the utilization of dietary urea (Ludden et al., 2000b). Further investigation on effects of chronic administration of NBPT in vivo is warranted. Some herbs e.g. melon (Cucumis melo) seed and neem (A. indica) seed cake were found to have the ability of suppressing the urease as well as protease activity in rumen (Makkar et al.,1980; Aggarwal et al., 1991), which opens a new vista in urea utilization and bypass protein technology.

India has a long tradition to use herbs for toning the human body and curing the diseases as per Aaurveda. In fact many herbs such as turmeric, jeera, ajwain, cardamom, coriander, hing, fenugreek seeds, kalongi, Tulsi, anwala etc are being used routinely as a food additive in human diet, which not only improves the food appeal but also improves the digestion and keeps away the ailments. Similarly, herbal preparations are being used for the livestock too. Active principles of herbs needs identification, charactization and accurate standardization as the concentration and type of active ingredients depend upon many factors such as location, maturity etc. However, keeping in view their undisputed benefits, the herbs are being used as powder or the extract for both human and animals as such preparations may contain some primary as well as secondary compounds. There is a strong need to purify such compounds so that these can be used effectively as feed additives as well as medicines acceptable to consumers and showing the potency

A herbal preparation containing nearly thirty two herbs is in vogue and popularly known as Batisa. It is being used at the level of 30 to 50 g/day to improve the appetite of animals, maintained on poor quality roughages for prolonged period. This kind of mixture helps in curing different types of indigestion by augmenting the protozoal mass, bacterial population and increased absorption of nutrients. Such mixtures, recommended only for 6-8 days supplementation, are popular even outside the country due to their effectiveness. There are several other preparations to cure the diseases and to remove the parasites in animals.

Herbal or botanical additives are being used in human diets in India and other several countries since ages as to keep the human fit and healthy. Such botanical ingredients or their extracts have also many applications in animals and these are being used for this purpose extensively through out the length and breadth of the country in spite of the fact that these are not considered strictly nutritional feed ingredients or pre mixtures. The documentation of knowledge about such herbal products is limited; however, their potential as feed additive has been recognized at international level. Therefore, such additives have been taken into consideration while defining the additives in animal diet by the international community while formulating the Codex code. Newly established European Food Safety Authority (EFSA) is going to put in place a new range of feed additives regulation, which will include most botanicals or plant extracts and plant essential oils. The main functions of botanicals cover:

- Pathogen control or resistance including antimicrobial and antifungal activity.
- Toxin tolerance, including mycotoxins tolerance and liver activity.
- Digestion aid, including stimulation of endogenous enzyme activity and N absorption as well as beneficial physiological and morphological effects.
- Pollution control, including manure odour and ammonia control and N binding activity.
- Antioxidant activity as in control of metabolic auto oxidative stress caused by blood born free radicals.
- Other effects such as stimulation or modification of immune response, increased feed intake, animal product pigmentation etc.
- Enhanced animal production in terms of growth and milk

Such feed additives, though less expensive and safe from public health points of view, need more exploration about the active ingredients and the mode of their action so that their potential can be explained in the field of animal production.

Bibliography

Aggarwal , N, Kewalramani, N., Kamra, DN, Agarwal, DK, and Nath, K. (1991) J. Sci. Food. Agric. 57: 147

Anthony, NB, Balog, JM, Staudinger, FB, Wall, CW, Walker, RD. and Huff, WE (1994) Effects of urease inhibitor and ceiling fans on ascites in broilers. 1. Environmental variability and incidences of ascities. Poultry Science 73: 801-809.

Arora and Madhu Mohini, (1984) Pashudhan 76

Arora SP, Thakur, SS Tripathi, AN, and Chhabra A. (1983) Influence of Galog on digestibility and milk production of Karan Swiss cows. Indian Vet. J. 60: 46-50

Barman, K and Rai, S.N. (2004a) Chemical composition, amino acid profile and tannin fractionation of certain Indian agro-industrial byproducts. Proc. XI Animal Nutrition Conference, Jabalpur (Abst No. 20)

Barman, K and Rai, S.N. (2004b) Comparative nutrient digestibility (in vitro) in cattle, buffalo and goats using different levels of tannin containing TMR and degrading products using HPLC. Proc. XI Animal Nutrition Conference, Jabalpur (Abst No. 73)

Barry TN and Duncan, SJ (1984) British J. Nutri. 654: 485- 491

Basset, R. (2000) Feed Mix. 8(6): 30- 32

Bhatta R., Krishnamurthy, U., and Mohammad F. (2000) Anim. Feed Sci Techno. 87: 263- 277.

Broudiscou LP, PaPON, y, Broudiscou, AF (2000) Anim. Feed Sci. Technol 87: 263-277.

Fenwick, GR, Proce, KR, Tysukamoto C, and Okubo K (1991) Saponins. In saponins in substances in crop plants. (EHD' Mello, CM Duffus and JH Duffus) Cambdrige, The Royal Society of Chemistry. UK

Francis G, Kerem, Z, Makkar, HPS and Becker, K. (2002) The biological action of saponins in animal system: A review. British J. Nutri. 88: 587-605.

Gahlot OP (1982) Pashudhan 68

Goeger, D.E., Cheeke, P.R., Schmitz, J.A. and Buhler, P.R. (1982) Effect of feeding milk from goats fed tansy ragwort (S. jacobaea) to rats and calves. Am. J. Vet. Res. 43: 1631- 1633.

Gunther, KD (1991) Kraftfutter 2: 80

Hussain I and Cheeke PR (1995) Effect of Yucca schidigera extract on rumen and blood profiles of steers fed concentrate or roughage based diets. Anim. Feed Sci. Technol. 51: 231- 242.

Kaur, H., Singh Birbal and Kewalramai, N. (1999) Phytoestrogenic content of some Indian fodders. Indian J. Dairy Sci. 652: 121-123.

Killeen GF, Madigen, CA Connolly, CR, Walsh, GA, Clark, C., Hynes, MJ., Timmins, BF, James, P., Headen, DR., and Power, RF. (1998) Antimicrobial saponins of Yucca schedigera and the implications of their in vitro properties for their in vivo impact. J Agril. and Food Chem. 46: 3178- 3186.

Kulkarni, MV (1976) Proc. Ist National Convention of Indian Council of Indigenous Vet. Med. New Delhi

Ludden PA, Harmon, DL, Larson, BT and Axe, DE (2000a) J. Anim. Sci. 79: 181-197

Ludden PA, Harmon, DL, Huntington, GB, Larson, BT and Axe, DE (2000b) I. Anim. Sci. 78: 188-198

Mader Tl and Brumm, MC (1987) Effect of feeding saarsaponin in cattle and swine diets. J. Anim. Sci. 65: 9- 15.

Miller, WJ and Wolin, MJ (2001) J. Dairy Sci. 84: 1445-1448

Lu CD and Jorgfensen NA (1987) Alfalfasaponins affect site and extent of nutrient digestion in ruminants. J. Nutri. 117: 919-927

Mahanta, PN, Bijwal, DL, Prasad, B and Gupta, PP (1983) Indian J. Vet. Med. 3: 73-78

Makkar, HPS, Sharma, OP, Pal, RN, and Negi, S (1980) J. Dairy Sci. 63: 785.

Makkar, HPS, Barowy, NK, Becker, K. and Degen, A. (1995) Anim. Feed Sci. Technol. 55: 67-76.

Makkar, HPS, Aregheore EM, and Becker, K (1999) Effect of saponins and plant extracts containing saponins on the recovery of ammonia during urea ammoniation of wheat straw and fermentation kinetics of the treated straw. J Agril Sci, Camb. 132: 313-321

Makkar, HPS and Becker, K (1996) Effect of Quillaja saponins on in vitro rumen fermentation. In saponins used in food and agriculture, pp 377-386 (GR Waller and Y. Yamasaki Ed) Plenum Press, N.Y.

Mohsin M and Pal, AK (1975) Isolation and estimation of phtoestrogens in Indian forage plants. Indian J. Anim. Sci. 45: 622-625

Odenyo, AA, Osuji PO and Karanfil, O.(1997) Effects of multipurpose tree (MPT) supplemtns on ruminant celiate protozoa. Anim. Feed Sci. Technol. 67: 169-180

Price, KR and Fenwick, GR (1985) Naturally occurring oestrogens in food- A Review. Food Additive Contaminants. 2: 73-106

Roy PK, Munshi, JD, and Dutta, HM. (1990) Effect of saponin extracts on morpho-history and respiratory physiology of an air breathing fish (Heteropneustes fossilis Bloch). J. Freshwater Biology. 2: 135-145.

Valdez, FR, Bush, LJ, Goetsch, AL, and Owens, FN. (1986) J. Dairy Sci. 69: 1568- 1575.

Wenk, C. (2002) Proc. International Symp. On Recent Advances in Animal Nutrition, 22 Nov. New Delhi, pp 140-21.

17
PROBIOTICS IN SMALL RUMINANTS

T. K. Dutta and S. S. Kundu

India has genetically diversified goat and sheep breeds, which are most suited to their respective native tracts after long adaptation. Goat and sheep are mainly habituated with browsing and grazing system of feeding. But the production potential is limited under browsing condition due to less availability of balance and optimum nutrition. In India, goat and sheep are mainly reared for meat, fibre, milk and skin production. India has second highest goat population ((123 million) (FAO, 2000) and fifth in sheep population (Singh and Karim, 2003). Under traditional system of feeding production potential of small ruminants is limited due to less utilization of conventional and non-conventional feeds. Probiotics, recently termed as direct fed microbial (DFM) has diversified use in domesticated animals (like small and large ruminants, pig and poultry) and in human beings. In the present paper, discussion will be focused on the beneficial effects of probiotics in small ruminants. During pre-ruminant stage lactic acid bacteria could be more beneficial for improving growth and immunity status of kids or lambs. Yeast culture (Saccharomyces cerevisiae) or fungal culture (Aspergillus orygae) may improve the rumen fermentation pattern, growth and milk production of small ruminants.

In the past century, various microorganisms have been tested for their ability to prevent and cure diseases in animals and humans. Microorganisms have also been added to domestic animal feed to enhance growth. The concept of microbial manipulation in the gastro-intestinal tract was first appreciated by Metchnikoff (1907) who viewed the consumption of yoghurt by Bulgarian peasants as conferring a long span of life. The term "Probiotics" was first coined by Parker (1974) who described this as "microorganism or substance which contribute to the intestinal microbial balance". In 1989, Fuller defined the probiotic as "a live microbial feed supplement which beneficially affects the host animals by improving its intestinal microbial balance." The term probiotic means "for life" and has a contrast with the term antibiotic which means "against life".

At present, probiotics are classified as GRAS (Generally Recognised As Safe) ingredient by the US Food and Drug Administration. According to EEC directive 70/524, several microorganisms have been authorized as new additive for feedstuffs. Now it is generally accepted that certain viable microbial cultures beneficially affect the productive potentials of small and large ruminants, pig, rabbits and poultry. The species employed in probiotic preparation are mainly lactic acid bacteria like Lactobacillus acidophilus, L. bulgaricus, L. lactis, L. plantarum, L. salivarius, L. farciminis, Streptococcus thermophilus, Enterococcus faecium, E. faecalis, Bifidobacterium species, Bacillus subtilis, B. cereus, B. cereus toyoi, B. licheniformis, Pediococcus acidilactici; and yeast and fungal culture like Saccharomyces cerevisiae and Aspergillus oryzae etc. The effects generally observed with probiotics in animal nutrition are increased productive parameters and better sanitary conditions (Breul, 1998).

A large range of modes of action can explain those positive effects of probiotics and some of them are specific for a given micro-organism. Among probiotics, the case of Saccharomyces cerevisiae is interesting to consider, since yeast has been used for decades, as both preventive and therapeutic agent for diarrhoea and other gastro-intestinal disorders in humans. Yeast is also known to induce positive effects both in ruminant and non-ruminant species. Yeasts are eucaryotic micro-organism, and their properties are completely different from those of bacteria, which are prokaryotic micro-organism.

Mode of Action of lactic acid bacteria

Several mechanisms of lactic acid bacteria have been reviewed by Dutta et al. (2002), which include adhesion to the digestive tract to prevent colonization of pathogens, neutralization of toxins, bactericidal activity, prevention of amine synthesis and enhanced immuno-competence.

Competitive Attachment

It has been demonstrated that lactobacilli compete with coliform and other pathogenic organisms for the sites of adherence on the intestinal surface. The attachment is believed to support proliferation and reduce peristaltic removal of organisms. Muralidhara et al. (1977) have reported the competitive attachment between lactic acid bacteria and coliform in the intestinal tract. The ability of bacteria to adhere to squamous epithelial cells appears to depend on attraction between an acidic mucopolysaccharide forming the outer layer of bacterial cell wall and a similar coating on epithelial cells (Fuller and Brooker, 1974).

Antimicrobial Activity

Lactic acid bacteria have the potential in limiting the growth of pathogenic microorganisms in calves (Abu-Tarboush et al., 1996). The protective effect of indigenous gut flora has been confirmed against Salmonella, E. coli, Campylobactor foetus sub sp. Jejuni, Clostridium botulinum, and Mersinia enterocolitica. Streptococcus thermophilus suppressed the growth of pathogenic bacteria, Clostridium perfrigens and Salmonella entridides by 73.3 and 51.8 per cent respectively (Sikes and Hilton, 1987). Following possible mechanisms have been suggested to explain the anti-microbial activity of lactobacilli and streptococci.

- Adhesion to the intestinal wall preventing colonization by pathogens	Fuller (1989)
- Lowering of intestinal pH (due to production of H_2O_2 or organic acid)	Renner (1991)
- Competition of nutrients	Wilson and Perini (1988)
- Production of antibacterial substances	Renner (1991)
- Increase in phagocytic activity and immunoglobulin levels	Saito et al. (1981)

Enhancement of Immunity

Lactic acid bacteria have the capability to enhance the immunity by the animals. Phagocytic activity and immunoglobulin levels have been increased by probiotics (Raibaud and Raynaud, 1991). L. casei and L. plantarum given parenterally stimulate phagocytic activity (Saito et al., 1981). Pollmann et al. (1980) observed elevated levels of total serum protein, apparently globulin rather than albumin and WBC counts when the animal fed L. acidophilus. Lactobacilli could be important in the development of immunity in young animals, particularly during weaning when protection must be acquired against antigens likely to cause gut inflammatory reactions (Miller et al., 1985).

Translocation of Micro-organisms from the Gut

Lactobacilli can translocate and can survive for many days in the spleen, liver, lungs and lymph (Bianchi-Salvadori et al., 1988). In the animals pre-treated with lactic acid bacteria (L. bulgaricus and S. thermophilus), E. coli were absent in the lymph nodes and stimulate the immunity (Bourliouse, 1986).

Prophylactic and Therapeutic Effect of Lactic Acid Bacteria

Against Diarrhoea

Neonates of all species can suffer from a number of adverse environmental conditions soon after birth, including dampness, chilling, drought, inadequate milk and periods of separation from their dams. These conditions favour for non-beneficial bacteria to colonize the digestive tract and result in increased neonatal morbidity and mortality. In neonatal piglets and calves, probiotics aided in the prompt establishment of an animal-microbes relationship beneficial to the newborn's intestinal tract. These studies have demonstrated improved animal health and performance (Collington et al., 1988). Since Metchnikoff's early study data in several species have shown the ability of lactobacilli to suppress coliform growth. Viable lactobacilli feeding was shown to reduce the incidence of diarrhoea in young dairy calves (Abu-Tarboush et al., 1996). These findings contrast with those of other workers who have not observed benefits from feeding with L. acidophilus (Hatch et al., 1973). No mortality of kids of Barbari breed (2-13 weeks of age) was recorded under probiotics (Lactobacillus sporogens) supplemented milk replacers (Dutta, et al. 2003).

Against Mastitis

Greene et al. (1991) have attempted to treat clinical mastitis in dairy cattle with intra-mammary infusion of lactobacillus. They observed that lactobacillus cured 35.5% of infected quarters but milk somatic cell counts remained unchanged, and concluded that Lactobacillus product was not effective as an intra-mammary treatment for mastitis. In goat, mastitis is a common problem. Due to less efficiency of antibiotics in goat mastitis probiotics may be tried.

Anti-carcinogenic Activity

A number of available reports in the literature suggest that certain lactic acid bacteria, including L. acidophilus and Bifidobacterium species may have an anti-cancer roles, the specific evidence for this is not yet compelling. Epidemiological evidence and dietary studies have shown that supplementation of lactic acid bacteria may reduce the risk of colon cancer in both animals and herd-man (Friend and Shahani, 1984). Feeding of lactic acid bacteria inhibited the growth of tumor in mice when inoculated with tumor cells intra-peritoneally (Shackelford et al., 1983). They found similar results with L. bulgaricus and S. thermophilus.

Vaccine Adjuvant

In conjunction with studies that indicated LGG (Lactobacillus GG) increased intestinal immunity in children with rotavirus-induced diarrhoea, Isolauri et al. (1995) tested LGG as an adjuvant to an oral vaccine to rotavirus in children. There was an increase of rotavirus-specific IgM-secreting cells in the LGG group compared to placebo 8d post vaccination. LGG also increased IgA and IgM seroconversion when measured in paired sera prior to vaccination and 30d post-vaccination. This area may be explored extensively for higher efficiency of vaccines for small ruminants.

Aflatoxin detoxification

Aflatoxins (AF) represent a group of closely related difuranocoumarin compounds produced by the common fungal molds Aspergilus flavus and A. parasiticus. They are a group from fungal secondary metabolites that are recognized as being of economic and health importance and are potent hepatocarcinogens in several species of animals (Eaton and Callinger, 1994).

Their production can be influenced by several factors including temperature, water activity, pH, available nutrients and competitive growth of other microorganisms. Once foods are contaminated with aflatoxins there are only two options; either the toxin is removed or the toxin is degraded into less toxic or non-toxic compounds. It has been observed that many microorganisms are able to remove or degrade aflatoxins in foods and feeds (Marth and Doyle, 1979) which has been known as probiotic bacteria and they are used to balance the intestinal flora and to prevent several gastrointestinal disorders (Yoon and Byon, 2002).

The range of AFG_1 binding activity was from 33% to 53% and most efficient binding of AFG_1 was observed by L. acidophilus CU028 and L. brevis CU 06 which bound 50% and 53% of AFG_1 respectively. The range of AFG_2 binding activity was from 46% and most efficient binding AFG_2 was observed by L. acidophilus CU028 and L. casei CU 901 which bound 68% and 57% of AFG_2 respectively. The differences in the binding activities of AFG_2 between the strains showed statistical significance ($P>0.05$) (Byan and Yoon, 2003). Probiotic lactobacilli have been found to efficiently bind aflatoxins (EI Nezami et al., 1998), the aflatoxin binding of the tested strains was found to be variable. Carcinogen and mutagen binding by bacteria is thought to be by the bacterial cell wall (Thyagaraja and Hosono, 1994).

Digestive and Metabolic Activity as Influenced by Lactic Acid Bacteria

Feeding of bacterial preparations increased feed conversion efficiency and live weight gain which may be due to improved digestion performance or indirectly due to the suppression of gut pathogens.

Carbohydrates

It is feasible that extra-cellular enzymes of gut micro-flora supplement endogenous secretions, particularly in neonates when the digestive system is immature (Kiddar and Manners, 1978). Szabo (1979) observed estimated activities of lactase and lypase in the large intestine of conventional piglet compared with germ-free animals, but at the same time inactivation of some endogenous enzymes was also found by gut micro-flora. For example, higher levels of peptidase and disaccharidase activities were found in the small and large intestines of germ-free than in conventional piglets.

Fats and Cholesterol Metabolism

Improved fat digestibility in growing pigs was observed by Mason and Just (1976) under the suppression of gut bacteria by antibiotics. This suggested that fat metabolizing bacteria reduce the availability of dietary lipid to the host. Ratcliffe et al. (1985) proposed that microbial hydrogenation could increase the amount of stearic acid, which is less well absorbed than unsaturated fatty acids. Hypo-cholesteromic effects were reported on yoghurt culture with S. thermophilus and S. bulgaricus (Jaspers et al., 1984).

Mineral Metabolism

Supplementation of lactic acid bacteria increased the bioavailability of calcium, phosphorus, magnesium and zinc from all diets (Schaafsma et al., 1988). Consumption of lactic acid bacteria resulted into increased bone calcium and improved bone formation (Kaup, 1988). Research reports are not available in respect of efficacy of lactic acid bacteria for lactose tolerance, fats and cholesterol metabolism and mineral metabolism in sheep and goat. Therefore, this area needs to be attended under Indian condition.

Yeast and fungal culture: Mode of action and effect in small ruminant productivity.

Survivability in the GI Tract

Certain yeasts and aerobic fungi are normal inhabitants of the rumen but most species isolates were considered to be transient and non-functional, entering the rumen via the feed (Orpin and Soblin 1988). Dawson (1988) reported that in fermentors fed a ration consisting of 0.75 forage and 0.25 concentrate, the concentration of yeast cells for Yea-Sacc was consistently 3-6 times greater than could be accounted for by the yeast present in the supplements suggesting that some yeast replication was occurring. The concentration of rumen viable yeast increased when yeast culture was added to the diet of steers (McLeod et al., 1990). In another study by Newbold et al. (1990) it has been observed that there were increased counts of yeasts in rumen fluid 1 h after yeast culture addition. Numbers then fell by 61% after 6h, but remained two orders of magnitude higher than that of control animals. Viable yeast persisted in the duodenum and ileum of treated animals, at values 6.5 and 6.8 times higher than control. Durand–Chaucheyras et al. (1998) confirmed the fact that added Saccharomyces cerevisiae did not colonize the rumen of lambs and Kung et al. (1997) reported that yeasts were essentially washed out of ruminal continuous fermentors. Earlier Arambel and Tung. (1987) concluded that Saccharomyces cerevisiae was unable to maintain a productive population within the rumen ecosystem. The viability of yeast cells in the rumen has been considered crucial because El Hassan et al. (1993) reported that yeast cultures need to be both viable and metabolically active to have a full stimulatory effect on ruminal fermentation.

pH and Carbohydrate

An important factor in the stimulation of forage digestion by yeast culture may be the stabilizing effect of yeast culture on pH and the metabolism of readily fermentable carbohydrate (RFC). Cereal grains in ruminant rations provide substrates for rapidly growing ruminal bacteria (Streptococcus bovis) that produce large quantities of lactate (Slyter, 1976). It is reported that rumen pH is mainly associated with concentration of lactic acid in the rumen (Williams et al., 1991). Diets having RFC depressed ruminal pH which lead to reduction in number of cellulolytic bacteria (Thomas and Rook, 1981), impaired forage degradation (Williams, 1989).

The effect of yeast supplementation on pH stabilization seems to be strongly dependent on the type of diet tested. Generally higher rumen pH has been observed with yeast supplementation when control pH tended to be below 6. Fiem et al. (1993) reported that the effect of yeast culture on the rumen pH was more pronounced in sheep fed with a maize silage/cereal based concentrate diet (high sugars/starch content) than with grass hay and sugar beet pulp-based concentrate. pH stabilization is generally associated with decreased levels of lactic acid in rumen.

Nisbet and Martin (1991) have demonstrated that soluble components in A. oryzae and S. cerevisiae culture filtrate stimulated lactate uptake by Selenomonas ruminantium and Megasphaera elsdenii. For this reason in concentrate diet there is more cellulolytic activity due to addition of yeast culture. Mathieu et al. (1996) have found an increase of the pH with yeast only in faunated sheep and not in defaunaed sheep suggesting that protozoa are involved in the effect of saccharomyces cerevisiae on the increase of rumen pH.

Production of Growth Stimulating Factors

Yeast cells in the rumen may supply a chemical growth factor to the cellulolytic microorganisms (Offer, 1990). S. cerevisiae produces specific factors like B-vitamins or branched chain fatty acids to stimulate the growth of cellulolytic bacteria (Chademana and Offer, 1990). Callaway and Martin (1997) also reported that yeast culture provided soluble growth factor (i.e., organic acids, B-vitamins, and amino acids) that stimulated growth of ruminal bacteria that utilize lactate and digest cellulose.

Stimulation of brush border dissacharidases

Buts et al (1986) have shown that oral ingestion of Sacchromyces cerevisiae by human volunteers and weaned rats resulted in marked increases in the specific and total activities of brush border membrane disaccharidase including sucrase, lactase and maltase. This property could be interesting since diarrhoea is associated with a decrease of the intestinal disaccharides activities. Buts et al (1994) concluded that increased disaccharidase activities could be mediated by endoluminal release of polyamines (spermine and spermidine) produced by live yeast.

Anti-adhesive properties of yeast

Binding of pathogens to yeast cell wall induces a protective effect since the complex Sacchromyces cerevisiae/pathogen is then rapidly eliminated from the digestive tract (Gedek, 1989). Competition between yeast and pathogens for binding to intestinal cells could help explain the beneficial action of yeast, since adhesion is crucial to the expression of the cytopathogenic effect. Frequency of Salmonella typhimurium colonization was significantly reduced in broilers due to yeast treatment (Line et al., 1998) although Campylobacter colonization was not affected by yeast supplementation.

Increased Microbial Population

Production potential of yeast culture can be associated to their effect on the increased microbial population in the rumen. Addition of yeast culture resulted into increase in concentration of total anaerobic bacteria, but the increase was associated with fibre digesting and lactic acid utilising bacteria (Dawson, 1992). Yeast culture supplementation stimulates the growth of cellulolytic bacteria in the rumen (Newbold et al., 1995). It is particularly pronounced when forage containing diets are fed (Dawson, 1990). Combined culture of yeast (S. cerevisiae), lactobacilli and enterococci supplementation to the diet of steers enhanced the concentration of cellulolytic bacteria in rumen (5 to 40 times). Enhanced growth of rumen bacteria could result in enhanced microbial protein synthesis and increased contribution of the microbial population to the digestive process. Cell yields were increased by 7 to 63% when cultures of Ruminobactor amylophilus-1024 and Fibrobactor succinogenes-S-85 were treated with yeast. Total bacterial counts under in vitro condition were increased significantly ($P<0.01$) in viable culture supplementation groups (S. Cerevisiae-NCDC-47 and S. cerevisiae-NCDC-47 + L. plantarum-NCDC-25 + E. faecium-NCDC-124) when the substrate had high or medium concentrate. But, in high roughage groups no difference was recorded among treatment groups (Dutta et al., 2001). It has been suggested that an increased bacterial flora in animals fed S. cerevisiae is central to the action of yeast in the rumen (Wallace and Newbold, 1992).

Increase in the number of total culturable bacteria in the rumen appears to be one of the most consistently reported responses to yeast supplementation (Newbold, 1996). Increased levels of rumen protozoa following Saccharomyces cerevisiae ingestion were also reported (Miranda et al., 1996). Aspergillus fermentation extracts (Chang et al. 1999) and yeast cultures (Chaucheryas et al., 1995) have been shown to directly stimulate rumen fungi, which may improve fiber digestion. Saccharomyces cerevisiae supplementation was associated with an increased flow of microbial protein leaving the rumen and enhanced supply of amino acids entering the small intestine (Erasmus et al., 1992).

Ammonia Production and Microbial Protein Synthesis

One of the common observations associated with the addition of yeast culture to ruminants and in rumen simulating fermentors has been the reduction of rumen ammonia concentration (Sohn and Song, 1996). The concentration of ammonia was decreased by 10 to 35 per cent in vitro (Carro et al., 1992). Similar results have been reported by Chademana and Offer (1990) in vivo, suggesting an improved microbial capture of ammonia. Whereas, Moloney and Drennan (1994) reported that rumen ammonia concentration was not affected when yeast was included in low concentrate diet of steer, but was reduced when yeast was added to the diet having high concentrate.

Reduced ammonia levels have not been associated with decreased protein degradation or deamination (Williams and Newbold, 1990). Incorporation of ammonia into microbial protein was enhanced due to supplementation of yeast (Carro et al., 1992), which was confirmed by greater microbial yield and microbial true protein reaching the duodenum (Erasmus, 1991).

Total Volatile Fatty Acid and Their Proportions

Much of the work on the effects of microbial cultures in the rumen has involved the measurement of concentrations and proportions of volatile fatty acids (VFA) as indicators of microbial activity. Many workers have reported that VFA production is improved due to addition of yeast culture in ruminants. Yeast culture may alter the pattern of VFA production (Martin et al., 1989). In lamb, yeast culture addition along with sugar-beet pulp and rolled barley (0.8:0.2) and 60g soybean meal increased total VFA and acetate (Rouzbehan et al., 1994). Whereas in other study, yeast culture addition increased TVFA non-significantly and acetate:propionate ratio was decreased from 5.01 to 3.81 mainly due to increase in propionate (Newbold et al., 1990) in sheep. In lactating cow, Harrison et al. (1988) observed that there was higher production of propionate and reduction of acetate to propionate ratio due to supplementation of yeast culture. Similarly, enhanced production of propionate and reduction of acetate to propionate was reported by Martin et al. (1989) and Moloney and Drennan (1994).

Supplementation of commercial yeast to the high concentrate diet of steer reduced acetate and acetate to propionate ratio; molar proportion of butyrate and iso-acids were higher (Moloney and Drennan, 1994). Dawson et al. (1990) have reported that neither the yeast culture supplement nor the mixed microbial (yeast, lactobacilli and enterococci) supplement consistently alter the patterns of VFA production in the continuous cultures or in the rumen of steers.

Total gas and Methane Production

While carbon dioxide receives the most attention as a factor in global warming, there are other gases to consider, including methane, nitrous oxide (N_2O) and chlorofluerocarbons (CFCs). The rising concentration of methane is correlated with increasing populations and currently about 70 per cent of methane production arises from anthropogenic sources and the remainder from natural sources. Agriculture is considered to be responsible for about two-thirds of the anthropogenic source. Biological generation in anaerobic environments (natural and men made wet lands, enteric fermentation and anaerobic wastes processing) is the major source of methane. Agriculture also contributes about 21-25%,

60% and 65-80% of the total anthropogenic emissions of carbon dioxide, methane and N_2O respectively (Duxbury et al., 1993). The release of an estimated 205-245 Tg (10^{12} g) methane per year from agriculture sources is derived from enteric fermentation (80 Tg), paddy production (60-100 Tg), biomass burning (40 Tg) and animal wastes (25 Tg) (Watson et al., 1992). The removal of hydrogen by methanogenesis has been reported to increase the production of acetate (Wolin and Miller, 1988). Both propionate and CH_4 formation compete for the available hydrogen in the rumen as a result of fermentation. Yeast culture supplementation resulted into reduction of methane production in steers by 28% (Williams, 1989). The addition of yeast culture resulted in a lower methane production for medium concentrate diet, but in a higher for the high concentrate diet (Carro et al., 1992). Harrison et al. (1988) have shown that in vitro gas production was not affected due to yeast supplementation.

The effect of probiotic addition on total gas and methane production in small ruminants has not been studied precisely. This area requires work to confirm the effect of probiotics on methane and animal production.

Forage Degradation in Rumen

The theory that yeast culture inclusion stimulates appetite has been enthusiastically pursued. Chademana and Offer (1990) reported that addition of Yea-Sacc to concentrate/forage diets in which the proportion of concentrate ranged from 20 to 60 per cent of the diet consistently increased degradability of hay up to 24h (37.3 to 42.2 per cent), but had no effect on the 48h degradability.

Many workers have reported improvement in degradability patterns of nutrients either in vitro or in sacco due to supplementation of yeast culture (Williams et al., 1991; Newbold et al., 1995). Supplementing the high concentrate diet with yeast culture resulted in significantly higher DM and NDF degradabilities (Carro et al., 1992). Moreover, filter paper (cellulose) degradability (24h) tended to be higher for the vessels supplemented with yeast culture than for the control (33% Vs 27%). These results might suggest that yeast culture increased the population of fibre-degrading bacteria and/ or their activity. However, yeast culture had no significant effect on DM and NDF degradabilities with medium or low concentrate diet (Carro et al., 1992). In vitro digestibility of NDF was increased by yeast or yeast + white rot fungi (Armillaria heimii) treatment, with the yeast + fungi combination showed highest values in hay based ration. Strain variability of S. cerevisiae was observed on nylon bag degradability of straw and hay (Newbold et al., 1995).

Some effects of yeast culture on rumen fermentation

Effect	References
1. Moderated ruminal pH	Williams et al. 1991
2. Stabilized fermentation	Harrison et al., 1988
3. Altered VFA production	Harrison et al., 1988; Rouzbehan et al., 1994
4. Decreased ammonia concentration	Dawson and Newman, 1987; Carro et al., 1992
5. Increased concentrations of anaerobic bacteria and cellulolytic bacteria	Harrison et al. 1988; Dawson et al., 1990; Newbold et al. 1995
6. Enhanced microbial protein synthesis	Chademana and Offer, 1990
7. Reduced methane production	Williams, 1989
8. Increased concentrations of of yeast in the populations	Dawson et al., 1990
9. Decreased lactic acid concentration	Williams, 1989

Feed Intake and Nutrient Utilization as Influenced by S.cerevisiae

Nutrient supply to the animals has been improved due to yeast culture supplement at a fixed intake (Williams et al., 1990), but in farm trials, its effect on intake appears the most important cause of improved performance. In several studies it has been observed that yeast culture addition increased the feed intake in calves (Bonaldi et al., 1986; Hancock et al., 1994). However, some studies indicated no added advantage of yeast culture supplementation to lactating cows on DMI (Kung et al., 1997). Differences in response to added yeast might have been due to interactions among yeast, diet and stage of lactation.

A number of studies provided evidence indicating that live yeast cells enhances the digestive process in the gastrointestinal tract. Bhoi (1992) has shown that the fibre digestion was better in the combined culture of yeast and L.acidophilus in goats as compared to individual ones. Supplementation of S. cerevisiae increased the digestibility of protein, cellulose (Wohlt et al., 1991), fibre (Gomez-Alarcon et al., 1990), NDF and ADF (Kim et al., 1992). Similarly, Weidmeier et al. (1987) observed that supplementation of yeast culture increased hemicellulose and CP digestibility in ruminants. DM digestion in the rumen of dairy cows was increased receiving yeast culture (Gomez-Alarcon et al., 1987). Carro et al. (1992) reported that effect on digestibility is dependent on the forage to concentrate ratio, supplementation of yeast culture with high concentrate diet resulted in significantly higher DM and NDF digestibilities in rumen (Rusitech). However, on high forage diet yeast culture had no effect on DM, NDF and cellulose digestibility.

Some studies (Harrison et al., 1987; Chademana and Offer, 1990) revealed that DM digestibility was not changed by addition of yeast culture, suggesting that the effects of yeast on digestion may be very subtle and can not easily be identified in studies of total tract digestibility.

Response of probiotics on productive performance in small ruminants

Growth

In ruminants, higher growth is positively related with the higher rumen fermentation pattern and nutrient utilization pattern. Probiotics, either lactic acid bacteria or yeast culture, have beneficial effect on higher nutrient utilization. Significantly ($P<0.05$) higher weight gain and average daily gain (ADG) were observed in lambs fed complete rations supplemented with Yea-Sacc[1026], followed by Lactobacillus acidophilus and control (without probiotics) (Rao et al., 2003). Earlier similar observations were recorded by Rouzbehan et al. (1994) in lambs fed Yea-Sacc supplemented barley. Kmet et al. (1993) and Birch et al. (1994) also observed higher growth rates in lambs fed probiotics. The higher growth rate in Yea-Sacc supplemented ration might be due to increased flow of microbial protein leaving the rumen and an enhanced supply of amino acids entering the small intestine.

Milk production

Several workers have reported that supplementation of yeast culture to the lactating cows improved milk yield or FCM yield (Williams et al., 1991; Kung et al., 1997).

Teh et al. (1987) tested the effect of feeding yeast culture with or without added $NaHCO_3$ on lactating goats and found that both yeast culture and $NaHCO_3$ increased milk yield without an increase in DM intake. In the high producing cows, there was a 6% increase in milk production due to supplementation of viable mixed microbial feed additives (S. cerevisiae, Streptococcus faecium and Lactobacillus acidophilus), whereas there was no treatment effect in the low productive cows (Hoyos et al., 1987). Williams et al. (1991) have shown that there was interaction between diet composition and yeast culture regarding the DMI and milk yield, effects of yeast culture were greatest in diets containing 60:40 (concentrate:forage) ratio.

Some workers reported that milk yield was unaffected by the addition of yeast culture to the diet of cows (Erdman and Sharma, 1989; Higginbotham et al., 1994). Dawson (1993) stated that yeast culture supplements did not have equal beneficial effects with all types of diets, and it is currently not possible to define the dietary conditions that provide optimum response to yeast culture supplementation.

Teh et al. (1987) found that both yeast culture and $NaHCO_3$ increased milk fat per centage in early lactation goats. Other authors have also observed significant improvement in milk fat per centage of lactating cows due to supplementation of yeast culture (Putnam et al., 1997). Williams et al. (1991) have noticed that milk fat per centage slightly improved only in high concentrate diet (60%). Whereas, other authors did not record any difference in milk fat per centage due to yeast culture supplementation (Erdman and Sharma, 1989; Higginbotham et al., 1994).

Probiotics or direct fed microbial have great potential to enhance growth and immunity status of pre-ruminant kids or lambs. Lactic acid bacteria have specific function in digestive system and immunity of small ruminants. Whereas, yeast culture triggered the benefial effect on rumen fermentation and intestinal digestion. However, sporadic observations are available on the use of probiotics in small ruminants in India. India has diversified goat and sheep breeds, which has distinct differences among themselves in respect of phenotypic and genotypic traits. No systematic studies have been conducted in India to see the efficacy of probiotics in small ruminants. Following areas should be attended carefully before recommending probiotics for small ruminants in India.

1. During early stage of life, small ruminants are very susceptible to bacterial infection, in particular E. coli infection. Due to antibiotics resistance and cost factor probiotics have great opportunity to be used to save the life of early growing kids/lambs.
2. Immunity status of small ruminants during early and late stage of growth under probiotics feeding should be studied thoroughly.
3. Production potential of probiotics in terms of growth, milk and wool production and skin quality may be investigated thoroughly before recommendation of probiotics in small ruminants.
4. Small ruminants production under Indian condition is by and large dependent on browsing and grazing. Incriminating factors present in such feeds may be detoxified by use of probiotics. However, this area needs thorough investigation.

5. Most of the yeast culture works in high concentrate feeding regimen, therefore, suitable species or strain of yeast culture is to be identified for better efficacy under high roughage feeding or under grazing condition of Indian goats or sheep.

6. Use of probiotics should be tested for higher productivity keeping economics in mind in small ruminants under intensive and semi-intensive system of feeding, as many commercial farms of goats and sheep are coming up fast under intensive and semi-intensive system of feeding.

Bibliogrpahy

Abu-Tarboush, H.M., Al-Saiady, M.Y. and El-Din, A.H.K. 1996. Evaluation of diet containing Lactobacilli on performance, faecal coliform, and lactobacilli of young dairy calves. Anim. Feed Sci. Technol. 57:39-49.

Arambel, M.J. and Tung, R.S. 1987. 19th Biennial Conference on Rumen Function. Chicago, Illinois.

Bhoi, G. 1992. Growth performance and feed conversion efficiency in goat kids kept on dietary additive of L.acidophilus and S.cerevisiae. M.Sc. Thesis submitted to NDRI, Karnal.

Bianchi Salvadori, B., Camaschella, P. and Cislaghi, S. 1988. Effect of yogurt lactic acid bacteria and bifidobacteria on translocation of E.coli in the lymph system. Int. Symp. Intert. Microecol. Alghero.

Birch, K.S., Thomas, J.D. and Ross, T.T. 1994. Growth and carcass characteristics of newly received feeder lambs treated with probiotics and vitamin-E. Sheep and goat Res. J. 10:201-206.

Bonaldi, G., Buratto, L., Darsie, G., Didone, G.P. and Mondini, S. 1986. Use of S.cerevisiae and L. acidophilus in veal calves. Obiettivi-e-Documenti Veterinari. 7(1):49-53.

Bourliouse, P. 1986. Interet de lingestion volontaire de microorganisms:cas de la microflore du yaourt. Cah. Nutr. Diet. 21:204-208.

Bruel, S. 1998. Les probiotiques en alimentation animale. Med. Chir. Dig. 27:89-91.

Buts, J.P., Bernasconi, P., Van Craynest, M.P., Maldague, P. and De Meyer, R. 1986. Response of human and rats small intestinal mucosa to oral administration of Saccharomyces boulardii. Pediatr. Res. 20:192-196.

Buts, J.P., De Keyser, N. and De Reademaeker, L. 1994. Saccharomyces boulardii enhances rat intestinal enzyme expression by endoluminal release of polyamines. Pediatr. Res. 36:522-527.

Byun, B.R. and Yoon, Y.H. 2003. Binding of Aflatoxin G_1, G_2 and B_2 by probiotic Lactobacillus spp. Asian-Aust. J. Anim. Sci. 16:1686-1689.

Callaway, E.S. and Martin, S.A. 1997. Effects of a Saccharomyces cerevisiae culture on ruminal bacteria that utilize lactate and digest cellulose. J. Dairy Sci. 80:2035-2044.

Carro, M.D., Libzien, P. and Rohr, K. 1992. Influence of yeast culture on the in vitro fermentation (Rusitech) of diets containing variable portions of concentrates. Anim. Feed Sci. Technol. 37:209-220.

Chademana, I. and Offer, N.W. 1990. The effect of dietary inclusion of yeast culture on digestion in the sheep. Anim. Prod. 50:483-489.

Chang, J.S., Harper, E.M. and Calza, R.E. 1999. Fermentation extract effects on the morphology and metabolism of the rumen fungus Neocallimastix frontalis EB 188. J. Appl. Microbiol. 86:389-398.

Chaucheyras, F., Fonty, G., Bertin, G. and Gouet, P. 1995. In vitro utilization by a ruminal acetogenic bacterium cultivated alone or in association with an archea methanogen is stimulated by a probiotic strain of Saccharomyces cerevisiae. Appl. Environ. Micro. 61:3466-3467.

Collington, G.K., Parker, D.S., Ellis, M. and Armstrong, D.G. 1988. The influence of Probios or Tylosin on growth of pigs and development of the gastro-intestinal tract. Anim. Prod. 46:521-522.

Dawson, K.A. and Newman, K.E. 1987. Effects of yeast culture supplements on the growth and activities of rumen bacteria in continuous culture. J. Anim. Sci. 65 (Suppl.I): 452.(Abstr.)

Dawson, K.A. 1988. In: Biotechnology in the Feed Industry. Ed. T.P. Lyons, pp.101-112.

Dawson, K.A. 1990. Designing the yeast culture of tomorrow. Mode of action of yeast culture for ruminants and non-ruminants. In: T.P.Lyons (Editor), Biotechnology in the Feed Industry. Alltech. Technical Publications, Nicholasville, KY.pp. 59-78.

Dawson, K.A. 1992. Current and future role of yeast culture in animal production:A review of research over the last six years. Asia Pacific Lecture Tour on "Improving Nutrient Utilization while reducing pollution:New Dimensions Through Biotechnology", pp. 15-37.

Dawson, K.A. 1993. Current and future role of yeast culture in animal production: a review of research over the last six years. pp 269 (Suppl.) Proc. Alltech's 9th Annu. Symp. Alltech Tech. Publ., Nicholasville, KY.

Dawson, K.A., Newman, K.E. and Boiling, J.A. 1990. Effects of microbial supplements containing yeast and lactobacilli on roughage-feed ruminal microbial activities. J. Anim. Sci. 68:3392-3398.

Durand-Chaucheyras, F., Fonty, G., Bertin, G., Theveniot, M. and Gouet, P. 1998. Influence of feeding varying levels of yeast additive during digestive transit in lambs. Reprod. Nutr. Dev. 38:275-280.

Dutta, T. K., Kundu, S. S. and Sharma, D. D. 2001. Potential of probiotics supplementation on in vitro rumen fermentation and ^{35}S incorporation in microbial protein. Indian J. Anim. Nutr. 18:227-234.

Dutta, T. K., Kundu, S. S. and Sharma, D. D. 2002. Mechanism of action and health benefits of probiotics. Intas Polyvet, 3:14-23.

Dutta, T.K., Singh, Nawab, Rekhate, D.H., Reddy, T.J and Shettar, V.B. (editors). 2003. Final Report of NATP/RPPS-12 entitled "Utilization of by-products of pulses, oilseeds along with coarse cereals grains for intensive goat production" published by Central Institute Research on Goats, Makhdoom, Farah, Mathura, UP (India).

Duxbury, J.M. and Mosier, A.R.1993. Status and issues concerning agricultural emissions of green house gases. In: Agricultural Dimensions of Global Climate Change, Kaiser, H.M. and Drennen, T.W.(Eds), Dalray Beach, FI: St. Lucie Press, pp 229-258.

Eaton, D.L. and Callanger. 1994. Mechanism of aflatoxin carcinogenesis. Ann. Rev. Phamacol. Toxicol. 34:135-172.

El-Nezmi, H.S., Kankaanpaa, P., Salminen, S. and Ahokas, J. 1998. Physicochemical alterations enhance the ability of dairy starins of lactic acid bacteria to remove aflatoxin from contaminated media. J. Food protec. 61:466-468.

El-Hassan, S.M., Newbold, C.J. and Wallace, R.J. 1993. The effect of yeast culture on rumen fermentation: growth of the yeast in the rumen and requirement for viable yeast cells. Anim. Prod. 56:463.(Abstr.).

Erasmus, L.J. 1991. The importance of the duodenal amino acid profile for dairy cows and the impact of changes in these profiles following the use of Yea-sacc[1026]. Feed Compounder, 11:24-29.

Erasmus, L.J., Botha, P.M. and Kistner, A. 1992. Effect of yeast culture supplement on production, rumen fermentation and duodenal nitrogen flow in dairy cows. J. Dairy Sci. 75:3056.

Erdman, R.A. and Sharma, B.K. 1989. Effect of yeast culture and sodium bicarbonate on milk yield and composition in dairy cows. J. Dairy Sci. 72:1929-1932.

Fiems, L.O., Cottyn, B.G., Dussert, L. and Vanacker, J.M. 1993. Effect of a viable yeast culture on digestibility and rumen fermentation in sheep fed different types of diets. Reprod. Nutr. Dev. 33:43-49.

Food and Agricultural Organization of the United Nations (FAO). 2000. Statistical Databases.

Friend, B.A. and Shahani, K.M. 1984. Antitumour properties of lactobacilli and dairy products fermented by lactobacilli. J. Food Protec. 47:717-723.

Fuller, R. 1989. Probiotics in man and animals. Appl. Bacteriol. 66:365-378.

Fuller, R. and Brooker, B.E. 1974. Lactobacilli which attach to the crop epithelium of the fowl. American J. Clinical Nutri. 27:1305-1312.

Gedek, B. 1989. Interaktion zwischen lebeden Hefezellen und darmpathogen Escherichia coli keimen. In Okosystem Darm, Morphologie, Mikrobiologie, Immunologie, Muller, J., Ottenjann, R. and Seifert, J. (eds). Springer Verlag, pp. 135-139.

Gomez-Alarcon, R., Dubas, C. and Huber, J.T. 1987. Effect of Aspergillus oryzae (Amaferm) and yeast on feed utilization by Holstein cows. J. Dairy Sci. 70(Suppl.I):218.

Gomez-Alarcon, R.A., Dudas, C. and Huber, J.T. 1990. Influence of cultures of Aspergillus oryazae on rumen and total tract digestibility of dietary components. J. Dairy Sci. 73:703.

Greene, W.A., Gano, A.M., Smith, K.I., Hogan, J.S., Todhunter, D.A. 1991. Comparison of probiotic and antibiotic intramammary therapy of cattle with clinical mastitis. Bovine Practioner, 26:119-122.

Hancock, D.L., Brake, A.C., Montgomery, A.L., Dominey, J.R., Mattingly, C.A. and Cecava, M.J. 1994. Influence of yeast addition and compudose ® implantation on feeding performance and carcass characteristics of growing and finishing steers. J. Anim. Sci. Vol.72(Suppl.I)/J. Dairy Sci. Vol.77 (Suppl.I).

Harrison, G.A., Hemken, R.W., Dawson, K.A., Harmon, R.J., Newman, K.E. and Morehead, M.C. 1987. Yeast culture supplement in diets of lactating cows. II. Effects on liquid dilution rate and apparent digestibility. J. Dairy Sci. 70(Suppl.I):218.

Harrison, G.A., Hemken, R.W., Dawson, K.A., Harmon, R.J. and Barker, K.B. 1988. Influence of addition of yeast culture supplement to diets of lactating cows on ruminal fermentation and microbial populations. J. Dairy Sci. 71:2967-2975.

Hatch, R.C., Thomas, R.O., Thayne, W.V. 1973. Effect of adding Bacillus acidophilus to milk fed to baby calves. J. Dairy Sci. 56:682 (abstr.)

Higginbotham, G.E., Coller, C.A., Aseltine, M.S. and Bath, D.L. 1994. Effect of yeast culture and Aspergillus oryzae extract on milk yield in a commercial dairy herd. J. Dairy Sci. 77:343-348.

Hoyos, G., Garcia, L. and Medina, F. 1987. Effects of feeding viable microbial feed additives on performance of lactating cows in a large dairy herd. J. Dairy Sci. 70(Suppl.I):217.

Isolauri, E., Juntunen, M., Rautanen, T., Sillanaukee, P. and Vesikari, T. 1995. Improved immunogenicity of oral Dx RRV reassortant rotavirus vaccine by Lactobacillus casei GG. Vaccine 13:310-312.

Jaspers, D.A., Massey, L.K. and Luedecke, L.O. 1984. Effect of consuming yogurts prepared with 3 culture strains - on human serum lipoproteins. J. Food Sci. 49:1178-1181.

Kaup, S.M. 1988. Bioavailability of calcium on yoghurt and its relationship to the hypocholesterolemic properties of yoghurt. Disease Abstr. Int. B. 48:1959.

Kidder, D.E. and Manners, M.J. 1978. Conditions in the rumen. In. Digestion in the Pig. eds. Kidder, D.E. and Manners, M.J. Sciente Chnica, Bristol, pp. 33-46.

Kim, D.Y., Figueroa, M.R., Dawson, D.P., Batallas, C.E., Arambel, M.J. and Walters, J.L. 1992. Efficacy of supplemental viable yeast culture with or without Aspergillus oryzae on nutrient digestibility and milk production in early to mid-lactating dairy cows. J. Dairy Sci.75(Suppl.I):206.

Kmet, V., Flint, H.J. and Wallace, R.J. 1993. Probiotics and manupulation of rumen development and function. Archives Anim. Prod. 44:1-10.

Kung, Jr.L., Kreck, E.M., Tung, R.S., Hession, A.O., Sheperd, A.C., Cohen, M.A., Swain, H.E. and Leedle, J.A.Z. 1997. Effects of a live yeast culture and enzymes on in vitro ruminal fermentation and milk production of dairy cows. J. Dairy Sci. 80:2045-2051.

Line, J.E., Bailey, J.S., Cox, N.S., Stern, N.J. and Tompkins, T. 1998. Effect of yeast supplemented feed on Salmonella and Campylobactor populations in broilers. Poultry Sci. 77:405-410.

Marth, E.H. and Doyle, M.P. 1979. Update on molds; degradation of aflatoxin, Food Technol. Jan. 81-87.

Martin, S.A., Nisbet, D.J. and Dean, R.G. 1989. Influence of a commercial yeast supplement on the in vitro ruminal fermentation. Nutr. Rep. Int. 40:395.

Mason, V.C. and Just, A. 1976. Bacterial activity in the hind-gut of pigs. 1. Its influence on the apparent digestibility of dietary energy and fat. Z. Tierphysiol Tierernahr Futtermittelk 36:301-310.

Mathieu, F., Jouany, J.P., Senaud, J., Bohatier, J., Bertin, G. and Mercier, M. 1996. The effect of accharomyces cerevisiae and Aspergillus oryzae on fermentations in the rumen of faunated and defaunated sheep; protozoal and probiotic interactions. Reprod. Nutr. Dev. 36: 271-287.

McLeod, K.R., Karr, K.J., Dawson, K.A., Tucker, R.E. and Mitchell, Jr., G.E. 1990. Rumen fermentation and nitrogen flow in lambs receiving yeast culture and (or) monensin. J. Anim. Sci. (Suppl.1.1):73:266.

Metchnikoff, E. 1907. Prolongation of life. London, Heinemann. Miller, B.G., Phillips, A., Newby, T.J., Stokes, C.R. and Bourne, F.J. (1985). A transient hypersensitivity to dietary antigens in the early weaned pig:a factor in the aetiology of post weaned diarrhoea. Proc. 3rd Int. Seminar on Digestive Physiology of the Pig, Copenhagen, May, Nat. Inst. Anim. Sci., Denmark, pp.65-66.

Miller, B.G., Phillips, A., Newby, T.J., Stokes, C.R. and Bourne, F.J. 1985. A transient hypersensitivity to dietary antigens in the early weaned pig:a factor in the aetiology of post weaned diarrhoea. Proc. 3rd Int. Seminar on Digestive Physiology of the Pig, Copenhagen, May, Nat. Inst. Anim. Sci., Denmark, pp.65-66.

Miranda, R.L.A., Mendoza, M.G., Gonzalez, M.S. and Barcena, G.R. 1994. Effect of Saccharomyces cerevisiae and Aspergillus oryzae cultures and NDF level on ruminal fermentation. J. Anim. Sci. 72 (Suppl.I)/J. Dairy Sci. 77 (Suppl.I):299.

Moloney, A.P.and Drennan, M.J. 1994. The influence of the basal diet on the effects of yeast culture on ruminal fermentation and digestibility in steers. Anim. Feed Sci. and Technol. 50:55-73.

Muralidhara, K., Sheggeby, G.G., Elliker, P.R., England, D.C. and Sandine, W.E. 1977.Effect of feeding lactobacilli on the coliform and lactobacillus flora of intestinal tissues and faeces from pigs. J. Food Prot. 40:288-295.

Newbold, C.J., Williams, P.E.V., McKain, N., Walker, A. and Wallace, R.J. 1990. The effect of yeast culture on numbers and fermentation in the rumen of sheep. Proc. Nutr. Soc. 49:47A.

Newbold, C.J., Wallace, R.J., Chen, X.B. and Mclntosh, F.M. 1995. Different strains of Saccharomyces cerevisiae differ in their effects on ruminal bacterial numbers in vitro and in sheep. J. Anim. Sci. 73:1811-1818.

Newbold, C.J. 1996. Probiotics for ruminants. Ann. Zootech. 45: (suppl.) 329-335.

Nisbet, D.J. and Martin, S.A. 1991. Effect of a Saccharomyces cerevisiae culture on lactate utilization by the rumen bacterium Selenomonas ruminantium. J. Anim. Sci. 69:4628-4633.

Offer, N.W. 1990. Maximising fibre digestion in the rumen:The role of yeast culture. In: T.P.Lyons (Ed.). Biotech. in the feed Industry, 6th Animal Symposium, Alltech Technical Publication, Nicholasville, KY.

Orpin, C.G. and Joblin, K.N. 1988. The rumen anaerobic fungi. In The Rumen Microbial Ecosystem. Ed. P.N.Hobson. Elsevier Applied Science, London and New York, pp.129-150.

Parker, R.B. (1974). Probiotics, the other half of the antibiotics story. Anim. Nutri. Health. 29: 4-8.

Pollmann, D.S., Danielson, D.M. and Peo, E.R. 1980. Effects of microbial feed additives on performance of starter and growing finishing pigs. J. Anim. Sci. 51:577-581.

Putnam, D.E., Schwab, C.G., Socha, M.T., Whitehouse, N.L., Kierstead, N.A., Garthwaite, B.D. 1997. Effect of yeast culture in the diets of early lactation dairy cows on ruminal fermentation and passage of nitrogen fractions and amino acids to the small intestine. J. Dairy Sci. 80:374-384.

Raibaud, p. and Raynaud, J.P. 1991. Experimental data on the modes of action of pro-biotics. New trend in veal calf production. Proceedings of the International Symposium on veal calf production. Wageningen, Netherlands, 14-16 March 1990 [Edited by Metz, J.H.M., Groenestein, C.M.J., pp 269-275].

Rao, T.N., Rao, Z.P., Rama Prasad, J. and Prasad, P.E. 2003. Supplementation of probiotics on growth performance in sheep. Indian J. Anim. Nutr. 20:224-226.

Ratcliffe, B., Cole, C.B., Fuller, R. and Newport, M.J. 1985. The effect of yoghurt on performance and the gut microflora of baby pigs. Proc. Nutri. Soc. 44:88A.

Renner, E. (1991). Cultured dairy products in human nutrition. Bull. IDF, 255:1-24.

Rouzbehan, Y., Galbraith, H., Rooke, J.A. and Perrott, J.G. 1994. A note on the effects of dietary inclusion of lambs given diets containing unground pelleted molassed dried sugar-beet pulp and barley in various proportions. Anim. Prod. 59:147-150.

Saito, H., Tomioka, H.and Sato, K. 1981. Enhanced resistance of Lactobacillus against Listeria infection in mice. Med. and Biol. 102:273-277.

Schaafsma, G., Dekker, P.R. and deWaard, H. (1988). Nutritional aspects of yoghurt. II.Bioavailability of essential minerals and trace elements. Netherland Milk Dairy J. 42:135-146.

Shackelford, L.A.,Rao, D.R., Chawan, C.B. and Pulusani, S.R. 1983. Effect of feeding fermented milk on the incidence of chemically induced colon tumours in rats. Nutr. Cancer. 5: 159-164.

Sikes, A. and Hilton, T. 1987. Sensitivity of food brone bacteria (spoilage & pathogenic) to a methanol-acetone extract of milk fermented by Streptococcus thermophilus. J. Food Prot. 50:812-814.

Singh, K.K. and Karim, S.A. 2003. Emerging trends in meat production from sheep and its export potential. In: The Proceedings of Interaction Seminar on "Meat production and excport potential: Impact of globalization and quality concepts" organized at Central Institute for Research on Goats, Makhdoom, Farah, Mathura, UP (281 122). pp 51-59.

Slyter, L.L. 1976. Influence of acidosis on rumen function. J. Anim. Sci. 43:910.

Sohn, H.J. and Song, M.K. 1996. Effect of feeding yeast diets on the digestibility by sheep. Korean J. Anim. Sci. 38:578-588.

Szabo, J. 1979. Protein, carbohydrate and fat degrading enzymes in the intestine of germ free and conventional piglets. In: Clinical and Experimental Gnotobiotics. eds. Fliedner, T., Heit, H., Niethammer, D. and Pflienger, H., Gustav Fischer Verlag, Stuttgart, pp.125-128.

Teh, T.H., Sahlu, T., Escobar, E.N. and Cushaw, J.L. 1987. Effects of live yeast culture and sodium bicarbonate on lactating goats. J. Dairy Sci. 70(Suppl.1):200. (Abstr.).

Thomas, P.C. and Rook, A.F. 1981. In: W.Haresign and D.J.A.Cole (Ed.). Recent Developments in Animal Nutrition, pp. 157-183. Butterworths, U.K.

Thyagaraja, N. and Hosono, A. 1994. Binding properties of lactic acid bacteria from food borne mutagens. Food Chem. Toxicol. 32:805-809.

Wallace, R.J. and Newbold, C.J. 1992. Probiotics for ruminants. In: Scientific basis of the probiotic concept. (Ed. Fuller, R.), Chapman Hall, London.

Watson, R.T., Meira Filho, L.G., Sanhueza, E. and Janetos, T.1992. Sources and Sinks. In: Climate Change 1992. Houghton, J.T., Callander, B.A. and Van, S.K. (Eds), Cambridge : Cambridge University Press, pp 25-46.

Weidmeier, R.D., Arambel, M.J. and Walters, J.L. 1987. Effect of yeast culture and A. oryzae fermentation extract on ruminal characteristics and nutrient digestibility. J. Dairy Sci. 70:2063.

Williams, P.E.V. 1989. The mode of action of yeast culture in ruminant diets: A review of the effect on rumen fermentation patterns. Biotechnology in the feed industry. Proceedings of Alltech's fifth Annual Symposium (Ed. by Lyons,T.P.), pp.65-84, Nicholasville, USA. Alltech Technical Publications.

Williams, P.E.V., Walker, A. and MacRae, J.C. 1990. Rumen probiosis:The effects of addition of yeast culture (viable Yeast [S.cerevisiae] plus growth medium) on duodenal protein flow in wither sheep. Proc. Nutr. Soc. 49(2): 128A.

Williams, P.E.V. and Newbold, C.J. 1990. Rumen probiosis:The effects of novel microorganisms on rumen fermentation and ruminant productivity. In: W.Haresing and D.J.A.Cole (Ed.). Recent Advances in Animal Nutrition. Butterworths, London, pp. 211-227.

Williams, P.E.V., Tait, C.A.G., Innes, G.M. and Newbold, C.J. 1991. Effects of the inclusion of yeast culture (Saccharomyces cerevisiae plus growth medium) in the diet of dairy cows on milk yield and forage degradation and fermentation patterns in the rumen of steers. J. Anim. Sci. 69:3016-3026.

Wilson, K.H. and Perini, F. 1988. Role of competition for nutrients in suppression of Clostridium difficile by the colonic microflora. Infection and Immunity. 56:2610-2614.

Wohlt, J.E., Finkelstein, A.D. and Ghung, C.H. 1991. Yeast culture to improve intake, nutrient digestibility and performance by dairy cattle during early lactation. J. Dairy Sci.74: 1395-1400.

Wolin, M.J. and Miller, T.L. 1988. Microbe-microbe interactions. In: The Rumen Microbial Ecosystem (Ed. Hobson.P.N.) Elsevier Applied Science, London. UK. pp. 343-359.

Yoon, Y.H. and Byun, B.R. 2002. Antagonism against Helicobacter pylori and proteolysis of Lactobacillus helveticus CU 631 and strain identification. Asian-Aust. J. Anim. Sci. 15:1057-1065.

18
PROTECTION OF PROTEINS AND FATS

S. K. Sirohi ,T. K. Walli and S.K.Tomar

The feed shortage exist with regard to both protein as well as energy feeds. The problem is not only the feed availability, but also about the feed quality and the cost. Further, protein and energy density in the ration of dairy animals are low in developing countries, and hence are not able to meet the protein and energy requirements after calving, as DM intake during this period is low (NRC, 1989). This leads to substantial loss in body weight which adversely affects production and reproduction in dairy animals (Scott et al.,., 1995). To over come the problem of feed shortage, and to optimize nutrient supply to our bovine stock, no doubt, we have to generate newer feeds, but apart from that, we have to devise alternative technologies to increase nutrient supply through better utilization of existing and newer feeds. In this paper, two such nutritional technologies, i.e. by allowing ruminal escape of nutrients viz. bypass protein and bypass fat have been discussed, which may increase the efficiency of protein and energy utilization and also overcome the adverse effect of negative energy balance in dairy animals. The potential of these technologies for increasing the productivity of these animals has also been discussed.

BYPASS PROTEIN TECHNOLOGY

BACKGROUND

The discovery by Mc Donald (1954) that soluble dietary proteins are extensively degraded in to ammonia in the rumen and not utilize by microbes at the rate which they degraded. Subsequently the different studies revealed that proteins and amino acids administered post ruminally resulted in greater N retention as compared to when these are given directly in rumen led to attempts to find the ways and means of protecting soluble, high quality protein and limiting amino acids from microbial degradation within rumen.

Methods for Bypass protein

- Oesophageal groove Closure
- Post ruminal infusion

- Tannic acid treatment
- Formaldehyde Treatment
- Protection of amino acids
- Calcium salts of fatty acid coated proteins
- Heat Treatment

All the above mentioned methods for protecting proteins are used by different workers. The closure of oesophageal groove is a conditional reflex and is a normal function in young animals, but rarely occurs in mature animals. But some workers found that this can be activated by the presence of salts of copper, silver, zinc and sodium in the mouth which can use to supplement protein protecting from microbial digestion (Orskov and Benzie, 1969). Similarly proteins and amino acids are administered directly to duodenum or abomasum instead of being as a part of the protein. Tannic acid is also used by different workers to protect protein because tannins have greater affinity towards protein and forms complex which can only be solubilized in acidic pH (Hatfield, 1973). The main draw back of this treatment is that some condensed tannin protein complexes are not broken even in acidic pH. Chatterjee and Walli, 2003 treated protein meals directly with formalin. They found that treatment with formaldehyde at 1.2 g/100g CP is optimum for mustard and groundnut cake without any adverse effect on post ruminal digestibility of cake protein. After treating the cake with formalin, it is kept under air tight condition in polythene bags for few days. In this process, the amino group of proteins gets attached to aldehyde group of formaldehyde to form methylene bridges, which are resistant to ruminal pH, but get dissociated in the acidic pH of abomasum. Another approach for protection of amino acids gained importance after methionine is recognized as a first limiting amino acid for wool growth, body weight gain and milk production. Then subsequent interest developed in protecting lysine when it was discovered to be the second limiting amino acid for growing cattle and lactating cattle. The most commonly used procedures include lipid protected product, carbohydrate surface coated product, lipid/pH –sensitive polymer coated product and use of analogs and derivatives of methionine. In lipid protected product matrix of DL-methionine coated with calcium salts of long chain fatty acids, lauric acid and butylated hydroxytoluene (BHT) are important. BHT is used as a preservative for fatty acid and this product contains about 65 % methionine. Carbohydrate surface coated methionine is produced in the form of pellets. Pellets in core contain DL methionine and are starch coated with several thin layers of ethyl cellulose and stearic acid. The final product contains a minimum of 85 % methionine, 8.5 % non structural carbohydrates, 1.5% ash and 0.5% crude fat with some little moisture content.

A lipid/pH-sensitive polymer coated methionine contains about 75 % DL-methionine. These are also pellets consist of a core DL-met plus ethyl cellulose which is covered with a coat of stearic acid containing droplets of poly(2-vinylpyridine-co-styrene).Other approach in ruminants is the use of analogs and methionine derivatives. Amino acid (AA) derivatives are free AA to which a chemical blocking group has been added to the alpha –amino group or in the acyl group has identified. Common examples are isopropyl-DL-met, t-butyl-DL-met, N-stearoyl-DL-met and capryl-caproylic-DL-met. The extent of ruminal bypass is greater in longer chain alkyl ester rather than shorter. Amino acid analogs are produced from the substitution of an alpha –amino group of the AA with an on-nitrogenous group such as a hydroxyl group. The most studied AA analog is met hydroxy analog 2-hydroxyl-4-methylthio butanoic acid (HMB).Sklan and Tinsky (1993) used calcium salts of long chain fatty acids to coat meal protein in different cakes. In physical treatment several workers used heat treatment to increase the bypass value (Deacon et al., 1988). Heat treatment is combination of time and heat which decreases the rumen solubility of proteins by creating crosslinkages both within or among peptides chain and to carbohydrates. However, high temperature for long time renders protein less digestible due to Maillard reaction between sugar aldehyde and free amino groups. Jet sploding and extrusion methods are commonly used by workers. In Jet sploding high temperature (315degree centigrade) is given for short period while in extrusion heat is given along with steam. Among technologies formaldehyde treatment and encapsulated protected protein seems too useful and feasible in our conditions. In our country lot of work has been carried out on formaldehyde treatment technology and this technology has proved its beneficial role in dairy animals even at low production level. However feeding of encapsulated amino acid in dairy animals is new area which needs more research in our condition.

Performance of Animals on Protected Proteins

Trials were conducted in India by different workers revealed better growth and lactation performance by animals. A significant increase in growth rate was reported by Mudgal (1979), Gupta and Walli (1987), Kumar and Walli (1994); Tiwari and Yadav (1994), Chatterjee & Walli (2003) on feeding of formaldehyde treated GN cake and/or mustard cake in goats and crossbred cows. Increase in growth rate reported as high as 25-30 percent in comparison to control diet. Lactation studies were also carried out in dairy animals to see the effect of formaldehyde treated cake on milk production by different workers. Sampath et al., (1997) reported significantly higher FCM yield in lactating crossbred cows fed formaldehyde treated GN cake (7.8 vs 9.4 kg/d). Similar trend was reported Garg et al., (2003) and Chatterjee & Walli (2003) in crossbred cows and buffaloes by and Sahoo and Walli (2002) in Goats. Recently a trial conducted under NDRI/NDDB collaborative project on feeding of formaldehyde treated mustard cake showed 15% increase in milk production over control in crossbred cows(Walli and Sirohi 2004a).In another trial on feeding of roasted soybean to crossbred cows under NDRI/ American Soybean Association collaborative project also shown increased milk production to the tune of about 10% (Walli and Sirohi 2004b).Some trials were conducted on extrusion technology by Yugandharkumar et al.,, (1994) to reduce the protein degradability in GN cake, Soybean meal and Sunflower cake.

Benefits of protein protection

- Utilization of low quality protein can appreciably improved
- Higher the UDP, higher is the availability of intact amino acids
- More amino acid flux is available for tissue protein synthesis
- Increased flow of NAN at abomasum
- Increased efficiency of N utilization and N balance
- Increased growth rate and feed conversion efficiency
- Net nutritional value of particular dietary protein can be increased

BYPASS FAT TECHNOLOGY

Background

The genetically superior cows and buffaloes with respect to milk production require better inputs, especially the nutrients supplying energy and protein precursors, in order to exploit their potential fully with regard to milk production. In the developing countries, the energy density of the rations generally fed to high yielding dairy animals is lower than actually required, as fibrous crop residues also constitute part of their diet. Hence, these diets are unable to meet the energy requirement of such animals, since we can't over feed the animals with such types of feeds, because of the limitations of the DM consumption. The feeding of rations having lower energy content can adversely affect the productive and reproductive performance of these animals.

Adding fat to dairy rations can affect productive efficiency of dairy cows through a combination of caloric and non caloric effects. Caloric effects are attributable to greater energy content and energetic efficiency for lipid compared to carbohydrate or protein with the overall benefit being increased milk production. Non caloric effects are caused by benefits from added fat that are not directly attributable to its energy content or increased milk production. Examples of non caloric effects include improved reproductive performance, and altered fatty acid profile of milk. Non caloric benefits related to milk quality.

Dietary fats ingested by the animals are hydrolysed in rumen to glycerol and fatty acids. While the glycerol is fermented to propionic acid, the unsaturated fatty acids are either partially or completely biohydrogenated to increase the quantity of saturated fatty acids leaving rumen. Inclusion of fat in the diet can increase its energy density, because the energy value fat is 2.25 times higher than carbohydrate or protein. But inclusion of unprotected fat in the ration of ruminants is not recommended, for the simple reason that this fat causes inhibition of rumen fermentation, especially, the cellulose fermentation, which is the most important activity of rumen microbes. Also, the higher level of fat in the diet could prove toxic to rumen microbes. This ultimately results in lower DM intake and lower milk production by the animals (Palmquist and Jenkins, 1980). The level of unprotected fat in the total diet should not exceed 4% (Palmquist, 1988).

This problem can however be easily overcome by feeding protected lipids to ruminants. By protecting the lipids using some physical or chemical agents, these lipids do not under go lipid hydrolysis or bio-hydrogenation in rumen, but bypass rumen and digested in the lower tract. Feeding of protected lipids to dairy animals increase the energy density of the diet without compromising fibre digestion in rumen (Scott et al.,, 1995). Apart from increasing the energy intake of the animals, there is an added advantage of feeding protected unsaturated fat to cows, as the milk produced by such cows shall have higher unsaturated fatty acids in milk fat, which makes a softer butter, and is also safer for humans, especially the heart patients. Bypass rumen fat can be supplemented to get designer milk with higher content of long chain unsaturated fatty acids for human beings (Gulati et al.,, 2001).

The Technology:

Fats can be protected from ruminal biohydrogenation by several ways:

i. Encapsulation with formaldehyde of protein-fat complex in crushed oilseeds by formaldehyde. This method did not prove to be that effective. Hence, an alternative method of protecting the dietary fatty acids from ruminal degradation and hydrogenation was proposed, based on the

ii. Conversion of fatty acids into Ca- salt of fatty acids.

iii. Prilled fatty acids, in which saturated fatty acids are liquefied and spraying the mixture of fatty acids under pressure into a cooled atmosphere , resulting in dried Prilled fatty acids , which are inert in rumen

iv. Fatty acyl amides are known to be resistant to ruminal biohydrogenation.

v. Crystalline fat is generally made up of saturated fatty acids; these do not melt at rumen temperature and thus, are resistant to ruminal hydrolysis.

vi. PUFA fed in small quantity may get hydrogenated and try to remove hydrogen ions from rumen, so that, the extra fat given later, is not subjected to biohydrogenation.

Out of all these methods, the calcium salt of fatty acids is the most commonly used method, as the method may be cheaper and more effective. Generally, two methods are used for the production of calcium salt of fatty acids, viz. Fusion Method and Double Decomposition Method.

(a) Fusion method

In this method, oils and fatty acids are heated with Calcium oxide or Calcium hydroxide in the presence of catalyst, in a closed vessel at a required temperature and pressure. Water produced in reaction and the added water is driven off as steam and the resulting product is a hard mass of calcium saponified salts or bypass fat.

(b) Double decomposition method

This method requires heating of the known quantity of fat supplement in metal container, followed by addition of an alkali (aqueous sodium hydroxide solution) in the melted fatty matter with constant stirring till the fatty acids are dissolved completely. After saponification, the heating is stopped. While the contents are still warm, calcium chloride solution is added slowly to the water soluble sodium soap with constant stirring, which ultimately causes precipitation of calcium soaps. Excess water is then removed by filtration. The calcium-soap is dried at low temperature and the lumps are broken and ground, to be used as bypass fat.

At present, India is importing protected fat or may be some industries have hooked up with some foreign firms for the manufacture of this product. However, the indigenous methodologies for the protection of fat and the development and scaling of the technologies are being tried at many research centers in the country, including NDRI, Karnal. Different byproducts from edible/non-edible oil industries and other unconventional oil supplements have been tried, for the protection of their fat and for the preparation of bypass fat by the above two methods. The purpose of trying to make use of non-conventional and non edible fat sources is to make the technology of bypass fat commercially viable and cost effective.

Effect of Feeding Protected fat

(a) Rumen studies and nutrient digestibilities :

Results of an in vitro trial on various oil supplements viz. Karanj oil, Kusum oil, Palm fatty acid(PFA), Mahaua oil , Acid oil(A.O) and Soapstock (S.S), converted into inert fat, showed that at 5% level of supplementation DMD was at par with control diet (wheat straw and concentrate in a ratio 60 : 40). However at 10 % level, values decreased slightly (Sirohi et al.,, 2002). However, Reddy et al., (2001) reported that in vitro DM digestibility and in Sacco DM disappearance were not adversely affected by inclusion of calcium soap of palm oil even up to 15% level in sheep ration. The in vivo trial, using rumen fistulated buffaloes, supplemented with A.O, S.S, PFA and Karanj oil indicated that protected fat can be included in the ration upto 7 percent without affecting the rumen fermentation parameter like TVFAs , NH3-N, TCA-N and Total-N and nutrient digestibilities (Sirohi et al., 2002). Similarly, Elliot et al.,, (1996) did not observe any effect of feeding Prilled fat or and calcium salt of fatty acids on rumen fermentation characteristics or nutrient digestibility.

Several workers have reported that dry matter intake; total tract digestibility of DM and other nutrients remains unaltered on feeding of bypass fat supplements to dairy animals (Schauff and Clark 1989; King et al.,, 1990; Elliot et al.,; 1996 and Avilla et al.,, 2000).

(b) Effect on Milk Yield and Milk Composition:

With regard to feeding of protected fat supplements to dairy animals, several workers have observed that milk yield as well as milk fat is enhanced (Herman son, 1989; East ridge and Firkins, 1991).Savoini, et al., (1992) found though there was an increase in milk yield, there was a decrease in fat, protein and intermediate chain fatty acids content in milk, on feeding calcium soaps of fatty acids to dairy cows. Klein et al.,. (1989) observed that milk fat content was not affected by crystalline supplementation. But there was a significant decrease of C8- C16 fatty acids while stearic acid and oleic acids increased. The decrease in milk protein content was also observed by Fellin et al.,, (1989) and Lebzien et al., (1992) on feeding of protected fat to dairy cows. Both these groups of workers observed increase in milk yield, but while Fellin et al., (1989) found increase in fat content also, Lebzien did not observe any change in fat content of milk.

Studies carried out by Garg and Mehta (1998a,b,c) and Mishra and Thakur (1999) on lactating dairy animals showed that milk yield and milk fat content significantly increased by feeding protected fat supplements to these animals. Sarwar et al (2003) studied the effect of feeding saturated fat on milk production and composition in crossbred dairy cows in early lactation in Pakistan. The diets containing 2.5, 3.5 and 4.5 % bypass fat caused significant increase in 4 % FCM yield of these animals. Purshothaman (2004) found significant increase in 4 % FCM yield in cross bred cows fed calcium salts of palm fatty acids, when the protected fat supplement was given at 4% level over concentrate mixture. There was also a substantial increase in the unsaturated fatty acids viz. oleic, linoleic and linolenic acid. Bisen (2004) found significant increase in milk yield and FCM yield in lactating goats fed calcium salts of fatty acids. The above author also observed increase in milk fat, but there was no change in milk protein, although there was a decrease in some intermediate chain fatty acids in milk fat.

(b) Effect on reproduction

Feeding of bypass fat has been shown to have another beneficial effect, as it also increases the reproduction efficiency. Several hypothesis have been put forth to explain the positive effect of protected fat on reproductive performance of the animals. The direct effect could be that the supplementation of bypass fat could reduce the detrimental effects of negative energy balance, which would increase both lactation as well as reproductive performance. Improved energy balance could result in an earlier return to postpartum ovarian cyclicity (Palmquist and Jenkins, 1980).Since the feeding of bypass fat invariably results in increased blood cholesterol concentration, it in turn, increases the plasma progesterone concentration, which can improve the fertility of the cow (Staples et al., 1998). Supplemental fat also improving the fertility through the reduction in PGF 2a and /or by modifying circulating concentration of insulin, GH and enhance the synthesis of IGF-1 in ovarian cell (Williams and Stanko, 1999).

Benefits of Fat protection

- Positive energy balance during early stage of lactation
- Ketosis can be prevented in lactating animals
- Increase in milk production and FCM yield
- To alter the fatty acid composition of milk and meat
- For increasing the supply of essential fatty acid
- Increasing the flow of unsaturated fatty acid at the duodenum
- Improved reproduction efficiency

Bypass protein technology and the feeding of protected fat certainly has relevance under our situations as the diet are generally low in energy content and it is not possible to meet the energy and protein requirement of high yielding animals as such. However, the technology needs to be commercialized for taking the benefits of protected nutrients.

Bibliography

Bisen, D.K (1994) Production response of lactating goats fed calcium soaps of long chain fatty acids protected protein supplemented diets. M.V.Sc Thesis, NDRI Deemed Univ., Karnal

Chatterjee, A and Walli, T.K. (2003). Economics of feeding formaldehyde treated mustard cake as bypass protein to growing calves. Indian J. Dairy Sci. 56(4):241-244

Deacon, M.A, DeBoar, G and Kennelly, J.J (1988) Influence of jet spolding and extrusion on ruminal and intestinal disappearance of canola and soybeans. J. Dairy Sci. 71(3):745

Eastridge, M.L and Firkens, J.L (1991) Feeding hydrogenated fatty acids and triglycerides to lactating dairy cows. J. Dairy Sci. 74:2610-2616

Elliott, J.P., Drackly, J.K. and Weigel, D.J (1996) J. Dairy Science 76(6): 1031-1039

Fellin, A., Barcarolo, R., Tutta, C., Tapparo, F and Tapparo, M (1989) Changes in milk composition of milk fat after feeding fats to cows. Scienza-e-tecnica-lattiero-casearia. 40 (4):288-298

Ferguson, K.A., Hemsley, J.A. & Reis, P.J. (1967). Aust. J. Sci., 30: 215.

Garg, M .R. and Mehta, A.K. (1998b). Effect of feeding bypass fat on feed intake, milk production and body condition of Holstein Friesian cows. Indian J. Anim. nutr., 15 (4): 242.

Garg, M. R.; Sherasia, P.L.; Bhanderi, B.M.; Gulati; S.K. and Scott, W. T. (2003). Effect of feeding rumen protected protein on milk production in lactating cows. Indian J. Dairy Sci. 56(4): 218-222.

Garg, M.R. and Mehta, A.K. (1998a). Effect of feeding bypass fat on feed intake milk production and body metabolism and composition of lipids in the rumen of sheep. J. Agri. Sci., (Camb), 101:97.

Garg, M.R. and Mehta, A.K. (1998c). Effect of feeding bypass fat on feed intake, milk production and body condition of Holstein Friesian cows. Indian J. Anim. Snutr., 15(4): 242.

Gulati, S.K, Ryde, I, Kaur, R, Scott, T.W, Garg, M.L, Sherasia, P.L and Singh, D.K (2001) Role of protected nutrients in sustainable milk production. In "Proc. of Anim. NutritionConf..Nov.9-11, 2001

Gupta, H.K and Walli, T.K (1987) Indian J Anim.Nutr.4:94-99

Hatfield, E.E (1973) Treating proteins with tannins and aldehydes.page171 in Effect of processing on the nutritive value of feeds. Nat. Acad. Sci., Washington DC

Hermanson, J.E (1989) Feed intake, milk yield and milk composition by replacing unprotected fat Ca soaps for dairy cows. Anim. Feed Sci. and Technology, 22 (3):193-203

Jakhmola, R. C. and Mishra, R. K. (2000) Feeding strategies using unconventional feeds. Proc. III Biennial Conf. ANA on Livestock feeding new millennium. HAU, Hisar.

King, K.R, Stock dale, C.R and Trigg, T.E (1990) the effect of blend of dietary unestrified and saturated long chain fatty acids on the performance of dairy cows in mid lactation. Aust. J. Agric. Research 41:129-139

Klein, F., Giesecke, D., Propstmeice, G and Burg Staller, G (1989) Crystalline fat in rations for high yielding dairy cows in early lactation. Effect on fatty acid pattern of milk fat. Zuchtungskunde 61(2):131-140

Kumar, V and Walli, T.K (1994) Effect of feeding urea treated wheat straw supplemented with HCHO treated GN cakes on growth performance of crossbred calves.Indian J. Anim.Nutr. 4:29-33

Lebzien, P., Daenicke, R., Rohr, K (1992) Effect of Ca soap of palm oil fatty acids on milk yield and milk composition. Iandbauforschung-velkenrode 42 (2): 85-88

McDonald, I.W (1954) the extent of conversion of food protein to microbial protein in the rumen of sheep. Biochem.J. 67:400

Mishra, S and Thakur, S.S (1999) Effect of feeding protected mustard oil on rumen fermentation, milk production and milk fat composition in dairy cattle. Ph.D. Thesis NDRI Deemed univ., Karnal

Mudgal, V.D and Senger, S.S (1980) Effect of feeding protected and unprotected protein on growth rate and and body composition in goats. J. Nuclear Agric. & Biol. 9:19

Oke, B.O and Loerch, S.C (1989) J. Anim. Science (Supp.1) : 67:538

Orskov E R & Benzie D (1969). Studies on the oesophageal groove to prevent the fermentation of food in the rumen. British Journal of Nutrition 23:415-420

Palmquist, D.L (1988) The feeding value of fats . In Feed Science, (Eds) E.R. Orskov , Elsevier Publ., Amsterdam, The Netherlands pp: 293a

Palmquist, D.L and Jenkins, T.C (1980) Fat in lactation ration Review, J. Dairy Sci. 63 : 1

Reddy, Y.R, Krishna, N and Rao, E.R (2001) In vitro and in sacco evaluation of rations supplemented with varying levels of dietary bypass fat in sheep. Indian J. of Anim. Nutr.18(3):243-247

Sahoo,B and Walli,T.K (2002). Comparative nutrient utilization ,productive performance and feed efficiency of lactating goats fed on low and high bypass protein supplemented with or without molasses as energy source.Proc. of IV Bienniel ANA conference held at WBUA&F.Sci., Kolkata,Nov.22-24,2002 pp: 169.

Sampath,K.T, Prasad,C.S, Ramchandra,K.S, Sundareshan,K and Subarao,A (1997) Effect of feeding undegraded dietary protein on milk production of crossbred cows.Indian J. Anim.Sci. 67(8):706

Sarwar, M., Sohaib, A., Khan, M.A and Mahr- Us-Nisha (2003) Asian Aust. J. of Anim. Science 16 (2) :204-210

Savoini, G, Polidori, F, Dell-Orto,V, Lanzani, A., Bondiolli, P and Fedeli, E (1992) Calcium soaps and free fatty acids in dairy cow nutrition, effects on milk yield and yuality. World Review of Animal Production 27(2):43.49

Schauff, D.J and Clark, J.H (1989) J. Dairy Science, 72 : 917

Scott, T.A., Shaver, R.D., Zepda , L., Yandell, B and Smith, T.R (1995) J. Dairy Sci. 78: 2435-2451

Sirohi, S.K , Walli, T.K, Thakur, S.S and Malik Raman (2002) Development and evaluation of technology for fat protection from unconventional resources. NDRI Annual Report pp:18

Sklan, D. and Tinsky, M. (1993). Production and reproduction response by dairy cows fed varying undegradable protein coated with rumen bypass fat. J. Dairy Sci., 76: 216-223

Staples, C.R., Burke, J.M and Thatcher, W.W (1998) Influence of supplemental fats on reproductive tissues and performance of dairy cows. J. Anim. Science 81 : 856-871

Tiwari,D.P and Yadav, I.S (1994) Effect on growth ,nutrient utilization and blood metabolites in buffalo calves fed ration containing HCHO treated cake. Indian J. Anim. Sci.64(6):625

Walli, T.K and Sirohi, S.K (2004a) Evaluation of heat treated (Roasted) soybean on lactating crossbred cows. Project report :NDRI/American Soybean Association Collaborative Project, NDRI, Karnal.

Walli, T.K and Sirohi, S.K (2004b). Evaluation of formaldehyde treated rapeseed meal with respect to enhancement in milk production in crossbred cows. Project report: NDRI/ NDDB Collaborative project, NDRI,Karnal

Williams, G.L and Stanko, R.L (1999) Dietary fat as reproductive nutraceuticals in beef cattle. In proceedings of the American Society of Animal Science pp:1-12

YugandharKumar, M , Ramaprasad,J and Krishna,N (1994) Effect of heat, formaldehyde or extrusion cooking on rumen protein degradability of rapidly degradable supplements in crossbred cattle. Indian J. Dairy Sci. 47:459

19
UMMB SUPPLEMENT TO STRAW BASED DIET

M.R. Garg and B.M. Bhanderi

India has the largest population of cattle and buffalo in the world and ranks number one in milk production. The country produces about 90 million tonnes of milk per annum with an annual per capita consumption of 240 g/day. Growth in milk production has been about 4 percent. Indian milk production comes from buffalo milk (approx. 54 percent), cow milk (approx. 42 percent) and the balance (4 percent) is from small ruminants (sheep and goats). The basis for Indian milk production is the millions of non-descript cows and buffaloes in rural areas, fed mainly on crop residues and agro-industrial by-products. The mainstay of the feeding system in India is fibrous feed (straws and stovers), which forms the bulk of ruminant diets. These fibrous feeds are deficient in protein, energy and minerals, with poor palatability and digestibility, but have the advantage that the ruminants thriving on these feeds do not compete with the human food. The low quality of these fibrous feeds coupled with the non-availability of protein meals or their availability at a very high cost in developing countries, lead to the use of non-protein-nitrogen sources such as urea for overcoming the deficiency of nitrogen in fibrous feeds, thus enhancing their digestibility, intake and nutrient availability through optimisation of rumen fermentation (Makkar, 2003). The availability of grains as energy supplements is limited and if available, major quantity of grains is used for feeding monogastric animals, mainly poultry.

Leave aside production, such low quality feeds without additional supplements cannot support even body maintenance of the animals. One of the methods of increasing utilization of straws and stovers is the supplementation of deficient nutrients in the form of fermentable N, energy and minerals, ensuring thereby enhanced microbial growth in the rumen, which in turn enables the ruminants to consume more straw (Garg et al., 2003). Several workers have shown increased intake or digestibility, or both, when the straw is supplemented with urea, molasses and minerals (Pathak and Ranjhan, 1976; McLennan et al., 1981). Spraying these additives on the straw is not a viable option due to the risk of urea toxicity and problems of distribution, handling and storage of molasses under field conditions. Various treatments-physical, chemical, physiochemical and biological have also been tried to improve intake and utilization of nutrients from poor quality roughages. Physical-wafering, chopping, grinding, milling, steaming under pressure, irradiation, soaking, boiling, etc. and chemical treatments - alkali, ammonia, acids and gases - to break down lignocellulosic compound have been tried, but with variable success. All these treatments have some or the other drawback. Improper use may lead to accidents and cause severe economic loss, especially in the case of urea. An excessive amount of urea or faulty treatment of roughages treated with it may harm, or even kill animals due to ammonia toxicity. To obtain appropriate use of urea, various methods have been tried worldwide.

The problem of feeding urea to animals has been overcome in India to certain extent by the introduction of urea and molasses based feed supplements in the form of urea-molasses mineral block (UMMB) licks, developed by the National Dairy Development Board (NDDB), Anand, India (Kunju, 1986a,b). Several researchers had previously reported the usefulness of UMMB licks for supplementing crop residue-based diets for large and small ruminants (Leng, 1983; Sansoucy, 1986, 1995). The slow ingestion of urea provided through such licks ensures its efficient, non-toxic utilization. However, the formulation, packaging and feeding of UMMB licks required critical attention, to ensure their regular and proper use by the farmers.

NDDB first introduced UMMBs to farmers in the year 1983, when they were prepared by using a "hot process" technique. However, because of the high cost of the production process and its inefficiency, these licks were not very popular with farmers. This was exacerbated by cost increase, which resulted in a rise from Rs. 5 to Rs. 20 for a 3 kg block between 1983 and 1994.This stimulated further research and development work to improve the production technology. This paper describes some of the benefits of using UMMBs and gives a brief introductory description of the "hot process" used for UMMB production. It then summarizes the research undertaken at NDDB for standardizing the formulation of UMMBs and for developing means for their large-scale production by the "cold process". It also deals with UMMB packaging, quality control and long-term storage, and examines the licking behaviour of animals presented with these blocks under field conditions.

PRODUCTION ASPECTS OF UMMB TECHNOLOGY

Acceptance of any product greatly depends upon its manufacturing process, cost of production, shelf life, convenience of use, etc. Various problems in production were encountered when UMMB technology was first introduced, affecting acceptance by farmers. NDDB spent a substantial amount of time and money in standardizing UMMB production technology, to ensure that the product is in presentable form. For the benefit of institutions and individuals engaged in the production of UMMB, experiences with UMMB production at different times and stages is described below:

The hot process

The ingredients used for the production of blocks by the hot process are given in Table 1. These were produced by steam heating molasses mixed with other ingredients, in a double-jacketed insulated vessel. After heating for 150 to 180 minutes at 130°C, the material was removed from the vessel, weighed in aliquots of 3 kg, put into moulds and allowed to harden. Although these hot process blocks were distributed to farmers for nearly ten years, they were never used regularly. This was probably due to inefficient extension and marketing, coupled with costs, which quadrupled between 1983 and 1993, in contrast to the price of feed concentrates, which only doubled over the same period.

Other related problems included the high cost of plant maintenance and fuel, unreliable equipment with frequent breakdowns, high labour demands and the difficulties of manually weighing the hot material. The blocks were also highly hygroscopic: at 60 percent relative humidity, blocks would deliquesce in storage and form a liquid mass.

Table 1. Composition of hot process blocks

Ingredients	Percentage
Urea	15
Molasses	45
Mineral mixture	10
Calcite powder	8
Sodium bentonite	3
Cottonseed meal	15
Common salt	4

Source: Garg et al., 1998.

The cold process formulation

As an alternative to steam heating the ingredients, adding gelling agents such as calcium and magnesium oxide, calcium hydroxide, cement, di-ammonium phosphate etc. helps to solidify the block material (Sansoucy, 1986; Sansoucy et al., 1988; Tiwari et al., 1990). This technique is referred to as the "cold process".

Initially, four formulations were tried by incorporating minor changes in ingredients suggested by Sansoucy (1986). Molasses, to which common salt and urea were added, was mixed in a vertical mixer for five minutes, after which calcium oxide was added and the ingredients were mixed thoroughly for a further ten minutes. The material was then transferred to the moulds to solidify overnight. After storage for one week, the blocks were offered to animals that were fed a crop-residue-based diet. Each animal licked 250 to 350 g of block per day. Encouraged by these observations, the evaluation of UMMB licks was extended to cooperative dairies. However, it was noted that by four to six weeks after production the blocks had become very hard and were only licked sporadically. The production of blocks using this formulation was thus discontinued.

To overcome this hardness problem, the proportion of bran was increased to 30 percent and calcium oxide was reduced to 6 percent during winter (maximum temperature, 22°C; minimum temperature, 8°C; relative humidity, 40 to 60 percent). Based on temperature and humidity data, formulations for summer, winter and rainy seasons were standardized. Blocks were produced in different seasons using the respective formulation and stored for four weeks before being fed to animals in the different agro-climatic zones.

After conducting rumen studies, feeding trials on growing and lactating animals were conducted for four to six weeks under controlled conditions at various farms where the level of animal production was medium to high. Before distribution of the product, farmers were given an explanation and demonstration of its use. Different animals were selected at random in various villages. Initial and final milk yield and fat yield were recorded after two weeks of preliminary feeding. Results of some of these field trials are shown in Table 2. Increased straw intake and fat yield were reported by most of the farmers. It was observed in field trials that the animals licked the blocks in sizable quantities, depending on the composition of their basal diet. In general, each 3 kg block lasted for one week per animal.

Following the farm trials, block licks were offered to individually kept village animals in different areas, and the level of acceptance ranged from 30 to 60 percent. It was felt that some of the village animals, because of their low to medium levels of production and access to sufficient green forage (e.g. lucerne), might not be tempted to lick the UMMB.

It appeared that the animals' poor acceptance of the blocks could be due to high pH and an unpleasant taste. The pH was between 10.5 and 11.5 when the level of calcium oxide was between 6 and 7 percent. In view of this, further investigations were carried out to vary and improve block formulation. By using various organic acids – citric, tartaric, boric, etc. it was possible to reduce the pH from 11.5 to 8.5, but the cost was prohibitive. Phosphoric acid also reduced the pH when incorporated at greater than 2 percent in the formulation, but it affected the solidification of blocks, especially during summer. When the blocks were too soft, they were licked rapidly and had to be removed to avoid urea intoxication in the animals.

Table 2. The observations on response of feeding UMMB lick in villages

S. No.	Village	CF (kg/d)	UMMB (g/d)	Milk yield (kg/d) Pre-lick	Milk yield (kg/d) With lick	Fat (g/day) Pre-lick	Fat (g/day) With lick
1.	Alwa	2.0	410	4.8	5.9	330	450
2.	Punadhara	2.0	352	4.0	4.8	270	340
3.	Fulgenamuwada	1.0	382	2.4	3.5	160	280
4.	Hirapura	2.0	300	4.2	5.2	350	480
5.	Bamroli	2.0	320	3.6	4.2	270	380
6.	Dehgam	2.0	285	4.3	4.7	310	350

Source: Kunju, P.J.G. (1988)

On studying the reaction of different gelling agents with molasses, it was felt that the gelling action of calcium oxide involved two steps. First, its reaction with moisture from the molasses, and, second, its reaction with the carboxylic group of organic acids present in molasses (predominantly aconitic acid). Apparently, the latter reaction was primarily responsible for block solidification.

Based on the above observations, moisture content in the moisture-contributing ingredients (molasses, urea, salt, etc.) was partially bound by brans, clays and mineral mixture at the first mixing and calcium oxide was added later. A smaller amount of calcium oxide was then required for solidification. By using guar meal powder along with the brans and clays, it was possible to reduce the proportion of calcium oxide to 4 percent. Subsequently, the pH was brought down to between 7.5 and 8.0 by adding phosphoric acid and sodium di-hydrogen phosphate. Using the latter two ingredients, several other formulations were developed that had pH of between 7.5 and 8.0. The blocks produced in this way were readily licked by 95 percent of village animals in Gujarat, Rajasthan and Karnataka. At present, UMMB licks are manufactured without using guar gums. Instead, calcium and magnesium oxides are added in the formulation at 4 and 2 percent, respectively. At the end, phosphate buffer is added to bring the pH down to between 8 and 8.5 (Table 3).

Table 3. Composition of cold process UMMB formulation

Ingredients	Percentage
Urea	6
Molasses	45
Mineral mixture	6
Deoiled rice bran	14
Rice polish fine	13
Calcite oxide	4
Magnesium oxide	2
Phosphate buffer	10

MANUFACTURING OF UREA MOLASSES MINERAL BLOCKS

NDDB, in association with an industry partner, has developed a device for manufacturing UMMBs that is capable of mixing the ingredients thoroughly and efficiently. It is mobile and comprises a 300-litre stainless steel vessel with a diameter of 150 cm. It has a rotor in the centre on which specially designed scrapers and mixing worms are fixed at an angle to ensure thorough mixing of the materials (Garg et al., 1998). The speed of the rotor can be adjusted to suit the scale of operations. A sliding door is provided at the bottom of the vessel. After mixing, the material is discharged into a stainless steel tray for transfer into moulds or a pressing device. Using this method, it is possible to produce approximately 500 blocks in one eight-hour shift. In view of its mixing efficiency, micronutrients, deworming agent and vitamins may also be added as desired.

A pressing device for UMMB licks

Originally, the UMMB mixture was filled into moulds or egg crates and left overnight to solidify. To produce 500 blocks per day required 500 moulds, at a cost of approximately Rs. 250 000. To reduce this cost, a rotary, pneumatically controlled pressing device was developed, that costs approximately Rs. 200 000. After mixing, the material is weighed in aliquots of 3 kg and pressed in a rectangular stainless steel die. The blocks pressed in this manner maintain their shape and solidify without the need for moulds or egg crates.

Packaging of Blocks

Since block licks are hygroscopic, proper packaging is very important and should be moisture proof to maintain the quality of the blocks. Bags made of different materials were evaluated; they included polythene sheet, multifilm (low density/high density), PET laminated film (aluminium foil/PET film/polythene sheet) and high molecular weight high-density (HMHD) sheet. Considering their cost, sturdiness and impermeability, HMHD bags were found to be the most suitable.

A WOODEN DISPENSER FOR UMMB LICKING

Since most of the animals in developing countries are underfed, they tend to bite blocks, which might lead to over-ingestion and result in inefficient utilization or urea toxicity. To avoid this problem, a specially designed wooden dispenser has been developed for this product to facilitate licking. It can be kept in front of the animals or fixed on the wall of mangers at a convenient point for easy access by the animal. Since the product is in the form of a hard block and the biological system of the animal helps in regulating the intake, no case has so far been reported of urea toxicity under farm or field conditions, in spite of its wide use in different States. At present, for manufacturing UMMBs by the cold process, ten commercial plants in the dairy cooperative sector and two in the private sector have been established in different states. Annual production has been between 300 000 to 400 000 UMMBs of 3-kg each.

EFFECT OF UMMB FEEDING ON DRY MATTER INTAKE

When considering the dry matter intake (DMI) of fibrous feed, the primary limiting factors are its digestibility and the rate at which it is broken down to particle sizes that can pass through the reticulo-omasal orifice (Preston and Leng, 1984). The fine grinding of fibrous feeds would facilitate its passage into the lower tract, but its digestibility in the lower tract is decreased. Hence, it is ideal if the fibrous feeds are fermented in the rumen and broken down to particle sizes that can facilitate the flow and facilitate its digestibility. Increase in intakes of dry matter (DM), organic matter (OM), crude protein (CP), neutral-detergent fibre (NDF) and acid-detergent fibre (ADF) with UMMB lick supplementation has also been supported by several researchers (Manget Ram, 1989; Mohini, 1991; Gupta and Malik, 1991) (Tables 4 and 5). With UMMB supplementation, straw DMI increased by 30 to 50 percent in different experiments.

Table 4. Account of Daily Straw And Ummb Intake And Straw Dm Digestibility Coefficient In Two Groups

Group DOMI**	Body weight (kg)	UMMB intake (kg)	Straw intake** kg/100kg B.Wt.	g/w $^{0.75}$ (kg)	digestibility coneficient	Straw DM through straw (kg/100kg B.Wt.)
I	224.0 ± 14.2	---	1.27 ± 0.08	48.77 ± 2.43	48.54 ± 1.06	0.619 ± 0.03
II	228.4 ± 12.4	0.44 ± 0.04	1.95 ± 0.06	75.55 ± 1.79	48.65 ± 1.20	0.986 ± 0.05

**$p < 0.01$

EFFECT OF UMMB FEEDING ON DIGESTIBILITY AND NUTRIENT BALANCES

Digestibility increased (Table 5) due to increased rates of rumen fermentation, mediated through a larger population of microflora and increased cellulolytic activity. Straw OM digestibility was around 40 to 45 percent under unmanipulated conditions. With UMMB supplementation, digestibility increased to 50 percent (Manget Ram and Gupta, 1988). Mohini (1991) observed significant enhancement in the digestibility of nitrogen-free extract (NFE) with UMMB lick in paddy-straw-based diets. Digestibility of ADF was enhanced from 37.4 percent to 41.3 percent with UMMB licks supplementation with wheat straw, while NDF digestibility increased much more than ADF, i.e. from 42.6 to 51.8 percent. DM and OM digestibility increased from 44.0 and 45.22 percent to 50.0 and 53.0 percent, respectively, by UMMB licks supplementation (Tiwari et al., 1990). Based on these observations, it can be safely concluded that supplementation with UMMB licks boosted the digestibility of basal diets based on low quality forages.

EFFECT OF UMMB FEEDING ON RUMEN FERMENTATION

The important feature in utilization of nutrients in ruminants is the anaerobic fermentative digestion. Therefore, to increase the efficiency of nutrient utilization or productivity, there is need for actions that maintain an environment conducive to better microbial activity in the rumen. The major requirements for obtaining better microbial activity and cell production in the rumen are:

- supply of enough nitrogen
- supply of enough ATP and
- supply of enough minerals and monomers

The primary limiting factor with straws is N deficiency – insufficient N to ensure adequate ammonia in the rumen fluid (Kunju, 1988; Manget Ram, 1989; Srinivas and Gupta, 1991; Srinivas, 1991). When supplementation in the form of UMMB lick was provided, the ammonia-N (NH_3-N) in the rumen fluid increased to optimum (Manget Ram and Kunju, 1986; Kunju, 1988; Manget Ram, 1989; Mohini, 1991). NH_3-N concentration increased substantially from 76 mg/l to 239 mg/l after UMMB-lick supplementation with a paddy-straw-based diet. When NH_3-N in the rumen increases, the lick consumption diminishes proportionally (Garg et al., 1990). The ammonia level is believed to be a biosystemic control of lick intake by the animal (Kunju, 1988). Manget Ram (1989) observed significant ($P<0.01$) difference in rumen NH_3-N level when wheat straw was supplemented with either concentrate mixture or UMMB lick. The NH_3-N levels in rumen fluid were 223 mg/l and 183 mg/l, respectively, for UMMB lick or concentrate supplementation. Even at this high level of rumen NH_3-N, blood NH_3-N rose only to 1.27 mg/100 ml, which indicated no toxic effect of urea through UMMB licks (Table 6). Total N and trichloracetic acid (TCA)-precipitable N did not differ significantly between concentrate and UMMB lick supplementation. Equal TCA-precipitable N for both the supplements indicated equal microbial yields (Gupta et al. 1970; Manget Ram and Gupta, 1986, 1987; Manget Ram, 1989). When preformed amino acid sources increased in the UMMB block, the NH_3-N content was not significantly different from the concentrate-supplemented group, which indicated that NH_3 released from UMMB licks was used with the same efficiency as that from concentrate supplementation (Mohini, 1991).

With increased DMI, the volatile fatty acid (VFA) concentrations increased when lambs consumed UMMB supplement along with a basal diet of wheat straw. A small but insignificant shift in the VFA proportion towards higher propionate production was also observed (Sudana and Leng, 1986). It was calculated that for 100 mg ammonia per litre of rumen liquor, the total VFA (TVFA) level should be around 25 mM/l. When UMMB was fed, the level of ammonia was 112–195 mg/l and TVFA concentration was 48–54 mM/l (Kunju, 1988). TVFA production was significantly higher ($p<0.01$) with concentrate supplementation than with UMMB supplementation with paddy-straw-based diets, compared with feeding paddy straw alone (Mohini, 1991). Rumen turnover also increased with UMMB supplementation, which indicated rapid DM digestion due to effective colonization by the rumen microflora (Manget Ram and Gupta, 1988; Manget Ram, 1989; Mohini, 1991; Srinivas, 1991). Sixty percent of the straw DM disappearance was achieved in 48 hours by supplementing UMMB licks alone with straw-based rations. Bacterial production rate as g/day DOMI was considerably higher with UMMB supplementation compared with concentrate supplementation. Nevertheless, the percentage efficiencies of N incorporation in cattle were 30.83 and 29.54 for concentrate and UMMB-supplemented groups, respectively (Manget Ram, 1989). In buffaloes, N incorporation efficiencies were only 23.31 and 17.78 percent for concentrate and UMMB-supplemented groups, respectively (Mohini, 1991). In contrast, protozoan production rate was about halved in UMMB-supplemented groups when compared with concentrate-supplemented groups. This could be due to a partial defaunating effect of either UMMB lick ingredients in general, or sodium bentonite in particular (Manget Ram, 1989; Mohini, 1991). The amino acid composition of ruminal bacteria showed higher serine, glycine, threonine, alanine and arginine, and lower lysine, while most of the amino acids were similar for protozoa, except for lysine, when animals were supplemented with either UMMB lick or concentrate mixture (Manget Ram, 1989). The overall conclusion, based on rumen parameters, was that the UMMB licks could invariably and effectively replaced concentrate supplementation at maintenance level.

EFFECT OF UMMB FEEDING ON MILK PRODUCTION

In India, the effect of feeding UMMB lick on milk production was studied extensively at NDDB, both in buffaloes and crossbred cattle. Twenty Surti buffaloes in their second and third lactation were divided into four groups of five animals each. The first group was fed on rice straw and cattle feed. The second group received the same ration plus UMMB. The third group was given cattle feed equal to 80 percent of that given to first group, with UMMB lick. The fourth group was given cattle feed equal to 60 percent of the first group, along with UMMB and 1.0 kg bypass protein. It was observed that the economic gains in the fourth group were remarkable. The animals on an average licked 350, 570 and 370 g/day UMMB lick in the second, third and fourth groups, respectively. The fat-corrected milk yields were 7.38, 8.07, 6.99 and 7.19 kg (120 days), respectively, for groups 1 to 4 (Kunju, 1986a, b).

In lactating Jersey and crossbred Jersey cows, milk yields were tested by substituting 50 percent of green fodder with rice straw. Animals in-group I were fed green fodder ad lib and concentrate at 40 percent of milk production. Animals in groups II and III were fed half the green fodder of group I, but with concentrate similar to group I. In addition, group II was offered rice straw ad lib, while group III was provided free choice of UMMB lick along with ad lib rice straw. Fat-corrected milk production was 10.45, 10.00 and 10.84 kg/day for groups I, II and III, respectively, with body weight changes of +0.187, -0.245, +0.035 kg/day. Thus, the block lick supplementation could maintain milk production in both Jersey and their crosses in group III without loss of body weight with 50 percent reduction of green fodder DM and ad lib feeding of rice straw. It was noticed that the supplementation increased the net return over feed cost by Rs 2.42 per day per animal (1985 values).

Kunju (1988) reported on successful village trials with UMMB supplementation for milk production. It was observed under field conditions that each 3 kg block lick lasted for one week per animal. At six villages (situated in Kaira District Cooperative Milk Producers Union Ltd, Anand, Gujarat, India), the milk yields were enhanced in animals when given free access to UMMB licks. Not only milk yields, but also fat percentages were enhanced. Increased straw intake and fat yield (Table 2) were reported by most of the farmers. On average, each farmer benefited by Rs 2–3 per day. Many farmers reported improvement in the general health of animals on supplementation with block licks compared with feeding straw alone. Increased straw intake was reported by all farmers, with simultaneous improvement in milk yield and fat percentages (Dave and Choudhary, 1986).

ADVANTAGES OF FEEDING UMMB LICKS TO ANIMALS

- Stimulates rumen fermentation, thereby, increases straw intake by animals.
- Increases microbial protein synthesis and supply at abomasum level, giving higher productivity.
- Improves daily milk (by 0.5–1.0 kg) and fat (by 0.3–0.5 percent) yields.
- Increases lactation length.
- Maintains health and reproductive functions.
- Improves growth rate of animals on straw-based diets.
- No risk of urea toxicity.

FACTORS AFFECTING UMMB LICKING BY ANIMALS

- Level and type of concentrate supplementation.
- Level and type of basal ration, which includes leguminous and non-leguminous green fodder and dry fodder such as crop residues or hay.
- Type of animal (species and breed).
- Physiological stage, such as growth, lactation or non-lactation (dry).
- Method of dispensing UMMBs.
- Extent of availability of UMMBs.
- UMMB hardness.

POINTS TO BE REMEMBERED FOR MAXIMIZING GAIN FROM UMMB FEEDING

- Dispense the UMMB in front of the animal in a proper way.
- Initially, the licking of UMMB by Zebu cattle and buffalo will be slow.
- Needs an adaptation period of 1–2 weeks.
- Do not discontinue the block.
- Use the block as a lick only.
- Do not spray water on the block for licking.
- The UMMB lick should be protected from dung, urine and rain.

Shortage of feeds and fodders, in terms of both quantity and quality is a major problem for developing countries like India in meeting the nutritional requirement of livestock. The unpredictable pattern of rainfall and recurring droughts also adversely affect agronomy and livestock. Despite the increased reliability of long-term weather forecasting, droughts lead to large economic losses among animal rearing communities. During such prolonged dry periods, only feed resources available are crop residues and highly lignified fibrous materials. The feeding of such material is energetically wasteful. However, if supply of the essential nutrients required for growth of microflora is made available by supplementation with UMMB licks, intake and digestibility of fibrous feed can be improved significantly. As a result, growth and milk production can be enhanced significantly with very little input cost. As a result, growth and milk production can be enhanced significantly with very little input cost.

Table 5. Digestibility Coefficient Of Various Nutrients In Two Groups

Group	DM*	OM*	CP**	EE	CF	NFE
I	48.54 ± 1.06	48.98 ± 1.21	---	48.91 ± 1.56	42.96 ± 0.94	62.54 ± 1.80
II	53.35 ± 1.05	53.85 ± 1.39	50.30 ± 1.62	49.22 ± 0.82	43.28 ± 0.71	64.15 ± 2.61

*p<0.05; **p<0.01

Table 6. Different N Constituents In Blood Plasma In Two Groups

Group	Total N** (g/100 ml)	NH_3-N** (mg/100 ml)	Urea-N** (mg/100 ml)
I	1.822 ± 0.02	0.29 ± 0.03	4.29 ± 0.21
II	2.165 ± 0.02	1.27 ± 0.04	17.56 ± 0.36

**$p<0.01$

Bibliography

Dave, A.S. and Choudhary, K.M. (1986). Observations in villages on animal lick feeding. Mehsana District Co-operative Milk Producers' Union Ltd., Mehsana. Cited in Kunju, 1986b.

Garg, M.R., Sanyal, P.K. and Bhanderi, B.M. (2003). Urea molasses mineral block supplement in the ration of dairy animals-Indian experiences: In: FAO Publication: Urea Molasses Multinutirent Blocks- Simple and effective feed supplement technology for ruminant agriculture (H.P.S. Makkar and M. Sanchez, Eds.).

Garg, M.R. and Gupta, B.N. (1992). Asian-Australasian Journal of Animal Science, 5: 39–44.

Garg, M.R., Mehta, A.K. and Singh, D.K. (1998). World Animal Review, 90: 22–27.

Garg, M.R., Tripathi, A.K. and Kunju, P.J.G (1990). Indian Journal of Animal Nutrition, 7: 55.

Gupta, B.N. & Malik, N.S. (1991). Indian Journal of Animal Science, 61: 113.

Gupta, B.N., Khan, S.A. and Murthy, V.N. (1970). Indian Veterinary Journal, 47: 773.

Kunju, P.J.G (1986a). Urea molasses block lick: a feed supplement for ruminants. pp. 261–274, in: M.N.M. Ibrahim & J.B. Schiere (eds). Rice straw and related feeds in ruminant rations. Proceedings of an International Workshop, Kandy, Sri Lanka, 24–28 March 1986.

Kunju, P.J.G (1986b). Asian Livestock, 11: 154–157.

Kunju, P.J.G (1988). Asian-Australasian Journal of Animal Science, 1(4): 233–239.

Leng, R.A. (1983). The potential of solidified molasses-based blocks for the correction of multinutritional deficiencies in buffaloes and other ruminants fed low quality agro-industrial by-products. pp. 135–150, in: The use of nuclear techniques to improve domestic buffalo production in Asia. Vienna: IAEA.

McLennan, S.R., Wright, G.S. and Blight, G.W. (1981). Australian Journal of Experimental Agriculture and Animal Husbandry, 21: 367.

Makkar, H.P.S. (2003). Efficient utilization of crop residues and enhanced animal productivity through feeding of urea molasses multinutrient blocks: Experiences of some Asian, African and Latin American countries. Paper presented at NDDB, Anand, November 19-20, 2002.

Manget Ram. (1989). Effect of supplementing straw-based diet with urea-molasses mineral block licks on rumen fermentation pattern, nutrient utilization and growth in crossbred cattle. Ph.D. Thesis, Kurukshetra University, Kurukshetra, India.

Manget Ram and Gupta, B.N. (1986). Journal of Nuclear Agriculture and Biology, 15: 179.

Manget Ram and Gupta, B.N. (1987). Indian Journal of Animal Nutrition, 4: 223.

Manget Ram and Gupta, B.N. (1988). Journal of Nuclear Agriculture and Biology, 17: 100.

Manget Ram and Kunju, P.J.G. (1986). Indian Journal of Animal Nutrition, 3: 244.

Mohini, M. (1991). Effect of urea molasses mineral block supplementation to straw based diets on fibre degradability, rumen fermentation pattern and nutrient utilization and growth in buffalo calves. Ph.D. Thesis, National Dairy Research Institute, Karnal, India.

Pathak, N.N. and Ranjhan, S.K. (1976). Indian Journal of Animal Science, 46: 515.

Preston, T.R. and Leng, R.A. (1984). Supplementation of diets based on fibrous residues and byproducts. p. 373, In: F. Sundstol and E. Owen (eds), Straw and Other Fibrous Byproducts as Feed. Amsterdam, the Netherlands: Elsevier.

Sansoucy, R. (1986). World Animal Review, 57: 40–48.

Sansoucy, R. (1995). World Animal Review, 82: 78–83.

Sansoucy, R., Aarts, G. and R.A. Leng. (1988). Urea-molasses blocks as a multinutrient supplement for ruminants. pp. 263–279, in: Sugar cane as feed. FAO Animal Production and Health Paper, No. 72.

Srinivas, B. (1991). Effect of modified urea molasses mineral block supplementation to straw based diets on rumen fermentation pattern and milk production in crossbred cattle. Ph.D. Thesis. National Dairy Research Institute, Karnal, India.

Srinivas, B. and Gupta, B.N. (1991). Indian Dairyman, 43: 260.

Sudana, I.B. and Leng, R.A. (1986). Animal Feed Science and Technology, 16: 25.

Tiwari, S.P., Singh, V.B. and Mehra, V.R. (1990). Animal Feed Science and Technology, 29: 333–338.

20
MINERAL MIXTURE PREPARATION

M. Parthasarathy

To sustain the livestock productivity minerals need to be supplemented in the ration because their presence in the feed and fodders may not be sufficiently inadequate to fulfil the animals requirements. However, during the course of minerals supplementation care must be taken about the minerals already present in the animal ration. For adequate mineral nutrition, general supplementation of mineral mixture in the concentrate mixture is advised. Normally, concentrate mixture is recommended to be mixed with 2% mineral mixture alongwith 1% common salt to ensure the availability of all the macro - and micro minerals to the animals as per their requirements. However, in case of high availability of minerals from dietary components, the level of mineral mixture from dietary components can be reduced. In case of deficiency or toxicity for a particular mineral in a specific zone, composition of mineral mixture may be manipulated accordingly.

Requirements of mineral mixtures (BIS 1992)

1. All ingredients used shall be of high quality and shall be free from any substances harmful to cattle.
2. The mineral mixture shall be in the powdered form thoroughly mixed and completely homogenous.
3. The mineral mixtures shall be free from adulterants, insects or visible fungus infestation and undesirable odour.
4. Mineral mixtures shall be free from spores of Bacillus anthracis and Clostridium species.

Characteristics of a mineral mixture (Mudgal et al., 2003)

1. Calcium - phosphorus ratio should not substantially exceed 2:1
2. Formulation should be sufficiently palatable to allow adequate consumption in relation to requirements.
3. The particle size must allow adequate mixing without segregation.
4. High quality mineral salts should be used to ensure biological availability

of each mineral element. Salts containing high fluorine concentrations should be avoided.

5. Mineral mixture of good quality bearing ISI mark should be used.

The prevention and correction of mineral deficiencies

Successful procedures for the prevention and control of all mineral deficiencies (and many mineral toxicities) have been elucidated (Underwood and Suttle, 1999). The procedure of choice varies greatly with different elements, climatic environments, animal species and economic conditions.

1. Continuous direct methods

Hand-fed animals can best be supplemented by mixing the required minerals with the feed offered. When adequate trough time or space is allowed, variation in individual consumption is not pronounced and the amounts included should not exceed average mineral requirements. The precise amounts and proportions of supplementary minerals required will depend on the nature and degree of the deficiency and the form and intensity of production. Where individual animals productivity is very high, husbandry conditions are intensive and farm labour costs are high, it is usual to purchase mixed feeds compounded to contain the required minerals in adequate quantities and with sufficient margin of safety.

Where the husbandry conditions are less intensive and farm labour is more plentiful and less costly, the same results can be achieved by home mixing and only those minerals known to be needed are added.

2. Free - access mineral mixtures

The most widely used method of supplementation is the provision of mineral mixtures in loose ('lick') or block form. Common salt is a vital ingredient of such supplements because it is palatable and attractive to most animals. Individuals are relied to consume sufficient for their needs where supplies are freely available and to seek it out actively where it is less accessible. So long these mineral mixtures contain 30-40% salt, they are consumed in amounts sufficient to meet the needs of livestock for other minerals (McDowell et al., 1993). However, individual variation in consumption from licks or blocks can be marked (Bowman and Sowell, 1997). Seasonal variation in mineral consumption can also occur, but intakes are more uniform from granulated than from block sources of minerals (Rocks et al., 1982).

3. Slow - release methods

The efficacy and costs of administering minerals to individual animals can be improved by using large doses in relatively inert, slowly mobilized forms. The administration of heavy pellets (Millar and Meads, 1988), glass bolus (Millar et al., 1988) or particles of the mineral such as copper oxide, which are retained in the gastro-intestinal tract, act as slow - release sources. A bullet consisted of cobaltic oxide (60%) and finely divided clay remains in the reticulo-rumen for months or years, slowly dissolving and supplying cobalt to the rumen bacteria. A soluble glass bolus which is not susceptible to coating. A steady supply of cobalt can be introduced through a introduction of soluble glass bolus which is not susceptible to coating (Zervas, 1988).

Leguminous fodders, oil cakes and animal products are rich sources of minerals. Supplementing rations with good quality mineral mixtures is most convenient. Preparation of a mineral mixture is based on the target species, cost and availability of ingredients and percentage absorbability of mineral elements. One such formula for preparing a mineral mixture is (Ranjhan, 1991) suggested in Table 1.

Table 1. Formula for mineral mixture preparation

Ingredient	Parts
Sterilized bone meal, fine powdered	45
Ground limestone	10
Dicalcium phosphate	12
Common salt	30
Yellow oxide of iron	0.5
Potassium iodide	0.25
Starch	0.75
Sodium carbonate	0.75
Sodium thiosulphate	0.75

To every 100 kg of the mixture add finely powdered 50 g of cobalt chloride, 250 g copper sulphate, 300 g of manganese sulphate and 300g of zinc sulphate. The mineral supplement should be added at the rate of 2% of concentrate mixture to protect animals against possible mineral deficiencies.

Several ingredients can be blended into a mineral mixture based upon them availability and cost. Ingredients for mineral mixture for dairy cattle and poultry as suggested by BIS (1992) are presented in Table 2.

Table 2. Ingredients for mineral mixture

Ingredients
Bone meal
Calcined bone meal
Ground limestone
Dolmite lime
Oyster shell grit
Dicalcium phosphate
Magnesium carbonate
Magnesium oxide
Manganous dioxide
Manganous sulphate
Zinc carbonate
Zinc chloride
Zinc sulphate
Zinc oxide
Potassium iodide (stabilized)
Sodium iodide
Potassium iodate
Cupric sulphate
Cupric chloride
Ferrous sulfate
Ferrous carbonate
Cobalt sulphate
Cobalt chloride
Common salt

Common ingredients of mineral supplements and their actual mineral content are presented by Underwod and Suttle (1999) and elemental absorption coefficients for dairy cattle on dry matter basis are given in NRC (2001).

Two types of mineral mixtures were advocated for preparation containing salt (I) and without salt (II) for supplementing cattle feeds by BIS (1992) and are presented in Table 3.

Table 3 : Requirements (%) of mineral mixtures

S.No.	Characteristic	Type I (with salt)	Type II (without salt)
1.	Moisture, Max.	5	5
2.	Calcium, Min.	18	23
3.	Phosphorus, Min.	9	12
4.	Magnesium, Min.	5	6.5
5.	Salt (as sodium chloride), Min.	22	-
6.	Iron, Min.	0.4	0.5
7.	Iodine (as KI), Min.	0.02	0.026
8.	Copper, Min.	0.06	0.077
9.	Manganese, Min.	0.1	0.12
10.	Cobalt, Min.	0.09	0.012
11.	Fluorine, Max.	0.05	0.07
12.	Zinc, Min.	0.3	0.38
13.	Sulphur, Max.	0.4	0.5
14.	Acid Insoluble ash, Max.	3	2.5

Source: Mudgal et al., 2003

CATTLE LICKS

Cattle licks shall be in the form of blocks or bricks and sufficiently hard and strong so as not to crumble during handling (ISI, 1974). The block may have a hole at one end to facilitate ‘pegging’ to keep them above ground level or be provided with embedded rope for the purpose of hanging. Cattle licks may be prepared with varying sizes and weights (25 kg block, 2 kg brick and 100 g pet licks), may be either plain or mineralized. Specifications for cattle lick preparation for animal consumption are suggested by ISI (1974).

Table 4. Requirements of cattle licks (% DM basis)

S.No.	Characteristic	Plain	Mineralized licks
1.	Chloride (as NaCl), Min.	94	94
2.	Iron, Min.	-	0.13
3.	Iodine, Min.	-	0.003
4.	Copper, Min.	-	0.035
5.	Manganese, Min.	-	0.20
6.	Cobalt, Min.	-	0.001

Manipulation of mineral supplements

Mostly minerals are blended in ionized salt form in the mineral mixture based on their availability to animals. Manipulation of minerals in the pre-chelated form in the mineral mixture improves their availability. Chelated mineral supplements are being manufactured in UK, USA and Canada and India. The chelating ligands used as EDTA and proteinates of the mineral ion which functions as mineral sequestering agent. It carries the mineral ions at the absorption site and make them more absorbable. Naturally occurring chelates are hemoglobin, cytochrome, vitamin B_{12} etc. Chelate mineral supplements were reported to improve milk production, butter fat production and improved reproductive performance of repeat breeders (Ashmead, 1991; Roshanlal, 1990). A technology has been developed to prepare copper, manganese and zinc chelates using casein as an organic ligand (Parnerkar and Prasad, 1991) and another with soyprotein (Dinh and Chhabra, 2002). Use of chelated forms of trace elements are not always cost - effective than simple inorganic sources. Chelation may be useful for one element (e.g. chromium) does not guarantee its usefulness for others (Underwood and Suttle, 1999).

Over feeding of mineral mixtures

The provision of minerals in excess of the animal's requirement is not only economically wasteful but also confers no additional benefit on the animal and can be harmful. Excess of phosphorus and magnesium has been reported to cause death from urinary calculi (Hay and Suttle, 1993) while an excess of copper causes toxicity in sheep. There can be no justification for the purchase and use of 'Shotgun' mixtures of minerals, which are desired to cover a wide range of environmental and feeding regimens. The shotgun approach can be dangerous because it disturbs the mineral balance. Furthermore, the surplus minerals are excreted and few such as phosphorus and copper can cause environmental pollution (Underwood and Suttle, 1999).

False claims on mineral mixtures

The manufacture and sale of ready - mixed mineral mixtures by reputed firms is a legitimate and desirable business of value to farmers. However, every farmer should be on guard against exaggerated claims of advertising propaganda and should critically examine claims in the light of the particular mineral needs of stock under local conditions.

Precautions while selecting ingredients

1. Calcium containing mineral supplements are known to contain ground limestone, steamed bone flour and dicalcium phosphate. If rock phosphate is given to animals it is important to ensure that it is free from flouride other which may otherwise cause toxicity (ISI 1974).
2. Lack of sulfur in the diet can be corrected by the inclusion of elemental sulfur, sodium sulphate or calcium sulphate, but improvements in animal production is likely to be of limited value of rumen - degradable nitrogen or energy is not corrected. (Maynard et al., 1979)
3. Bone meal should be free from microorganisms such as B. anthracis, Cl. botulinum, C. chauvoei and C. septicum (ISI, 1979).

Thus, it can be concluded that mineral mixture supplementation in the animal ration is vital to optimize animal production and reproduction. Mineral deficiencies causes not only retarded animal growth and productivity as well as animal health and reproduction. Precautions should be taken about the correction of mineral deficiency as many mineral in excess of their requirement can also cause toxicity. The mineral mixture and its ingredients should be of high quality and free from adulterants.

Bibliography

Ashmead, H.D. (1991) Proc. 1st International Animal Nutrition Research workers conference for Asia and Pacific, Bangalore, India.

BIS (1992) Mineral mixtures for supplementing cattle feeds - specification (Third Revision) Bureau of Indian Standards, New Delhi.

Bowman, J.G.P. and Sowell, B.F. (1997) Delivery method and supplement consumption by grazing ruminants a review. Journal of Animal Science 75: 543-550.

Dinh, K.V. and Chhabra, A. (2002) Proc. IV Biennial Conference Animal Nutr. Assoc. Kolkata, India.

Hay, L. and Suttle, N.F. (1993) Urolithiasis. In: Aitken, I.D. and Martin, W.B. (eds.) Diseases of sheep 2nd edn. Blackwell Scientific London.

ISI (1974) Specification for calcined bone meal as livestock feed supplement. Indian standards Institution, New Delhi.

ISI (1979) Specification for bone meal as livestock feed supplement (First revision) Indian Standards Institution New Delhi.

ISI (1979) Specification for common salt and cattle licks for animal consumption. (First Revision). Indian Standards Institution, New Delhi.

Maynard, L.A., Loosli, J.K. Hintz, H.F. and Warner, R.G. (1979). Animal Nutrition Tata McGraw Hill Publ. Co., New Delhi.

McDowell, L.R., Cornad, J.H. and Hembry, F.G. (1993) Minerals for grazing ruminants in tropical regions, 2nd edn. Animal Science Department, University of Florida, Gainsville, USA.

Millar, K.R. and Meads, W. J. (1988) Selenium levels in the blood, liver, kidney and muscle of sheep after the administration of iron / selenium pellets or soluble glass boluses. Newzealand Veterinary Journal 36: 8-10.

Millar, K.R., Meads, W.J. Albyt, A.T. Scahill, B.G. and Sheppard, A.D. (1988) The retention and efficacy of soluble glass boluses for providing selenium, cobalt and copper to sheep. Newzealand Veterinary Journal. 36: 11-14.

Mudgal, V.D., Singhal, K.K. and Sharma, D.D. (2003) Advances in diary animal production. 2nd edn. IDBC, Lucknow, India.

NRC (2001). Nutrient requirements of dairy cattle. National Academy Press, Washington DC, USA.

Parnerkar, S. and Prasad, T. (1991) Proc. 1st International Animal Nutr. Res. Workers Conference for Asia and Pacific, Bangalore, India.

Ranjhan, S.K. (1991) Chemical composition and nutritive value of Indian feeds and feeding of farm animals. ICAR, New Delhi, p. 22.

Rocks, R.L., Wheeler, J.L. and Hedges, D.A. (1982) Labelled waters of crystallization in gypsum to measure the intake of loose and compressed mineral supplements. Australian Journal of Experimental Agriculture and Animal Husbandry 22: 35-42.

Roshanlal (1990) Effect of trace mineral supplements on growth and reproductive performance of animals. Ph.D. Thesis. NDRI, Karnal, India.

Underwood, E.J. and Suttle, N.F. (1999) The mineral nutrition of livestock. 3rd edn. CABI Publishing Wallingford, U.K.

Zervas, G. (1988) Use of soluble glass boluses containing Cu, Co and Se in the prevention of trace element deficiencies in goats. Journal of Agricultural Sciences, Cambridge 110: 155-158.

21
FEED PROCESSING FOR PIGS

R. Bhar and N. N. Pathak

Despite improvement in the production of food grains in India, there appears to be no serious approach in ration formulation for the pigs because pig husbandry is yet in the hands of economically weaker class of human population in most parts of the country. The most disappointing situation is the lack of appropriate planning for the development of pigs. For the development of any livestock production strategies demand and supply system should be given high priority, which has not yet been taken seriously and swine farming has been advocated in almost all the states. In Indian situation pig farming without scavenging may not be remunerative in most part of the country due to very low price of pork. Feeding under organized farming alone costs about 65 to 85 per cent of the recurring expenditures. Among the food grains the cereal grains are still and now a days coarse grains like maize, jowar, bajra, barley and minor millets are comparably priced with wheat and coarse rice. Under such situation it is rather difficult to visualize a grain based cheaper balanced diet for growing- finishing pigs in most part of the country where pork is quite cheap. The other factor to be considered for pig production is the growth potential in local, crossbred (local x exotic) and exotic pigs. There is great difference in the rate of body weight gain during growing finishing period in the three categories of pigs. Even the growth performance of common exotic breeds like Large White Yorkshire, Landrace, Middle White Yorkshire, Saddleback and others has reduced significantly due to rearing for several generations in the agro-climatic conditions of the Indian states. The average growth performance of local (desi), crossbred and exotic pigs is in the range of 200-300, 250-400 and 300-600 g, respectively during the growing-finishing period after weaning at 8 weeks of age. However, for the feeding of such pigs there is no feeding standard; and for all practical purpose, standards suggested by National Research Council (NRC) of National Academy of Sciences, USA is being used. Since the pig production has not yet become remunerative in most part of the country, the production has to be continued on the diets composed of greater proportions of as far as possible low fibre agro-industrial byproducts like molasses, brewers grains, tapioca byproducts and sal seed meal etc.

For the development of pig production in the country an All India Coordinated Research Project on pigs (AICRP on pigs) was started in 1970 with coordinating unit at the Indian Veterinary Research Institute, Izatnagar. At initial stage emphasis was given on the adaptation and breeding of two exotic breeds, i.e. Landrace and Large White Yorkshire, at different centres in the country and only after spending 12-15 years it was realized in late eighties of the previous century that objective has to be shifted for research for evolving economical rations. However, before this shift, need of evolving economic rations utilizing greater proportion of various agricultural byproducts and industrial wastes was realized and since then several studies were being conducted (Ranjhan et al.,1971, 1972; Pathak and Ranjhan, 1972, 1973,1981[a,b] Jain et al., 1978; Rao and Prasad, 1980; Agarwal et al. 1982; Pathak et al. 1983; Garg and Pathak, 1983, 1986; Kumar and Barsaul, 1988; Bauza et al.,1990; Bhar et al., 1996,2000, 2001, 2002; Soren et al.,2003, 2004, Saikia,2004). During the period an obnoxious aquatic weed, water hyacinth (Echornia crasipes) was also used in the diets of pigs (Pathak et al.,1979,1980; Talukdar et al., 1984). In view of the greater fibre tolerance of adult pigs fresh slurry of biogas plant has also been used successfully for the partial replacement of brans in the swine rations..

For optimum feeding of pigs both processing and balanced formulations are important aspects. In India very simple feed processing technologies like grinding, soaking and cooking are commonly used by the pig rearing families.At some places pelleting has also been introduced on small scale due to limited market. In countries with advanced pig farming some other methods of feed processing are also used. A brief description of common fed processing methods are as follows :

1.Grinding

Grinding is a process of particle size reduction of feeds. It increases the surface area; exposing a larger area to the digestive enzymes in the alimentary tract. While feeding a total mixed ration, it is important to grind ingredients to a uniform particle size to prevent sorting by the pig. Grinding of feedstuffs could be fine, medium and course in accordance with the permeability of particle through specified hammer mill screen of 1/8 – 3/16", 1/4 – 3/8" and 1/2" or larger, respectively.

Young pigs appear to perform better on finely ground feed. Feed intake is reduced along with the improvement in feed conversion efficiency (Wu and Allee, 1984). However, Ohh et al. (1983) did not find any improvement on the performance of pig on reduction of particle size of sorghum. Conversely, some other studies showed improvement in nutrient digestibilities by feeding finely ground sorghum (Owsley et al. 1981) and maize (Anon.2000) as compared with a medium or coarsely ground grain. Similar benefit of decreasing the particle size even of sun cured alfalfa meal was observed by Nuzback et al. (1982) in gestating sows. An increase in incidence of gastric ulcers is also noted as feeds become more finely ground. A medium fine grinding is, thus, generally recommended for the processing of feed for pigs. The recommended fineness for grinding various grains are medium for maize, medium to course for wheat, fine to medium for sorghum, and fine for barley and oats (Ensminger and Parker, 1984).

2. Heat treatment

Heating some feedstuffs (soybeans, tuber crops etc) has been shown to improve pig performance by eliminating certain toxins, destroying enzyme inhibitors, or making certain nutrients more available to the pig. Heat processing methods include either heat only (dry heat); or heat and moisture (wet cooking) with or without pressure. Excessive heat can cause reducing carbohydrates such as glucose to react with free amino groups to form a bond (Maillard reaction) that is not hydrolyzed by digestive enzymes (Pond and Maner, 1984). The time, temperature and method of heating process may affect the digestibility and availability of amino acids.

Pigs fed roasted milo had improved average daily gain and gain per unit of feed (Veum et al. 1972) and Jensen (1978) reported an improvement in palatability and efficiency of feed conversion in weanling pigs fed a diet containing roasted corn. Soybeans must be heat-treated for effective use by swine. The major objectives of processing soybeans are (1) to destroy the trypsin inhibitor, (2) to destroy the urease enzyme, (3) to inactivate the toxic hemaggluten and (4) to increase the nutrient availability.

Micronzing is another process of dry heating grains to 300°F for 20 seconds. The dry heat is supplied by infrared radiation. Microwaves with 3 x 108 to 3 x 1011 cycles per second are used. The micronizing process ruptures the cell wall and causes partial gelatinization of the starch, which increases its availability. Micronization of certain hard-shelled grains, such as milo, may improve growth rate and feed efficiency as Yang et al.(1975) indicated that micronizing sorghum increased growth rate from 6% to 18% and improved feed efficiency. However, Sasse et al. (1975) reported a reduction in growth rate with no effect on feed efficiency when micronized sorghum was fed to pigs. Ewan (1979) also did not find any added advantage of feeding micronized corn to weanling pigs. But

Luce et al. (1974) reported an improvement in feed conversion without any effect on average daily gain in growing-finishing pigs fed reground micronized milo.

3. Soaking and reconstitution

Soaking is one of the most common practice followed by the small and marginal pig rearers. It improves the acceptability and palatability of feed. Soaking of barley in water hydrolyzed 35-59% phytate phosphorus (Takemasa and Hijikura, 1983). Soaking or germination in barley decreased soluble or total beta-glucan content (Svihus et al., 1997; Mandal et al.,2004). Reconstitution is a process of conditioning the grains to raise its moisture content to 25-30% and storing in anaerobic condition for approximately 21 days. It results in disruption of the protein matrix of the grain. Soaking followed by reconstitution removes or inactivate some toxic substances. Different factors that influence the effects of reconstitution includes: grain to water ratio, time and temperature (85-90°C, optimum) and interaction with other dietary ingredients.

4.Pelleting

It is a mechanical hot or cold process of densification of ground grains or composite feed. It could be done with or without application of moisture or steam. Optimum temperature for hot pelleling is 65-70°C. Pelleting of composite concentrates diets improves feed utilization and increases rate of gain by at least 4 to 5% (Vanschoubroek et al., 1971; Hogberg et al., 1980). Moist heat and / or pressure in the pelleting process may increase the digestibility of starch and overall DE value of the diet (Seerley et al., 1962). Other advantages of pelleting include reduced dustiness, reduced storage space, less feed wastage, less loss due to wind blowing, and reduced sorting of the diets by the pigs. Crane et al. (1972) reported a marked decrease in the incidence of salmonella when pigs were fed pelleted feed.

5. Extusion

Extusion is the process of forcing feedstuffs through a restricting die under pressure that generates heat from friction. Mercier and Feillet (1975) found maximum expansion at 170-200°C with improved a-amylase digestibility for raw starch from 18% to 80%. However, Allee (1976) reported that extruding milo did not improve growth rate or feed efficiency in weanling pigs.

6. Paste and slurry feeding

Paste feeding is similar to liquid feeding, but water and feed are mixed at a ratio of 1:1 to 1.5:1.0, forming a paste/ slurry material. This material is delivered on demand through a self-feeder. Performance is generally improved in growing-finishing pigs fed a paste diet as compared with a dry diet. However, no benefits have been observed for feeding a paste diet to weanling pigs (Hogberg et al., 1980). Average daily gain and feed intake are substantially increased (10 to 15%) with little improvement noted in feed conversion when feeding a paste diet to growing pigs (Teague et al., 1970)

Effect of different processing methods on the performance of pigs have been reviewed by different workers (Hogberg et al., 1980; Danielson and Crenshaw, 1991; Holden and Zimmerman, 1991; Liptrap and Hoghberg,1991). To summarize all such studies, it must be recognized that the direction and magnitude of response to a particular set of processing conditions is never completely predictable, due to differences in pigs, agronomic practices, harvesting management, and crop variety. Above all economics (cost) of processing vis-a-vis its effect on pig performance plays a significant role in selecting the processing technique to be followed for formulation of diets for pigs.

Formulation methods of complete feed (ration) for pigs

Different feed ingredients, after necessary processing, are used for the formulation of diet/rations for pigs. Considering the potentiality of a particular breed, its production phase and requirements, different rations are formulated. Before attempting to balance a ration, following major points should be considered:

(a) Availability and cost of different feeds, (b) moisture content, (c) nutrient composition of feeds, (d) quality of feeds, (e) method of processing of the feed, and (f) the nutrient requirements and allowances, etc.

While formulation of diets pig producers must have some ideas about the substitution of one feed with other. Several rations have been formulated through the substitutions of costlier conventional energy and protein sources with relatively cheaper conventional or unconventional energy and protein sources (Agarwal,1971; Pathak and Rajhan,1973, 1981[a,b]; Pathak et al.,1979, 1980; Talukdar 1979; Agarwal et al. 1982, Anon.1985,1999,2000; Bhar et al., 1996,1997, 2000, 2001, 2002; Saikia, 2004). In using the feed substitution (Table 5), the following facts should be recognized (Ensminger and Parker,1984):

1. that, for best results, different ages and groups of animals within classes should be fed differently as per requirements.

2. that, individual feeds differ widely in feeding value as barley and oats vary widely in feeding value due to difference in hull and kernel content.
3. that, the substitutions are based primarily on supply and price; grains and grain by-products and or/protein supplements could be used interchangeably.
4. that, the feeding value of certain feeds is materially affected by preparation, say, cooking of potatoes and other tubers crops would improve its feeding value.

The comparative values of feeds shown in the substitution table (Table 5) are not absolute, rather, they are reasonably accurate approximations based on average quality feeds and reported feeding.

The ideal ration is one that will maximize production at the lowest cost. A costly ration may produce phenomenal gains in pigs, but the cost per unit of production may make the ration economically infeasible. Likewise, the cheapest ration is not always the best since it may not allow for optimum production. Therefore, the cost per unit of production is the ultimate determinant of the best ration. Awareness of this fact separates successful producers from marginal or unsuccessful ones.

Following four steps should be taken in an orderly fashion in order to formulate an economical ration:- (A) Find and list the nutrient requirements and/ or allowances for the specific animals to be fed, (B) Determine what feeds are available and list their respective nutrient compositions, (C) Find out the cost of the feed ingredients under consideration, and (D) Consider the limitations of the various feed ingredients and formulate the most economical ration.

Formulation of the ration may be accomplished by different methods viz. (i) the Pearson's square method, (ii) the simultaneous equation method, (iii) the 2 x 2 matrix method, (iv) the trial-and-error method, and (v) the computer method. The respective methods in detail could be referred in different text books (Pond and Maner, 1984; Ensminger and Parker, 1984; Pathak and Ranjhan, 1988, Pond et al.1995).

Maximum profit formulation

With the maximum profit procedure, both the nutritional requirements and the animal's performance are considered. Basically, the formulation contains all known feeding and nutrition inputs and animal production outputs. In this method we utilize feedstuffs based on cost and composition, animal performance (e.g.

daily weight gain or litter size; weight at birth and weaning). The animal product output is treated as an income and price of feed as an expense. The objective is to maximize the profit. This type of formulation requires knowledge of the maximum daily feed/DM intake of the pigs, production response to nutrient intake and daily nutrient requirement for maintenance.

Least cost formulation

Diet formulation using least-cost techniques is used extensively to minimize the cost of the diet. Once the appropriate equations are set up properly any linear programming software package can be used to solve the diet formulation problem. After a solution is obtained, it is up to the nutritionist to evaluate and verify that the solution conforms with nutritional knowledge (i.e., the diet will be palatable to the animal, that it does not contain nutrients and other substances in toxic amounts and that it attain the objective of formulation). The steps for a least cost diet formulation has been given in details in different text books (Ensminger and Parker, 1984; Pond et al., 1995). When many different feed ingredients are used, and other than the two major nutrients (energy and proteins) are also considered in formulation of an economic ration then computer model (Nath et al.2002) will make the formulation job very easy.

Ration formulations

The pigs may be classified into the following categories for the purpose of feeding.

1. Pre-weaned piglets

In India weaning is practiced at 6 to 8 weeks of age. The nursing ability of dams decreases significantly after 4 weeks of farrowing and piglets require supplemental feeding. A composite diet of about 20-22 per cent protein and 3300-3500 (kcal/kg) DE is used as a pre-starter or creep ration. However, the BIS (1987) specification for CP is 20% and ME is 3360 kcal/kg diet and NRC (1979) has divided the pre-weaning piglets feeding into two phages i.e., 1-5 kg and 5-10 kg body weights with CP requirements of 27 and 20% and ME of 3600 and 3400 kcal/ kg diet (or DE of 3700 and 3500 kcal/ kg diet). The rations of such high protein and energy content is offered to piglets from 2nd week of age up to weaning.

2. Growing phase

This is a period from weaning to about 45 kg body weight in fast growing European pigs, 35 kg in crossbreds and 25 kg in Indian local pigs. The diets should contain about 16-18% CP and 3100-3300 kcal DE under the Indian condition. However, the BIS (1987) specification for ME is 3170 kcal/kg along with this 18% CP and NRC (1979) specification of CP is 18, 16 and 14% for 10-20, 20-35 and 35-60 kg body weight along with similar ME (/DE) value of 3200 (/3300)kcal/kg diet in all the three phages of body weight.

3. Finishing phase

This period extend upto about 70, 60 and 50 kg body weight in exotic, crossbred and indigenous Indian pigs for economical return and production of good quality carcass. The diets should contain about 15-16% protein and 3000 to 3100 kcal DE per kg feed. BIS(1987) specification for CP and ME is 16% and 3170 kcal/kg finisher diet and NRC specification for more than 60 kg live weight is 13% CP along with the ME of 3200 (DE of 3300) kcal per kg diet

4. Breeding pigs

Balanced diets containing about 15% proteins and 3100 kcal DE per kg feed has been found adequate to support optimum breeding in pigs. Feeding should be restricted to control obesity which is highly undesirable for the breeding pigs, both boars and sows. BIS (1987) specification for breeding pigs is similar to that of finisher pigs. NRC (1979) specified the CP and ME (/or DE) of 12 % and 3200 (/or 3300) kcal/ kg diet for bred gilts and sows, young and adult boars.

Standard pig rations

Several diets have been formulated for development of different standard rations for creep, grower, finisher pigs. These could be used judiciously in exotic, crossbred or in the native Indian breeds with reference to their respective rate of production. Economics always plays a vital role in application of the respective diets either as a complete feed or as supplementary feeding under semi intensive (and /or scavenging) system of management. Formulation of rations could be further classified as per the ingredients used:

1. Cereal based diets

a) Conventional cereal based (>20% cereals)

b) Conventional low cereal by-product based (<20% cereals)

c) Non conventional cereal based viz. minor millets, ragi, kodo etc.

2. Grainless diets

3. Non-conventional diets

a) High molasses or liquid molasses, protein supplemented diets

b) Salseed meal, tapioca waste, kitchen/hotel waste based diets

c) Biogas plant slurry etc.

Ingredient composition of conventional diets have been presented in different tables. Number of experiments have been conducted to replace the conventional energy and protein sources of these rations by the unconventional feed ingredients. Different conventional energy sources of the standard rations have been successfully replaced partially by molasses (Pathak and Ranjhan, 1981; Garg et al., 1986), salseed meal (Agarwal, 1971; Pathak and Ranjhan, 1973), by kitchen wastes (Saikia, 2004), etc. Similar successful efforts have been made to repalce the conventional protein sources of standard rations by unconventional protein sources viz. replacement of groundnut cake by water washed neem seed kernal cake (Anon, 1985) and by urea ammoniated neem seed kernal cake (Bhar et al., 1997).

Efforts were also made to replace the complete compounded rations partialy or completely. Standard grower, finisher and breeder diets were successfully repalced with chaffed partially wilted water hyacinth @ 20-60% (Pathak et al.1979, Talukdar, 1979; Talukdar et al., 1984), grower ration by green berseem @ 25% (Bhar et al., 1996) and kitchen wastes @100% (Saikia, 2004).

i) Creep/pre-starter rations

On introduction of creep mixture (Table 1) at 7th to 14th day age in the diet of exotic, crossbred or Indian native suckling piglets, they could attain a body weight of 10-14, 8-12 and 5-8 kg, respectively at about 56 days of age. The creep mixture No. IV is being fed to the crossbred (Landrace x Desi) piglets under AICRP (2004) on pigs. The creep ration No. I was fed to Large White Yorkshire piglets which supported 300 g body weight gain per day with a 2.9 feed: gain ratio (Pathak and Rajhan, 1972), Adequate amount of good quality protein of animal origin is very important for balancing the rations. The creep ration should be of best among different pig rations; and CF, total ash and acid insoluble ash in the ration should not exceed 5, 8, and 4%, respectively (BIS, 1987).

ii) Grower rations

Grower rations (Table 2& 3) may contain lower level of cereal grains and animal proteins. The conventional cereal grains could be replaced fully or partially by the minor millets/or by grain processing byproducts and several agro-industrial waste materials. BIS (1987) specified maximum level of CF, total ash and acid insoluble ash in the ration at 6, 8, and 4%, respectively.

iii) Finisher rations

The finisher pigs could be reared on high fibre (8-12% CF) (Ranjan et al.1971, 1972) and lower energy containing palatable diets (Table 4) and CP % of the diet could be reduced even to 14%; thus, the scope of rearing finishing pigs on grainless rations containing lower level of animal protein has been demonstrated in several studies. However, BIS (1987) specified CF, total ash and acid insoluble ash in the ration maximum up to 8, 8, and 4%, respectively.

iv) Ration for pregnant and lactating sows

The rations suggested for the finisher pigs may be fed to the breeding sows and gilts with higher levels of vitamins. Experiments conducted at IVRI, Izatnagar (Pathak and Ranjhan,1972) have shown that 2-2.5 kg of meals may be sufficient for pregnant sows. In the case of gilts 3 kg mixture may be fed. Higher amount of meals may cause embryonic mortality. The rest of the feeding may be done with good quality succulent feeds viz. berseem, lucerne etc.

For lactating sows 3.5 kg of meals with an average 0.2 kg meal per piglets in the litter may be sufficient to meet the nutritional requirements of lactating animals.

v) Ration of boars

Breeding boars may be fed finisher ration @ of 2.5 kg per head per day. The rest of the ration may be a green.

Table 1: Composition of some creep mixture

Ingredients	% in the rations						
	I[a]	II[b]	III[b]	IV[c]	V[d]	VI[d]	VIII[d]
Ground yellow maize	46	40	40	60	40	30	20
Barley flower	-	-	-	-	-	10	10
Skimmed milk	-	10	-	-	10	10	10
Groundnut cake	20	10	20	20	30	30	30
Til cake	-	10	10	-	-	-	-
Fish meal	10	10	10	8	6	6	6
Wheat bran	10	10	10	10	-	-	-
Molasses	10	6	6	-	10	10	10
Brewer's yeast	2	2	2	-	2	2	2
Mineral salt	1.5	1.5	1.5	1.5	1.5	1.5	1.5
Salt	0.5	0.5	0.5	0.5	0.5	0.5	0.5

* Vitamin premix could be added as per manufacturers specification

[a] Pathak & Ranjhan (1972),[b] Ranjhan S.K. (1981) , [c]AICRP on pigs (2004)

[d] Sagar and Pathak (1987)

Table 2: Composition of cereal based grower rations.

Ingredients	% in the ration											
	I[a]	II[a]	III[a]	IV[b]	V[b]	VI[c]	VII[d]	VIII[d]	IX[e]	X[e]	XI[f]	XII[f]
Maize	60	30	10	30	30	50	35	18	35	17.5	40	20
Minor Millet	-	-	-	-	-	-	-	-	-	-	20	20
Groundnut cake	20	20	20	20	20	10	17 (DOGNC)	12 (DOGNC)	-	-	20	20
SESBM	-	-	-	-	-	-	-	-	10	10	-	-
Wheat bran	10	40	60	40	-	32.5	40	62	10	10	10	15
Rice bran	-	-	-	-	40	-	-	-	-	41.0	-	15 (DORB)
Fish meal	6.5	6.5	6.5	6.5	6.5	5.0	6	6	6	6	8	
(or FM)	8											
(or FM)												
Bone meal	1.0	1.0	1.0	1.0	1.0	-	-	-	-	-	-	-
Chalk	1.0	1.0	1.0	1.0	1.0	-	-	-	-	-	-	-
Min. Mixture	1.0	1.0	1.0	1.0	1.0	2.0	1.5	1.5	1.5	1.5	1.5	1.5
Salt	0.5	0.5	0.5	0.5	0.5	0.5	0.5	0.5	0.5	0.5	0.5	0.5
Calculated/ Estimated values:												
CP%	20	20	20	18	18	17.2	20.3	19.0	19.0	18.2		
DE(Mcal/kg)	3.2	3.1	2.9	3.0	3.0	3.2	3.2	2.9	3.4	2.7		
ME (Mcal/kg)	2.6	2.6	2.4	2.5	2.5	2.6	-	-	3.2	2.6		
Performance :												
Growth rate(g/d)	470	430	350	340	260	-	288	275	348	323		
Feed: gain	3.8	4.1	4.0	4.3	4.2	-	3.4	3.5	5.3	5.7		

Vitamins could be added as per manufacturers specification.

[a]Rajnhan et al. (1971), [b] Chhabra et al.(1971), [c] Pathak and Ranjhan (1972), [d] Bhar et al. (2001), [e]Soren et al.(2004), [f] Sagar and Pathak (1987); DOGNC is solvent extracted groundnut cake; FM is the meat meal and SESBM is the Solvent extracted soybean meal.

Table 3: Composition of the low cereal and non-cereal based grower rations

Ingredients	% of the ration								
	I[a]	II[a]	III[a]	IV[a]	V[a]	VI[a]	VII[b]	VIII[b]	IX[c]
Yellow maize	10	-	-	10	-	10	-	-	-
Rice Polish	-	-	70	60	35	30	-	-	-
Ground nut cake	20	20	20	20	10	10	7	-	30
SESBM	-	-	-	-	-	-	-	7	-
Til cake	-	-	-	-	10	10	-	-	-
Wheat bran	60	70	-	-	35	30	85	85	60
Fish meal	7.5	7.5	7.5	7.5	7.5	7.5	6.0	6.0	7.5
Mineral mixture	2.0	2.0	2.0	2.0	2.0	2.0	1.5	1.5	2.0
Salt	0.5	0.5	0.5	0.5	0.5	0.5	0.5	0.5	0.5

Vitamin premix could be added as per the manufacturers specification.

[a] Ranjhan, S.K.(1981), [b] Bhar et al. (2002), [c] Ranjhan et al. (1972); SESBM is the Solvent extracted soybean meal.

Table 4: Composition of the finisher ration for the pigs.

Ingredients	% of the ration													
	I [a]	II [a]	III [a]	IV [a]	V [a]	VI [a]	VII [b]	VIII [b]	IX [b]	X [c]	XI [c]	XII [c]	XIII [c]	XIV
Yellow maize	40	25	20	-	-	-	35	18	-	30	20	-	-	
Barely	-	15	-	-	-	-	-	-	-	-	-	-	-	
Sorghum / Bajra	-	-	-	-	-	-	-	-	-	20	20	-	-	
Milo	-	-	20	-	-	-	-	-	-	-	-	-	-	
Wheat bran	30	-	20	75	50	40	50	71	92	18	18	65	40	
Rice bran	-	-	-	-	-	-	-	-	-	-	-	-	25	
Rice Polish	-	30	10	-	25	25	-	-	-	-	-	-	-	
Ground nut cake	12	12	12	17	17	17	7	3 (solv.)	-	15	15	10	10	
Til cake	10	10	10	-	-	-	-	-	-	-	-	-	-	
Fish meal	5.5	5.5	5.5	5.5	5.5	5.5	6.0	6.0	6.0	5.0	5.0	5.0	5.0	
Molasses	-	-	-	-	-	10	-	-	-	10	10	18	18	
Mineral mixture	2.0	2.0	2.0	2.0	2.0	2.0	1.5	1.5	1.5	1.5	1.5	1.5	1.5	
Salt	0.5	0.5	0.5	0.5	0.5	0.5	0.5	0.5	0.5	0.5	0.5	0.5	0.5	

Vitamin premix could be added as per the manufacturers specification; [a] Ranjhan, S.K.(1981), [b]Bhar et al. (2000), [c] Sagar and Pathak (1987);

Table 5: Some unconventional feed sources for pigs, their relative value, safe level of replacement for conventional grain (energy)/oil cakes (protein supplements).

Feed stuff	Relative value (%)*	Level of inclusion of energy/protein sources (%)**
Energy sources:		
Tapioca	85	27
De-oiled rice bran	66	25
Sweet potatoes (raw)	20-25	27-41
Sweet potatoes (dehydrated)	90	27
Potatoes (raw)	25-28	20.5-41
Potatoes (dehydrated)	100	27
Jackfruit	-	50
Mahua flower	-	22-45%
Protein supplements:		
Cotton seed meal	85	8-9
Coconut meal	50	10-20
Linseed meal	80	5
Sunflower meal	90-95	8
Safflower meal		5-10
Til cake	49	10

* In comparison to cereal grain maize for energy and oilcake soyabean meal for protein source

** Replacement of energy and protein sources of standard ration for AICRP (pig) containing the following ingredients: Maize-35, Wheat bran-47, Soya bean meal-10, Fish meal-6, Mineral mixture – 1.5 and Salt-0.5%, respectively.

Bibliography

Agarwal, D.K. 1971. Effect of plane of nutrition on performance and carcass characteristics of Large White Yorkshire pigs. Ph.D. Thesis, IVRI, Izatnagar.UP

Agarwal, D.K., Pathak, N.N., Raina, B.L., Kumar, D., Sukh Deo and Chhabra, A.K. 1982. Note on the growth response of Landrace pigs fed diets containing high levels of wheat bran. Indian J. Anim. Sci. 52:1141.

Allee, G.L. 1976. Kansas State University Report of Progress 283:24.

AICRP. 2004. Annual Progress Report, Research Unit, Swine Production Farm, Livestock Production and Management Section, All India Coordinated Research Project on Pigs, IVRI, Izatnagar, UP.

Anonymous 1999. All India Coordinated Research Project on pigs. Annual progress Report (April 1998-March 1999). Directorate of Research, Assam Agricultural University, Khanapara, Gouhati-22 (Assam) p.27-29.

Anonymous, 2000. Effect of particle size of yellow maize (zia maize) on the growth performance, digestibility and carcass traits in crossbred pigs. All India Coordinated Research Project on Pigs. Annual Progress Report (April 1999- March 2000), Centre for pig production and research, Kerala Agricultural University, Manuthy, Thrissur-680651.p.13-16

Anonymous.1985.All India Coordinated Research Project on Pigs, Report for sixth five year plan period (April 1980 to March 1985), Indian Veterinary Research Institute, Izatnagar, UP p.13-16.

Bauza, R., Barlocco, N. and Cozzolino, D.1990. Use of rice bran in diets for fattening pigs. Effect of different levels of inclusion and zinc supplementation. Boletin de Investigation Facultad de Agronomia, Universidad de la Republica (25), p. 20. In: Nutrition Abstracts and Reviews (1992) 62: 5269 (Abstract).

Bhar, R, Murarilal, Pathak, N.N., Satya Paul and Bhatia, S.S. 1996. Nutrient utilization in adult boar fed on ration supplemented with green berseem. III Annual Conference of IAAVR and National Symposium on “Prospects of Livestock and Poultry Development in 21st Century”, CARI, Izatnagar, Feb. 23-24, p. 37.

Bhar, R., Chhabra, A.K. and Tiwari, C.B. 2002.Performance of crossbred (Landrace x Desi) finisher pigs fed on fish meal free diet, IXth Annual Conference of IAAVR and National Symposium on “Concepts in Sustainable Livestock Production and Health in New Millenium” at Nagpur, Feb. 4-5.

Bhar, R., Pathak, N.N. and Paul, S. 2000. Performance of crossbred (Landrace x Local Indian) finisher barrows fed on maize replaced wheat bran based diets. Asian Australasian Journal of Animal Sciences, 13: 1429-1432.

Bhar, R., Pathak, N.N. and Paul, S. 2001. Performance of crossbred (Landrace and Local Indian) grower pigs on maize replaced wheat bran and deoiled rice bran based diets. Indian J. Anim. Sci., 71: 168-168.

Bhar, R., Sastry, V.R.B., Gaur, G.K. and Satya Paul, 1997. Neem (Azadirachta indica) seed cake as protein supplement in the feeding of crossbred (Landrace x Desi) barrows. Proc. National Symposium of Animal Nutrition Association on Feeding Strategies for Eco-friendly Animal Production in India. Feb. 14-15, IVRI, Izatnagar, Abst. No. 175.

BIS. 1987. Bureau of Indian Standards. Indian Standard Specification for pig feeds (First Revision) IS : 7472-1986. Manak Bhavan, 9 Bahadur Sah Zafar Mar, New Delhi 110 002.

Chabra, S.S., Dhudapker, B. S., Ranjhan, S.K. and Gupta, B.S. 1971. Cited from Ranjhan S.K. (1981). Nutrient requirements and nutrition of pigs. In: Animal nutrition in tropics, 2nd revised edn. Vikash Publishing House Pvt. Ltd. New Delhi-10002, p. 367-381.

Crane, F.M. et al. 1972. Effect of processing on the nutritional value of feeds. National Academy of Sciences. Washington DC. p. 72-90.

Danielson, D.M. and Crenshaw, J.D. 1991. Raw and processed soybeans in swine diet. In: Swine Nutrition, Chapter 25, pp. 573-584. E.R. Miller, D.E., Ullrey, and A.J. Lewis (eds.) Butterwarth Heinemann, Boston, M.A.

Ensminger, M.E. and Parker, R.O. 1984 In: Swine Science. The Interstate Printers and Publishers. Inc. Illinois. p.151-199.

Ewan, L.C. 1979. Iowa State University (1979). Swine Research Report AS494J. Ames, IA : Iowa State University.

Garg, A.K.and Pathak, N.N.1983. Studies on feeding grainless ration to Landrace sows. Indian Journal of Nutrition and Dietetics, 20: 202-206.

Garg, A.K., Pathak, N.N., Anjaneyulu, A.S.R. and Lakshmanan, V., 1986. Utilization of cane molasses as source of energy in the diet of young pigs. Agricultural wastes, 17:225.

Hogberg, M., Mahan, D. and Seerley, R.1980. Physical forms of feed-feed processing for swine. In: National Pork Industry Handbook, No. 71. Cooperative Extension Service, Purdue Univ., West, Lafayette, Indiana.

Holden, P.J. and Zimmerman, D.R. 1991. Utilization of cereal grain by-products in swine feeding. In: Swine Nutrition, Chapter 25, p. 573-584. E.R. Miller, D.E., Ullrey, and A.J. Lewis (eds.) Butterwarth-Heinemann, Boston, M.A.

Jain,V.K., Sing, Jayal, M.M., Pathak, N.N. and Ranjhan, S.K. 1978. Utilization of fish meal as a source of animal protein in the diets of growing finishing pigs. Indian Vet.J., 55:617.

Jensen, A.H. 1978. Effect of certain processing methods or nutritional value of feedstuff for growing- finishing swine. Mimeo Urbana. University of Illinois.

Kumar, A. and Barsaul C.S.1988. A comparative study and economics of four rations in pigs. Indian Veterinary Journal 65: 172-173.

Liptrap, D.O. and Haghberg, M.G. 1991. Physical forms of feed : Feed processing and feeder design and operation. In: Swine Nutrition Ed. by MIller E.R., Ullrey, D.E. and Lewis, A.J., Butterworth-Heinemann, 80 Montvale Avenue, Stoneham, MA 02180 p 373-386.

Luce, W.G. et al. 1974. Oklahoma Animal Science Research Report, p.179, Stillwater, Oklahoma State University. Cited from Swine Nutrition Ed. by MIller E.R., Ullrey, D.E. and Lewis, A.J. (1991). Butterworth-Heinemann, 80 Montvale Avenue, Stoneham, MA 02180 p 373-386.

Mercier, C. and Fillet, P.1975. Cereal chem.52: 283. Cited from Mandal, A.B., Manwar, S.J. and Elangovan, A.V. 2004. Centre of Advanced Studies in Animal Nutrition, IVRI, Izatnagar - 243 122 (UP).p.47-54.

Mandal, A.B., Manwar, S.J. and Elangovan, A.V. 2004. Various methods of processing of feeds and forages. In: Feed and fodder processing and energy utilization in ruminants. Centre of Advanced Studies in Animal Nutrition, IVRI, Izatnagar - 243 122 (UP).p.47-54.

Nath, M., Elangovan, A.V., Mandal, A.B., Johri, T.S. 2002. Make feed poultry (version1.1.0) software for feed formulation. Central Avian Research Institute, Izatnagar - 243 122 Bareily (UP) India.

National Research Council 1979. Nutrient requirements of swine, No. 2 National Acad. Sci. Washington, DC.

Nuzback, L.J. et al. 1982. Report of progress 422. Kansas State University Agricultural Experiment Station. Manhattan, R.S.: Kansas State University.

Ohh, S.J. et al. 1983. Report of progress 442. Kansas State University Agricultural Experiment Station Manhattan: Kansas State University.

Owsley, W.F., Knabe, D.A. and Tanksley T.D. Jr. 1981. Effect of sorghum particle size on digestibility of nutrients at the terminal ileum and over the total digestive tract of growing –finishing pigs. J. Anim. Sci., 52: 557.

Pathak, N.N. and Ranjan, S.K. 1972. Effect of two levels of energy and protein intake on the weight gain of the pregnant Large White pigs, their litter size and litter performance. Indian J Anim Sci. 42:1048.

Pathak, N.N. and Ranjan, S.K. 1973. Utilization of salseed meal in the finishing ration of pigs. Indian J Anim. Sci. 43:424

Pathak, N.N. and Ranjan, S.K. 1988. Shukar Poshan. Indian Council of Agricultural Research, New Delhi.

Pathak, N.N. and Ranjhan, S.K. 1981[a].Effect of replacement of groundnut cake through mustard cake from the diets on the reproductive performance of pregnant Large White Yorkshire gilts. Indian J. Anim. Sci., 51: 575.

Pathak, N.N. and Ranjhan, S.K. 1981[b].Growth response and feed efficiency and carcass characteristics of Large White Yorkshire pigs fed ad lib. liquid molasses and protein supplement. Indian J. Anim. Sci., 51: 681.

Pathak, N.N. Garg, A.K. and Baruah, K.K. 1983. Reproductive response of Landrace sows fed grainless rations of agro-industrial by-products. Vetcol, Khanapara, 21:4.

Pathak, N.N., Srivastava, S.K. & Ranjhan, S.K. 1980. Nutritive value of water hyacinth (Eichhornia crassipes) for pigs. Indian J. Anim. Sci. 50: 886.

Pathak, N.N., Srivastava, S.K. and Ranjhan SK 1979[b]. A note on the growth rate and feed efficiency of Landrace pigs fed ad libitum water hyacinth and limited conventional feeds during growing- finishing periods. Indian J. Anim. Sci.49: 110.

Pond, W.G.and Maner, J.A. 1984. Swine production and nutrition, Westport C.T., AVI Publishing Co.

Pond W.G., Church, D.C., Pond K.R., 1995. Feed preparation and processing. In: Basic animal nutrition and feeding. 4th ed. John Wiley and Sows. New York.

Ranjan S.K., Shukla, V.P., Kumar, I., Pathak, N.N. and Joshi, B.C. 1972. Effect on growth rate and carcass composition in Large White Yorkshire pigs on various plane of nutrition during growing-finishing period. Indian J. Anim. Sci. 42:453.

Ranjhan , S.K.1981. Nutrient requirements and nutrition of pigs. In: Animal nutrition in tropics, 2nd revised edn. Vikash Publishing House Pvt. Ltd. New Delhi-10002, pp. 367-381.

Ranjhan, S.K., Gupta, B.S., Chhabra, S.S. and Dhudapkar, B.S.1971. Effect of various levels of crude fibre and energy in the rations of growing Middle White Yorkshire pigs. Indian Journal of Animal Sciences, 41: 373-376.

Rao, P.K. and Prasad, D.A.1980. Economic rations based on rice by-products for growing Large White Yorkshire pigs. Indian Journal of Animal Sciences, 50: 63-67.

Sagar, R.H. and Pathak, N.N. 1987. Feeding of pigs in tropics. In: Advanced animal nutrition in developing countries. Edited by U.B. Singh. Indo-Vision Pvt. Ltd. Ghaziabad, India, p. 423.

Saikia, P. 2004. Performance of crossbred pigs fed on kitchen and vegetable market waste. M.V.Sc. Thesis, Indian Veterinary Research Institute, Izatnagar, UP.

Seerley, R.W., Miller, E.R. and Hoefer, J. A. 1962. Growth, energy and nitrogen studies on pigs fed meal and pellets. J. Anim. Sci., 21: 829.

Sasse et al.1975. Procedings of the 23rd Annual Swine Short Course. Agricultural Science Technology Report No. T-5-111, Lubbock, TX: Texas Tech. University.

Soren, N.M., Bhar, R., Chhabra, A.K. and Mandal, A.B.2004. Utilization of energy and protein in local Indian crossbred gilts fed diets containing different levels of rice bran. Asian Aust. J. Anim. Sci., 17:674-677.

Soren, N.M., Bhar, R., Chhabra, A.K. and Mandal, A.B. 2003. Performance of crossbred gilts fed on diets with higher level of fat and fibre through addition of rice bran. Asian Aust. J. Anim. Sci., 16: 1650-1655.

Svihus et al.1979. Cited from Mandal, A.B., Manwar, S.J. and Elangovan, A.V. 2004. Various methods of processing of feeds and forages. In: Feed and fodder processing and energy utilization in ruminants. Centre of Advanced Studies in Animal Nutrition, IVRI, Izatnagar - 243 122 (UP).

Takemasa and Hijikura 1983. Cited from Mandal, A.B., Manwar, S.J. and Elangovan, A.V. 2004. Various methods of processing of feeds and forages. In: Feed and fodder processing and energy utilization in ruminants. Centre of Advanced Studies in Animal Nutrition, IVRI, Izatnagar - 243 122 (UP).

Talukdar, R.P. 1979. Nutritional studies on water hyacinth (Eichornia crassipes [Mart] solms) as a component of pig ration. Ph.D. Thesis, IVRI, Izatnagar., UP.

Talukdar, R.P., Pathak, N.N. and Ranjhan, S.K. 1984. Effect of ad libitum feeding of water hyacinth (Eichhornia crassipes) with restricted conventional feeds on nutrient utilization and reproductive performance of Landrace and Desi gilts. Indian J. Anim. Prod.,16:31.

Teague, H.S. et al. 1970. Animal Science Mimeo #201. Columbus, Off: Ohio Agricultural Experiment Station.

Vanschoubroek, F. et al. 1971. Nutr. Abs. Rev., 41: 1.Cited from Liptrap, D.O. and Haghberg, M.G. 1991. Physical forms of feed : Feed processing and feeder design and operation. In: Swine Nutrition Ed. by MIller E.R., Ullrey, D.E. and Lewis, A.J., Butterworth-Heinemann, 80 Montvale Avenue, Stoneham, MA 02180 p 373-386.

Veum, T.L., McFate,K.L.and Hedrick, H.B.1972. Roasted milo for growing-finishing swine. J. Anim. Sci., 35: 1111 (Abstr.).

Wu, J.F. and Allee, G.L.1984. Report of progress, agricultural experiment station. Manhattan, K.S: Kansas State University.

Yang, S.P. et al. 1975. Proc. of the 23rd Annual Swine Short Course. Agricultural Science and Technology Report No. T-5-111. Lubbock, T.X. Texas Tech. University.

22
PESTICIDE RESIDUES IN FEEDS

Subir K. Nag, Mukesh K. Raikwar, S.K.Mahanta and S.S.Kundu

A pesticide is any substance or mixture of substances intended for preventing, destroying or controlling any pest, including vectors of human or animal diseases, unwanted species of plants or animals causing harm during or otherwise interfering with the production, processing, storage, transport or marketing of food, agricultural commodities, wood or wood products or animal's feed stuff or substances intended for use as a plant growth regulator, defoliant, desicant or agent for thinning fruit or preventing the premature fall of fruit and substances applied to crops either before or after harvest to protect the commodity from detoriation during storage and transport.

As chemicals, pesticides are toxic xenobiotics which can be classified on the basis of different criteria such as the use, the chemical class, mode of action, and/or toxicity. However, the most common and convenient one is on the basis of use. Thus, they can be classified as insecticide, fungicide, herbicide, rodenticide, nematicide, acaricide, molluscicide, bactericide, algaecide etc. Each group includes several structurally different classes of chemicals.

In India 179 active ingredients of different pesticides including botanicals and microbial products are registered for use. On the basis of use pattern market share of insecticide in maximum (64%) followed by fungicide (20%), herbicide (12%) and others (4%). In case of crop wise distribution cotton occupies the largest share (52%) followed by rice (17%), fruits and vegetables (13%), plantation crops (8%), cereals, millets and oilseeds (7%), sugarcane (2%) and others (1%). The growth of pesticide market in India has been phenomenal. While only 2000 MT of pesticide was consumed in 1955, In 1994-95 the figure was 80000 MT. But after that there was decline in the consumption. In 1999-2000 only 54133 MT pesticide was applied (Agnihotri, 2000). The reduction may be attributed primarily due to ban or restriction on use of some organochlorine insecticides like aldrin, dieldrin, heptachlor, DDT, HCH (BHC) etc. which have higher application rates, and partially due to use of natural products like botanical pesticides, microbial pesticides and adoption of IPM Programme to some extent. There has also been a paradigm shift in the use of different chemical classes of insecticides. While up to 1997 organchlorines occupied about 72% share of total insecticides used in India, in 2002 their contribution was only 14.5% and organophosphates topped the list with 74% share. Synthetic pyrethroids covered 5% while natural product's contribution was only 2%.

Pesticides are essential and invaluable input in modern day agriculture due to the fact that pests, diseases, and weeds destroying 1/3rd of the crop or commodity during growth, harvesting and storage. Beside, these chemicals are inseparable for successful control of vectors of human and animal diseases. The use of pesticides is all likely to continue in the near foreseeable future despite the fact that various alternative methods of pest control are being promoted. Even in the IPM it is a major component. India is one of the largest producers and consumers of pesticides in South Asia.

However, pesticides are considered as doubly edged weapon. On the one hand they are indispensable to cope with the pressure of producing more and more from less and less by sophisticated complex scientific activity using modern high yielding varieties. On the other hand these molecules as most types of toxic xenobiotics, could be harmful as well. Being toxic substances many of them or their metabolites are reported to have carcinogencity, teratogenicity, mutagenicity, genotoxicity, neurotoxicity and many other adverse effects. Rapidly increasing use of pesticides often with inefficient technical advice has brought in its wake many environmental problems inimical to the interest of human beings. Over the years there has been a mounting fear and concern that indiscriminate and improportionate use of pesticides may lead to harmful and ill effects in human beings and animals and may have deleterious effect on the environment.

The use of pesticides leads to the residues on crop at harvest. The term 'Pesticide residue' may be defined as any specific substance in food, agricultural commodity, or animal feed resulting from the use of a pesticide. The term includes any derivative of a pesticide such as conversion product, metabolite, reaction product and impurities considered to be toxicological significance. Whenever pesticides are applied on a crop or commodity or on any substrate to control pests, diseases, weeds etc. they invariably leave toxic residues on the substrate on which they are applied. The amount of residues left depends on the nature of the chemical, dose and volume of application, nature of substrate and prevailing weather condition. The occurrence of pesticide residue in ecosystem may have a threefold impact on man, by reducing the reproductive capacity of his environment or by contamination of either his food or work environment. Man and animals are exposed to low level of pesticide residues in air, water and food chain for a prolonged period of time, which pose problem to all animals, birds and other organisms and also human being. Man is the ultimate consumer of pesticide. As we see in the pesticide cycle, residues of pesticides in the grains, pulses, oil and oilseeds, milk, ghee, coffee, fish, meat etc. is ultimately consumed by man. Through fodder, water, air and other foodstuffs pesticide residues reach animals and then through milk and/or meat products it is accumulated in the body of human being. This accumulation is five times higher in man in comparison to crops. The bioaccumulation and biomagnification of certain pesticide residues in human food chain is an important aspect of pesticide induced environmental pollution, which needs great attention.

The presence of pesticide residues has been detected in various items and in food chain. The level of pesticides is found to be at much higher level than expected, because of heavy contamination of environment. Problem of pesticide residues have been further aggravated because of ignorance of farmers and malpractices of pesticide dealers and retailers. Farmers at large in our country can not follow proper schedule of pesticide application and maintain the right dose of the chemical. Many a times they use pesticides in overdoses. They can hardly realise the hazards associated with pesticide residues particularly in fruits, vegetables and fodder crops which are consumed raw without any processing by man and animals. Among the different group of pesticides organochlorines are most persistent in nature. Being lipophilic they are deposited in body fat of man and animal. Such pesticides have an affinity for lipid material and are not easily biodegradable. So they cause contamination of animal of animal products like milk, meat, fish, egg, ghee, butter etc. Animal products contribute 70 - 90 % of the total oragnochlorinated pesticides in the diet of an Indian, particularly milk and milk products (Kannan et al., 1992). The residues of these pesticides in animal products also decline at a very slow rate even after the sources of contamination are eliminated. All the feed resources like cereal grains, oilcakes, brans, legume and nonlegume forage crops, crop residues are found to be contaminated with organochlorinated and other pesticides.

Sources of entry of pesticides in animal body system: There are three possible ways by which pesticides can enter into the animal body (Fig. 1). The main source of entry is the contaminated feed and fodder offered to animals for consumption. The feed materials may be contaminated by pesticides either at the time of cultivation of the crops in the field from which they have been prepared like oilseed crops (mustard, linseed, sesamum, cotton etc.) in case of oilseed cakes, cereals (paddy, wheat, maize, etc.) in case of straw, chuni and hay, or during the storage of the feed materials in the go downs particularly during rainy seasons. Green fodders and/or dual purpose crops like sorghum, maize, bajra, oat, berseem, cowpea, different grasses may act as direct source of contamination if pesticides are applied on them at the time of cultivation because many a times fodder crops after being treated with pesticides are fed to animals straight way without waiting sufficient time for the residues to go down below maximum residue limit. Pesticides are also used in a large scale for their useful properties to kill ectoparasites like ticks, mites, insects on the animal body. As a result they may enter into the animal body through skin pores when applied by drenching. Drinking water sometimes may also be a source of contamination although concentration may not be such as to worry about. After entry into the animal body pesticides are distributed in different tissues and organs. Since many of them particularly organochlorines and synthetic pyrethroids are lipophilic in nature, they have a tendency to accumulate in the adipose tissues and usually they do not get converted into water soluble metabolites. As the concentration in the fatty tissues exceeds a threshold level, the excess residues are tranlocated into the lactating glands of the animals from where they are secreted in the milk. Because of special position of milk in the diet of infants and children the presence of significant amount of residues in milk is undesirable. That is why residue limit for milk and dairy products tend to be more severe than those for other products.

Pesticide residues in feed, fodder, milk & milk products, fish and meat

Feed: Feed is one of the major source for the contamination of animal body with pesticide residues. As discussed earlier, feeds coming as by products of agricultural crops such as straw, oilseed cakes, chunnies are contaminated in the field in many ways directly or indirectly by pesticides. Apart from applying pesticide to the growing crops in the field, spraying of pesticide on feed

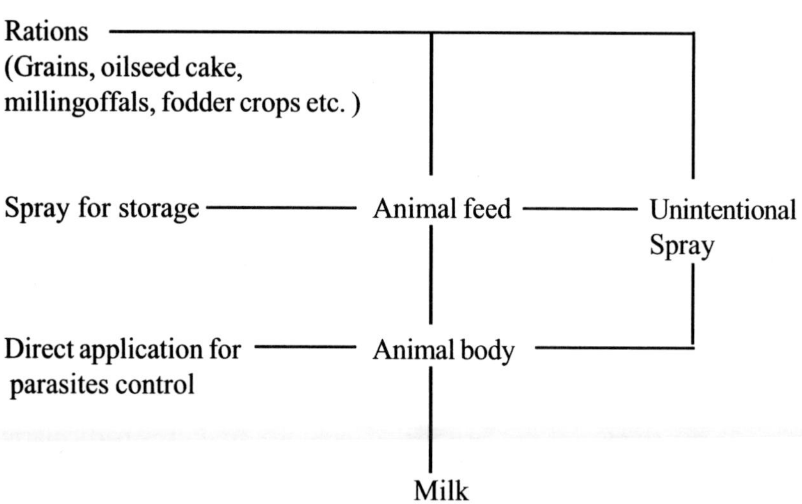

Fig. 1. Possible sources of contamination of animal body and animal products with pesticides.

concentrate bags in godowns for controlling storage pest is also a common practice which can also lead to contamination. The readymade feed concentrate sold in the market is actually a mixture of many grains and jaggery/molasses which many contain pesticide residues. Rice and wheat straw are one of the important feed materials used in India for cattle and buffaloes. Rice consumes second largest share of total pesticide (17%) consumed in India. Rice bran, a rich source of HCH and other residues is used as an ingredient in the readymade feed concentrate. Although wheat crop as such does not consume much pesticide but during the storage of wheat straw, air tied covered heaps are made on the ground in which soil was mixed with HCH in heavy dose to prevent to attack of termites. During summer months as temperature in the heaps rose very high (40-60^{0}C), HCH being volatile formed vapour and contaminated entired straw in the heap. Numerous example of the contamination of animals through animal feed have been reported in the literature (Back, 1970, 1975; Von Houweling et al. 1977). However public awareness of this did not become acute until 1974 when poly brominated biphenyls (PBD) were associated with an accident in Michigan in USA. The direct impact of this incident resulted in the destruction of 30,000 cattle and 6000 swine as well as sheep, poultry and dairy products. In USA (Pierson et al.1982) screening of random samples of feed comprising of grains, cereals, by products and miscellaneous for organochlorine insecticides like lindane, β-BHC, aldrin, dieldrin, pp^1-DDE, op^1-DDT, pp^1-DDD, pp^1-DDT, heptachlor, and its epoxide revealed average contamination levels of less than 10ppb.

In India studies to determine pesticide residues in different types of animal feed and fodder were very few. Few of them as available in the literature are discussed below. Shastri (1983) depicted results of monitoring of different categories of feed samples for organochlorine pesticide residues (Table-1).

Table 1. Pesticide residues in different categories of feed samples

S.No.	Product	Samples Screened	with residues	Above level	Residues in ppm	Insecticide
1	Poultry feed	37	36	-	0.13-5.33	DDT
2(a)	Cattle feed	13	11	-	0.23-2.0	DDT
2(b)	Ingredient	300	200	-	0.08-0.8	DDT
3.	Hay and other fodder	85	27	-	0.05-2.3	DDT
4.	Maize	11	11	-	0.13-5.7	DDT
5.	Wheat	7	7	-	0.30 -4.0	DDT
6.	Edible grain	15	15	-	0.13-0.96	BHC
7.	Cereals & Products	594	391	391	Tr-20	DDT, lindane, Endrin
8.	Pulses	161	49	49	Tr-10	BHC
9.	Oilseed	18	-	-	1.1-4.1	DDT

Singh et al. (1988) determined insecticide residues in wheat grains and straw arising from their storage in premises treated with BHC and DDT under malaria control programme in Punjab. All the 120 samples of wheat grains collected from BHC as well as DDT sprayed districts contained residues of both HCH and DDT, concentration of which varied from 0.01-5.18mg/kg and 0.01-2.14mg/kg respectively. Analysis of 40 wheat straw samples also showed presence of BHC (mean concentration 0.24 mg/kg) and DDT (1.35 mg/kg) residues in all the samples.

Analysis of 32 samples collected from local market of Lucknow revealed presence of α, β and γ isomer of HCH was found in all the samples and the mean concentration of total HCH was 0.393 ppm (Dixit et al. 1989). Residues of pp^1 DDE, op^1 DDT, pp^1 DDD and pp^1 DDT were also present in all the samples. Total DDT content was 0.236ppm. The level of aldrin was found to be 0.156ppm. Endrin, one of the most toxic organohlorines, was also present (0.02ppm) in all the feed samples along with endosulfan α-isomer (0.029ppm). Contamination of cattle feeds by DDT and HCH to the same extent was also reported earlier by Kaphalia and Seth, 1982). Dikshith, et al. (1989) in their attempt to quantify residues of different organochlorine pesticides in oilseeds used in the country found that mustard, groundnut and sesamum seeds obtained from Lucknow were contaminated with DDT to the extent of 130-3200ppb and HCH to the extent of 91-250ppb.

In another study conducted in Punjab by Battu et al. (1996) on monitoring of 105 samples of different feeds 100 and 80% contamination was found with residues of HCH and DDT respectively. Feed concentrates, straw and green fodder showed total HCH residues comprising α, β, γ and γ isomers up to 0.26, 2.28 and 0.69mg/kg and DDT residues up to 0.28, 6.70 and 0.35mg/kg respectively. The tolerable content of 0.02 mg/kg β-HCH and 0.10mg/kg ΣDDT in the feed samples (dry weight basis) were exceeded in about 35% samples, while those of α, β and γ HCH exceeded in about 3% samples.

Unnikrishnan et al. (1998) reported that BHC, DDT and endosulfan were detected in samples of cattle feed and feed ingredients collected from Bangalore. Total BHC content of the compounded feeds ranged from 0.0076-0.1197mg/kg, DDT ranged from traces to 0.01 mg/kg. The active isomer α–BHC constituted only a minor portion of total BHC content in most of these samples. In groundnut cake samples the predominant contaminant was DDT, while BHC was the major contaminant in compounded feed.

In a multilocational study conducted by AICRP (Pesticide residues) (Agnihotri, 1999) on straw to determine HCH and DDT residues it was revealed that out of 137 samples analysed, all sample excepting 10 samples from Bhubaneswar were contaminated with residues of HCH (range 0.01-0.568mg/kg). In addition, most of the straw samples also contained residues of DDT (range ND-0.35 mg/kg).

Limiting values are the concentrations of pesticides in feed and fodder if fed to lactating animals daily, the likely residues in milk will be less than their MRL values and safe for human consumption. The limiting value of DDT and HCH residues in feed for Indian buffalo (Bubalus bubalis) were calculated at AICRP (Pesticide residues), PAU, Ludhiana center, by feeding the buffaloes with green fodder and feed concentrates treated with different isomers of HCH, DDT and their analogoues. The intake of DDT and its metabolites through normal feed varied from 0.1-2.5mg/day, whereas other of total HCH varied from 0.3-3.2mg/day. Each buffalo was fed with treated diet for 100 days. Milk sample collected at different time intervals and analysed for insecticide residues. The concentration of pesticide in milk fed with DDT and its analogous increased rapidly during the first 10-20 days and then leveled off and plateaued during the remaining period of insecticide dosing. For HCH isomers, the plateau was reached within 5-15days of feeding. The transfer coefficient defined as "The percentage of daily intake of pesticide which is excreted in the milk each day after equilibrium conditions have reached" for α-HCH (12-15%), β-HCH (31-36%), β-HCH (2.7%) and γ-HCH (8.5%) (Kapoor and Kalra, 1997), most of the DDT isomers and its analogous (~5%) was higher in buffalo milk than in cow milk.

The limiting value of DDT complex, α, β, γ and γ isomers of HCH in feed and fodder for buffalo have been worked out to be 0.2, 0.3, 0.94, 0.03, and 0.1mg/kg (dry wt. basis). If the feed containing residues above the limiting values are fed to the lactating animals, it is likely to be passed to the milk. The limiting value of remaining organochlorinated and different other groups of pesticides are yet to be worked out.

Multilocational trial was carried out at 15 locations to determination the residues of DDT and HCH in feed concentrates. Out of 377 samples analysed, most samples contained residues of both HCH and DDT. The mean value ranging from <0.01 - 0.60 mg/kg for DDT and < 0.01 - 2.27mg/kg for HCH was found. The presence of residues of HCH and DDT present in straw and feed in almost all samples of different locations in amounts above the prescribed limit proved that they were a potential source of contamination in milk (Agnihotri, 1999).

HCH and DDT residues were monitored in certain dry fodder (pearl millet, wheat and barley) and fed concentrates (sesamum, mustard, and cottonseed cake) collected from Jaipur in Rajasthan (Gupta et al. 2000). No DDT residues was detected in any of the samples. However, HCH residues were present in the range of 0.3-1.73mg/kg in feed concentrates. In case of dry fodder wheat and barley had no residues of HCH but pearl millet samples were contaminated with HCH in the range of 0.06-0.11mg/kg.

In another study conducted at NDRI, Karnal (Prasad and Chhabra, 2001) it was found that contamination in feed concentrates and roughages was caused by BHC (73.3%), endosulfan (8%), heptachlor (8%) DDT (4.2%) and aldrin (2.6%).The content of BCH residues was highest in concentrate mixture followed by maize, groundnut cake, wheat bran, rice bran, cotton seed cake, barley, and mustard cake. Among the roughages it was highest in maize fodder followed by oat, berseem, wheat straw, lucerne, and paddy straw in the decreasing order. Among the different isomers of HCH, α and γ were more than β and δ. The two isomers of DDT (op^1 and pp^1) were present in all the forages and in most of the concentrate feeds as compared to fodders.

So far we have come across reports where feed and fodder samples were tested at different places only for DDT and HCH residues. But at IGFRI, Jhansi monitoring of diverse feed samples collected from different places of Bundelkhand is being done for residues of different group of pesticides viz organochlorines (OC), organophosphates (OP), carbamates and synthetic pyrethroids (SP). In concentrate feed sample. In case of organochlorines, DDT, HCH and endosulfan residues were found present in varying amounts in different concentrate feeds viz mustard seed cake, linseed cake, cotton seed cake, groundnut seed cake, sesamum seed cake and dry fodders like lentil straw, wheat straw, gram and oat chunni samples. The extent of contamination with different organochlorines varied from 28-100%. Among the organophosphates, chlorpyriphos, monocrotophos, quinalphos, malathion, phosphamidon were mainly detected in many concentrate feed and dry fodder samples. Among the carbamates only carbofuran was tested and was found only rarely. The extent of contamination with OPs varied from 20-90%. In case of synthetic pyrethroids, cypermethrin was found present in many samples, mostly in oilseed cakes and particularly in mustard seed cake and cotton seed cake even up to a concentration of 1.5mg/kg. Among others, fenpropathrin, cyhalothrin and fenvalerate were also detected in many samples. Oil seed cakes samples were more contaminated with residues of different pesticides than straw samples or chunnies. The extent of contamination of different feed samples with SPs varied from 30-100% (Nag and Raikwar, 2002, 2003).

In addition to HCH and DDT, residues of endosulfan and malathion were also detected in a limited number of feed concentrate samples out of a total of 17 tested by Kang et al. (2002) at Ludhiana (Punjab). Dicofol, an acricide organochlorine group, was also detected in two feed concentrate samples. Limiting value of β, γ and δ HCH and total DDT were exceeded in about 13, 6.5, 65 and 9.7% of animal feed samples on dry weight basis. However the results showed substantial decline in pesticide residues with respect to β-HCH and total DDT as compared to earlier report of 35% samples exceeding the limiting values of two insecticides (Battu et al. 1996). Feed samples collected from Jorhat district of Assam shown presence of lindane or γ-BHC (0.025-0.041mg/kg), β–endosulfan (0.0028mg/kg) and endosulfan sulfate (0.045-0.049mg/kg) residues in them (Deka et al. 2004).

Green fodder: Work on green fodder crops with respect to pesticide residues, their dissipation pattern and safety evaluation has been very limited. At IGFRI, Jhansi endosulfan, the recommended and commonly used insecticide in forage crops, was evaluated for persistence of residues and safe-waiting period following application at the recommended dose in fodder crops like sorghum, cowpea, lucerne and maize. The residual half-life around 3-4days and safe-waiting period around 9-14days have been recommended (Nag and Shah, 1999, 2001, 2002; Raikwar et al., 2003). Carbendezim, the systemic fungicide recommended and used in fodder crops was also evaluated for persistency in sorghum (Raikwar and Nag, 2004). Residual half-life of 6days was observed and safe-waiting period around 9-10days was recommended.

Gupta et al. (2000) monitored HCH and DDT residues in certain green fodder crops like pearl millet, guinea grass, mustard, fenugreek, oat, chinese cabbage and lucerne collected from Jaipur (Rajasthan) and they concluded that all the samples contained HCH residues above MRL. However, DDT residue was not detected in any sample. Prasad and Chhabra, (2001) analysed few green fodders such as maize, oat, sorghum, berseem and lucerne at NDRI, Karnal for organochlorine pesticide residues. According to their results, ΣHCH content was abnormally high ranging from 15-44 mg/kg DM basis, lowest in lucerne and highest in maize. ΣDDT and Σendosulfan residues ranged from 1.3-2.8mg/kg and 1.9-5.9mg/kg respectively. Fourteen green fodder samples collected from Ludhiana district of Punjab were evaluated for pesticide residues by Kang et al. (2002). All the 14 samples contained ΣHCH residues (range 0.03-0.82mg/kg) but in only 2 and 3 sample ΣDDT (BDL- 0.18mg/kg) and Óendsulfan (BDL-1.58 mg/kg) residues were detected. Among the OPs, malathion was found in 8 samples (BDL-4.35 mg/kg).

Sorghum, maize, bajra, oat and berseem collected from different places and locations of Bundelkhand region are being monitored for pesticide residues (Nag and Raikwar, 2002, 2003). About 20-60% samples were contaminated with different organochlorine pesticides like ΣDDT, ΣHCH and Σendosulfan ranged from Tr-2.8310mg/kg, 0.0067-0.0290mg/kg and Tr-0.6985mg/kg respectively. In case of organophosphates, contamination ranged from 0-60%. Phosphmidon, malathion, monocrotophos, chlorpyriphos and quinalphos were mainly detected. Synthetic pyrethroids particularly cypermethrin, cyfluthrin and fenvalerate were found present in some samples (20-60%).

Grasses like setaria, guinea, dinanath, sirsa, paragrass, Bothriochloa, hybrid napier and fodder cowpea collected from Jorhat district of Assam were analysed and no detectable residues of any pesticide was found (Deka et al. 2004).

Milk: Pesticides, which have an affinity for lipid materials and are not biodegradable accumulate in animal system. Such pesticides cause contamination of animal products like meat, milk, eggs, fish etc. The residues of these pesticides in animal products also decline at a very slow rate, even after sources of contamination are eliminated. Table-2 illustrates the relative potential of some pesticides as contaminants of animal products. Residue level of a particular pesticide found in milk is in direct proportion of transfer coefficient, following the ingestion of contaminated ration by lactating animals. OC pesticides such as DDT, dieldrin, HCH etc. have therefore been viewed as serious contaminants of bovine milk while the pesticides belonging to other groups are considered not to cause any significant residue problem. The residues of SPs and carbaryl have also been found to decline at a much faster rate than organochlorines. In view of these, the residues of OC pesticides are still detectable, though at very low levels, in dairy products in certain countries even through these pesticides have not been in use there for the last about 15 years.

Table 2. Transfer coefficient and rate of decline of certain insecticides in bovine milk following their ingestion.

Insecticide	Intake (mg/kg)	Transfer coefficient (%)	$T_{½}$ (days)
pp' DDT	25	5.1	53
Dieldrin	2	25.6	12
α–HCH	2	11.5	14
β-HCH	2	30.5	15
γ-HCH	17	22	6
Crbaryl	2000	0.16	0.7
Fenvalerate	454	0.44	2
-do-	1362	0.64	2
Deltamethrin	270	0.27	0.8

Kalra and Chawla (1985)

Contamination of bovine milk with organochlorine pesticides particularly with DDT and HCH was first reported in the 60's and 70's from Delhi area and Punjab (Agnihotri et al.1974; Dhaliwal and Karla, 1977.) Subsequently results of analysis of samples from Hyderabad (Laxminarayana, 1980), Bombay (Noronha, 1978) and Punjab (Sandhu, 1979, Karla and Chawala, 1983), Pondicherry (Adiroubane and Letchoumane, 1996), Himachal Pradesh (Kumar and Nath, 1996), Jaipur (Gupta et al., 1997) showed widespread contamination of milk samples with OC residues, particularly DDT and HCH. According to ICMR (1993) out of 2200 milk samples analysed all over India, 37% contained DDT and 42% HCH above MRL values.

According to report of AICRP (Pesticide residues) out of 487 milk samples collected from across the country and analysed for pesticide residues, DDT was detected in 86.5% samples of which 43.2% samples contained residues above the prescribed MRL of 0.05 mg/kg. High level of DDT residues were detected in samples of New Delhi (0.01-1.08mg/kg), Anand (0.18-25.6mg/kg), Ludianina (0.01-0.28mg/kg), Hyderabad (ND-0.25mg/kg), Rahuri, (ND-0.53mg/kg), Pusa (ND-0.17) and Coimbatore (0.01-0.43 mg/kg). In addition to DDT 89.7% samples were contaminated with HCH (80.3% with β-HCH)) out of which 77.8% of the samples had total HCH exceeding MRL of 0.1mg/kg on whole milk basis. However on the basis of β-HCH (active constituent of technical HCH) 80.3% milk samples were contaminated and only 31.6% samples exceeded MRL. All the four isomers of HCH were detected in the milk samples, among them the level of α-isomer was the highest followed by β, γ and δ. Maximum residues were detected in milk samples collected from Anand (1.12-5.12mg/kg) followed by Hyderabad (0.13-4.19mg/kg), Coimbatore (ND-0.70mg/kg), Jorhat (0.02-0.46mg/kg), Delhi (ND-0.39 mg/kg), Bangalore (ND-0.22 mg/kg) and Kanpur (0.01-0.21mg/kg).

A survey of dairy milk and milk products in and around Delhi was undertaken to monitor the levels of DDT and HCH by Mukherjee and Gopal (1993). The study revealed that pesticide residue levels in milk often exceeded the limits recommended by FAO/WHO expert committee. The 15 samples of dairy milk and 4 samples of milk products analysed had residue levels ranging from 0.022 to 0.166mg/kg for HCH and 0.042 to 0.382mg/kg for DDT (Table-3).

Battu et al. (2001) described a change in scenario with respect to contamination of bovine milk with pesticide residues. In 1999, analysis of 22 bovine milk samples from MILKFED depot of Ludhiana revealed that all were contaminated with lindane and values exceeded its MRL of 0.01mg/kg fixed under PFA rule. Most of the samples showed the presence of DDT at detection limit (0.005mg/kg). Further analysis of 24 samples in 2000 showed residues in 4 samples 2 of which exceeded its MRL. Lindane was detected in 12 samples all exceeding its MRL. In 2001 analysis of 10 samples showed no residues of DDT and lindane in 2 samples greater than MRL. Thus there was a decline in contamination of bovine milk with DDT and an increase in contamination with lindane residues.

Table 3. HCH and DDT residues in whole milk samples from different sources in Delhi

Sample	Frequency	ΣHCH (mg/kg)	ΣDDT (mg/kg)
Dairy milk (Zone 1)	4	0.058	0.197
Dairy milk (Zone 2)	3	0.080	0.104
Dairy milk (Zone 3)	3	0.069	0.193
Dairy milk (Zone 4)	3	0.086	0.108
Buffalo milk	2	0.166	0.220
Condensed milk	1	0.084	0.188
Cheese	1	0.110	0.345
Cream	1	0.132	0.382
Curd	1	0.022	0.042

Bovine milk samples collected from Tamilnadu Agriculture University Dairy farm and private vendors were evaluated for residues of chlorinated hydrocarbons by Vasanthi et al. (2003). Out of 69 samples analysed 84 and 24% of samples were contaminated with HCH and DDT, respectively. However, residues were below detectable levels.

Report about occurrence of residues of organochlorine in milk and milk products are numerous and some of them have been mentioned before. But presence of residues of other group insecticides like synthetic pyrethroids and organophosphates in milk are although rare but not uncommon because there has been a paradigm shift in the use pattern of insecticide. Earlier, mostly OCs were used but as a result of banning or restricting most of them, people have switched over to organophosphates, pyrethroids and other newer molecules like neonicotinoids. Among them pyrethroid group of insecticides are liophilic in nature although not much stable as the OCs.

Bovine milk sample collected from different places and locations of Bundelkhand region are being monitored for residues of different groups of pesticides viz, organochlorines, organophosphates, carbamate and synthetic pyrethroids. Milk samples of Jhansi, Banda, Lalitpur, Jaloun and Gwalior were contaminated with different OC compounds like ΣHCH, ΣDDT and endosulfan to the extent of 64-87%. But the concentration of pesticides were very low and mostly within their respective MRLs. Among the organophosphates, chlorpyriphos (0.0068-0.0279mg/kg), malathion (0.0122-0.0363mg/kg), quinalphos (0.0079-

0.0378mg/kg) were found present in many samples. The range of overall contamination with OPs ranged from 17-88%. Synthetic pyrethroids were found present most frequently and the range of contamination was 72-100%. Cypermethrin was predominant (0.2718-1.040mg/kg) followed by cyfluthrin (Tr-0.2187mg/kg), cyhalothrin (Tr-0.0706 mg/kg), fenvelarate (0.0144-0.2818mg/kg) and fenpropathrin (0.0074-0.0248 mg/kg). Deltamethrin was detected in very few samples (Nag and Raikwar, 2002,2003).

Kathpal et al. (2004) monitored bovine milk samples collected from cotton growing belt of Haryana (Hisar, Fatehabad, Sirsa). Out of 155 samples 138 were found contaminated. The HCH isomers were present in all samples (0.001-0.209mg/kg) but were above the MRL in only 5 samples. Total DDT residues were present in all samples (0.001-0.649mg/kg) of which 56 samples contained residues above MRL. Endosulfan and its sulfate (0.001-0.154mg/kg) was present in above MRL values in 29 samples. Chlorodane (0.001-0.037mg/kg) was detected in 23 samples. Cypermethrin and Deltamethrin were detected varying from 0.002-0.053 and 0.058-0.076mg/kg respectively. Only one sample with cypermethrin and two with deltamethrin were above their MRLs. Fenvalerate was detected in some samples. Among the OPs chlorpyriphos (0.001-0.027mg/kg) in 30 samples, monocrotophos (0.001-0.248mg/kg), quinalphos and methyl parathion were present in 16 samples. Four samples with monocrotophos and three with chlorpyriphos were above their MRLs.

Baby milk powder: Infant food collected from Ludhiana was found to be 100% contaminated with DDT, 90% of which were above the tolerance level (Shastry, 1983). Gupta et al. (1997), however, did not get any residues of DDT, α and δ-HCH in six milk powders collected from Jaipur. Only one milk powder was found to contain to β and γ-HCH. In the analysis of baby milk powder collected from Solan (HP), Hyderabad (AP), Trivandrum (Kerala), Kolkata (WB), and Bangalore (Karnataka), it was found that HCH was the major contaminant in baby milk powder (Agnihotri, 1999). The data on residues of DDT and HCH are presented in Table-4. The highest residues were detected in samples collected from H.P. (Solan). Among different isomers of HCH, β-isomer was found to be highest follwed by α, γ and δ. The presence of residues of HCH and DDT in infant food was of particular concern since new born children depend on them for a substantial period of time. In another multicenter collaborative study conducted by Kalra et al. (2001) in which 186 samples of 20 different infant formula collected from Mumbai, Pune, Mysore, Lucknow and Ludhiana were analysed to determine the level of DDT and HCH residues. It was observed that 70-94% samples were contaminated with DDT and HCH. The average concentration was 0.30 and 0.49mg/kg on fat basis for DDT and HCH respectively.

Table 4. DDT and HCH residues in baby milk powder

Brand No.	Centres and pesticide residues (mg/kg)						
	HP		Hyderabad		Kerala	West Bengal	Bangalore
	HCH	DDT	HCH	DDT	HCH	HCH	HCH
Brand I	3.774	1.470	0.578	0.226	0.251	0.522	0.225
Brand II	1.128	0.839	1.067	0.320	0.243	0.494	0.013
Brand III	1.886	0.344	0.415	0.042	0.354	0.142	0.081
Brand IV	2.863	0.468	0.458	0.021	0.241	0.694	0.071
Brand V	3.031	-	0.389	0.054	0.168	0.279	0.026

Ghee and butter: Before banning HCH and restricting use of DDT, the two insecticides contributed more than 50% of the total pesticides produced in India. Being liophilic in nature, these are likely to be deposited in fat enriched commodities such as edible oil, ghee, butter, etc. In a monitoring study conducted at Anand, Gujarat, by Shah et al. (1992) it was observed that 29 popular brand and 23 local brand ghee samples and 4 butter samples were contaminated with DDT and HCH isomers. The levels of ΣHCH and ΣDDT in ghee samples ranged from 0.02-4.96mg/kg and 0.02-7.62mg/kg with a mean of 1.84 and 2.38mg/kg respectively. The corresponding value for butter samples ranged from 0.86-3.68 and 1.65-5.84mg/kg with a mean level of 2.04 and 3.55mg/kg respectively. Of the total 52 ghee samples 6 and 35 samples exceeded extraneous residues limits with HCH and DDT respectively. In case of butter none exceeded the limit with HCH but all the 4 samples exceeded with DDT.

Out of eleven local butter samples collected from market of Jorhat in Assam three samples were contaminated with pp^{1}DDE (0.051-0.069mg/kg), β-HCH (0.049-0.058mg/kg), one each with pp^{1}DDT (0.055mg/kg), α-HCH (0.045mg/kg), α- endosulfan (0.078 mg/kg) and endosulfan sulfate (0.075 mg/kg).

Human milk : Not only bovine milk samples, human milk samples are also found contaminated with pesticide residues. Kathpal et al. (1992) detected DDT and HCH in human milk samples collected from Haryana, while Raha et al. (1999) found endosulfan in addition to DDT and HCH in human milk samples collected from Varanasi.

Kathpal et al. (2004) reported that 10 out of 11 samples of human milk collected from cotton growing belt of Hisar in Haryana were contaminated with HCH, DDT and endosulfan residues. Five samples contained HCH above MRL, eight contained total DDT above MRL and three showed endosulfan above MRL.

Monitoring of mother milk samples (51) for contamination due to pesticides such as organochlorines, organophosphates and synthetic pyrethroids were carried out at Solan in Himachal Pradesh (Gupta et al., 2001). Out of 51 samples 49 were found contaminated with ΣHCH residues (ND-1.285 mg/kg), all contained ΣDDT (0.074-2.412 mg/kg) and 9 samples contained dicofol (0.013-0.653mg/kg). Other organochlorines, organophosphates and synthetic pyrethroids were not present.

Poultry and Poultry feed: Chicken and eggs are favourite items in any non vegetarian diet and are vital source of animal protein. Samples of eggs, chicken and poultry feed were analysed for residues of HCH, DDT, aldrin and carbendazim, an important systemic fungicide, used for control of fungal diseases in the grain during storage (Agnihotri, 1999). In case of chicken samples of flesh, fat and different organs like liver, kidney and ovary were analysed separately to study the accumulation of residues in different organs. In case of eggs, only defective ones, which are likely to contain maximum residues were analysed. Residues of HCH, DDT, aldrin were either were non detectable or below the MRL. But residues of carbendazim were detected at 6.599mg/kg levels, which is much higher than it's MRL.

Most are the pesticides are non polar in nature and tend to accumulate in fatty tissues of animals. Analysis of chicken fat showed there was an accumulation of residues of HCH and carbendazim in fat samples. Samples of fat contained 2.723mg/kg HCH and 16.59mg/kg carbendazim. The relative concentration of aldrin and DDT in fat samples were 0.018 and 0.003mg/kg respectively. Accumulation of pesticide residues was highest in liver followed by kidney and ovary. In defective eggs there was no residue of DDT. However residues of HCH, aldrin and carbendazim were detected at the level of 0.004, 0.008, 1.176mg/kg respectively.

All poultry feed samples contained residues of HCH, DDT and carbendazim. The concentration of HCH residues varied from 0.020-2.410, DDT from BDL (below detectable level) to 0.281 and carbendazim BDL to 16.675mg/kg. The presence of high amount of residues in poultry feed particularly of carbendazim clearly shows that feed is the main source of residues in poultry birds and eggs. The source of carbendazim residues in poultry products was traced to maize grain treated with it to control fungal diseases during storage. DDT and HCH residues were present in almost all the constituents of poultry feed and can be taken as the main source of pesticide residues in poultry products.

Meat

Meat collected from Hyderabad, Izatnagar and Ludhiana was monitored for residues of organochlorine pesticides. Twentytwo out of 41 samples from Hyderabad contained residues of BHC in the range of traces to 2ppm. In case of Izatnagar samples all of the 18 samples were contaminated with DDT (0.20-2.23ppm). Samples from Ludhiana were contaminated to the extent of 25% with BHC, DDT and endrin (Shastri, 1983).

Egg

Chlorinated hydrocarbon contamination caused egg shell thinning increasing the chances of breakage in wild bird eggs, higher mortality at hatching and/or even caused congenital abnormality of the chicken leading to extirpation of species in wild ecosystem noticed as reported in several studies conducted in the USA (Wiemeyer, et al. 1978; Wilbur, 1978; Flickinger, 1979; Sticket et al. 1979a, 1979b; Blus et al., 1976b; Blus and Prouty, 1979). In a monitoring study of eggs, collected from Hyderabad, Mumbai, Pantnagar, Delhi, Izatnagar, and Ludhiana, it was observed that eggs were contaminated with organochlorines like DDT, BHC, lindane, endrin, and heptachlor to the extent of 25% to 100%. The concentration ranged from traces to 8 ppm (Shastry, 1983). Another study was conducted by Regupathy and Kuttalam (1992) to see the level of HCH and DDT residues in avian (Poultry hen, Country hen, Japanese Quail, duck, turkey) eggs in the Tamilnadu state. HCH was the predominant pollutant found to be present in nearly all of the eggs analysed and occurred at the level of 0.009-0.505mg/kg in wild birds, 0.014 - 0.048mg/kg in quails, 0.004-0.233mg/kg in poultry hen, BDL- 0.274mg/kg in country hen, BDL to 0.054mg/kg in ducks and 0.030mg/kg in turkey. DDT and its metabolites like DDE and DDD was not present in many samples and no samples contained residues of DDT exceeding its MRL of 1.25 ppm.

Fish

All the samples of fish of different species obtained from the markets of Ludhiana had residues of DDT ranging from 0.02-3.02mg/kg and HCH ranging from 0.03 to 1.12mg/kg. A five year monitoring programme was conducted in respect of endosulfan residues in large and small fishes collected from different markets of Kolkata and suburbs. Fifty seven percent were found to contain residues of endosulfan in the range of 0.01-0.03mg/kg. HCH, aldrin, endosulfan and DDT were also present in 60% samples from different districts of West Bengal (Saxena, et al. 2002).

Table 5. Extent of pesticide contamination in fish

Location	Year	Insecticide	Contamination %	Range (mg/kg)
Ludhiana	1983	DDT	100	0.02-3.02
		HCH (BHC)	100	0.02-1.12
Kolkata	1988-93	DDT	27	0.02-0.21
		Endosulfan	57.3	0.01-0.03

(Saxena, et al. 2002)

Chakraborty et al. (1996) monitored endosulfan residues in large and small fish collected from different market of Kolkata and suburbs. They found 227 fishes out of a total of 346 were contaminated with a concentration of 0.01 to more then 0.3 ppm.

Monitoring of fish samples for the presence of pesticide residues is also carried out by AICRP on Pesticide Residues. Reports published in 1999 said that fishes from Kerala were free from residues of DDT and endosulfan, however, 47% samples contained residues of HCH, which was in the range of Tr-0.25mg/kg (Agnihotri, 1999). In 2001 even HCH residues were not found in fish samples from Kerala. All the 37 samples collected from Assam also were free from DDT and HCH but 19% samples contained residues of endosulfan in the range of Tr-0.mg/kg. From Andhra Pradesh fish samples collected in 1999 were free from residues of DDT and endosulfan but contained HCH residues in the range of Tr-0.05mg/kg in 44% samples, which in 2001 reduced to trace levels (Table-6). In 2001 fish samples from West Bengal were highly contaminated, 75% samples contained residues of HCH, DDT and endosulfan and 29% samples had HCH above MRL. The frequency of contamination of fish samples from Coimbatore was high (87%) but the level of contamination was low (Saxena, et al. 2002).

Table 6. Contamination of fish samples with pesticide residues

Center	Year	Pesticides dectected	% Contamination	Residues
Vellayani	1999	HCH	47	ND-0.25
Vellayani	2001	None	0	-
Assam	1999	DDT	8.1	Tr
		HCH	2.7	Tr
		Endosulfan	18.9	Tr-0.721
Hyderabad	1999	HCH	44.4	Tr-0.05
		Endosulfan	11.1	0.01
Hyderabad	1999	HCH	21	ND-0.04
		Endosulfan	17	ND-0.05
Coimbatore	2001	DDT	75	ND-0.06
		HCH	87	ND-0.103
		Endosulfan	45.8	ND-0.038
Kalyani	2001	DDT	33.3	0.01-0.36
		HCH	66.7	0.02-1.57
		Endosulfan	16.6	0.08-1.25

(Saxena, et al. 2002)

Transfer of pesticide residues from feed to milk - Experimental evidence through feeding trials: A feeding study involving 16 lactating dairy cows was carried out in which mixtures of 5 pesticides (heptachlor epoxide, dieldrin, endrin, lindane and DDT) were fed at levels of approximately 0.05, 0.15, and 0.30ppm of each pesticide based on total feed consumption. Analyses showed that heptachlor epoxide and dieldrin transferred to the milk in much higher concentration than did the other pesticides. Next in order of concentration were endrin and lindane. Small but definite increases of DDT and TDE in the milk were noted with increased feeding levels of DDT, but the DDE concentration was apparently not affected by the feeding of DDT at these levels (Williams and Mills, 1964).

Witt et al. (1966) determined the level of DDT and its metabolites in milk of cows treated at the same dosage both for one day and six consecutive days in the following manner: i) intratracheal infusion of pp^{1}DDT; ii) alimentary exposure of a corn oil solution of pp^{1}DDT in a capsule; iii) an aged residue of technical grade DDT on alfalfa hay which had been pelleted; and iv) an intravenous infusion of pp[1]DDT. It was found that respiratory exposure of cows to DDT produced a lower rather than higher level of DDT and its metabolic products in the milk than alimentary exposures. Administration of DDT in the form of aged residues on alfalfa resulted in a higher residue level than when DDT was administered in solution in oil. Different routes of exposure resulted in different ratios of DDT, DDE and DDD in the milk. The predominant product resulting from intratracheal and intravenous (I.V.) exposure, which bypassed the rumen, was DDT but some DDD and DDE were produced from the longer term I.V. exposure. Alimentary exposure by means of DDT in oil solution produced predominantly DDT and DDD in milk. Alimantary exposure of DDT as an aged residue produced DDT, DDD and DDE.

The excretion of HCH residues in the milk of Indian buffalo after oral and dermal exposure was studied by Kapoor and Kalra (1988). Following the intake of 10, 25, 50 and 100mg of technical HCH for 100 consecutive days by different group of buffaloes, HCH esidues in milk showed an initial rapid rise but soon attained a dose dependent equilibrium. The transfer coefficient of HCH residues in milk fat at plateau showed an average value of about 15%. Half-life values for the rate of decline of HCH residues during post dosing period computed according to a two open-compartment model were 4.0, 4.1, 3.1 and 4.3 days for the rapid decline phase and 4.2, 7.2, 14.8 and 17.8 days for slow decline phase at dose levels of 10, 25, 50 and 100mg respectively. Dermal application of technical HCH to buffaloes also resulted in significant residues in milk. The proportions of α, β, γ and δ isomers of HCH in milk of buffaloes following oral and dermal routes of exposure were different. The proportion of γ-isomer in total HCH residues in milk was 5 and 33% following oral administration and dermal application respectively.

The transfer of DDT from feed to milk of goat was studied by Singh and Mudgal (1990). Six lactating goats, divided into 2 groups of 3 each were given 200 and 400mg of technical grade DDT containing 50% of active substances orally in a single dose. Milk samples were collected for 4 days and pooled. There was no significant variation between groups for milk yield and its chemical composition. Total DDT residues were 57.44 and 193.8ppm in pooled samples for single and double dose respectively.

Once again Kapoor and Kalra (1997) worked on transfer of HCH isomers from feed to milk of Indian buffalo Bubalis bubalis L. They fed 10mg each of α, β, γ and δ-HCH for 100 consecutive days to the buffaloes divided into four groups, another group was kept for control. The analysis of milk samples revealed that residues in milk after showing an initial sharp increase attained equilibrium level. The steady conditions of daily excretion of α, β, γ and β-HCH were attained in 15, 45, 15 and 15days and the transfer coefficients were 4.9, 36.6, 2.7 and 8.3% respectively. After termination of feeding with contaminated rations, the residues of γ-HCH declined at the fastest rate (half-life 1.5 and 3.0 for fast and slow decline phase respectively) followed by α, δ, β-isomers having half-life 2.2 & 3.8, 4.0 & 11.8 and 8.7 & 55.0 days for fast and slow decline phase respectively.

Surendranath et al. (1998) reported that cows maintained at the institute farm of NDRI, Bangalore, consumed through their feed, about 500μg of γ-HCH and 30μg of total DDT per day and excreted through milk about 80μg of β-HCH and 12μg of total DDT per day.

Feeding experiments of milking animals with pesticides was mostly confined with DDT, HCH and few cyclodienes like aldrin, dieldrin, heptachlor. However, endosulfan, the most important organochlorine insecticide of the cyclodiene group and still registered and used in many countries was not taken too much for feeding experiments to see its disposition kinetics, effect on animal performance and transfer of residues to milk. According to Indraninsigh et al. (1993) endosulfan residues could be detected in milk of only first day sample when fed to goats @ 1mg/kg body wt. for 28 days. Surendranath et al. (2000) could not detect any endosulfan residue in the milk of cattle even when fed with it for four weeks @ 50mg/day. Only traces of endosulfan sulfate were detected in the milk samples collected after one week of commencenment of experimental feeding trial. BHC was also fed @ 50mg/day for two weeks. Residues of BHC in the milk increased soon after dosing began and dropped sharply on discontinuation. Similarly feeding technical grade DDT increased the level of pp^{1}DDT in the milk.

At IGFRI, Jhansi, an experiment was conducted on excretion of residues through milk and performance of goats following oral administration of endosulfan (Nag et al., 2004) when fed @ 15 and 30mg/head/day for 25 consecutive days. Residues, comprising of α, β isomers and endosulfan sulfate, excreted through the milk and the concentration increased during the feeding period reaching its maxima in the samples taken on 25th day i.e. last day after commencement of feeding (0.194 and 0.282mg/kg for 15 and 30mg dose respectively). Thereafter, it started declining and reached the background level (around 0.065mg/kg) within 20 days after cessation of feeding. The transfer coefficient was, however, very less (0.57-0.85%). The rate kinetics of the decline phase followed the first order kinetics and statistical half-life of dissipation was almost same in both the treatment groups (8.67-8.88 days). There was no perceptible change in the utilization of nutrients, feed intake, milk yield and its composition and blood metabolites in the treatment group animals following ingestion of the pesticide.

In view of burgeoning population and the need to feed them all we have to produce more and more from less and less in the coming days. In other words, productivity has to be raised to the new heights and in this effort role of pesticides can not be ignored. Pesticides, as plant protection agents, are extensively used in agriculture, animal system, public health purposes and have become an integral part of agricultural productivity. Contamination of different food items, drinks, animal products etc. do take place due to pesticide residues as reported several times from different places during last three decades. This is not desirable because of the toxicity of the chemicals and the effect that they could exert on different organisms, animals including man because man is the ultimate consumer. However, many of the problems can be avoided or minimized if proper care is taken. The use of right chemical at the appropriate stage and at correct dose, use of right formulation and proper application tool, strict follow-up of the instructions, maintenance of safe waiting periods are some of the issues worth mentioning. The guidelines of Central Insecticides Board and Registration Committee under the Ministry of Agriculture, Govt. of India should be strictly adhered to and extension workers, plant protection persons should make farmers aware of them. Marketing of pesticides in rural areas should also come under strict vigilance. Feeds and fodders offered to animals grown for milk and meat should be monitored regularly for pesticide residues and samples containing residues beyond the permissible limits should be rejected or decontaminated. Green fodders, if sprayed with pesticides at the time of cultivation, should be allowed to remain in the field till the waiting period is over before offering to animals. If these things are taken care of, and with the ban/restriction of more persistent organochlorines like DDT, BHC, aldrin, dieldrin, heptachlor etc. the residue level in food, feed and animal products would be very less and below the permissible levels at any standards and our products would be competitive with those of the global partners in the new WTO regime.

Bibliography

Adiroubane, D. and Letchoumanae, S. 1996. HCH and DDT residues in bovine milk samples from Karaikal region of U.T. of Pondicherry. Pesticide Research Journal 8 (2) : 115-118.

Agnihotri, N.P. 2000. Pesticide consumption in agriculture in India - An update. Pesticide Research Journal 12 (1) : 150-155.

Agnihotri, N.P.1999. Pesticide safety evalution and monitoring. All India Coordinated Research Project on Pesticide Residues, Indian Agricultural Research Institute, New Delhi, pp. 104-111.

Battu, R.S., Singh, B. and Kalra, R.L. 1996. Seasonal veraation in residues of DDT and HCH in dairy milk in Punjab, India. Pesticide Research Journal 8 (1) : 32-37.

Battu, R.S., Singh, B., Chahal, K.K. and Kalra,R.L. 1996. Contamination of animal feed with residues of HCH and DDT. Pesticide Research Journal 8 (2) : 172-175.

Battu, R.S., Singh, Balwinder, Kang, B.K. and Chahal, K. K. 2001. Status of contamination of bovine milk with pesticide residues. In: Extended abstract of International Conference on Pesticides, Environment, Food Security organized by the Society of Pesticide Science, India, New Delhi from 19-23 November, 2001.pp- 265-266.

Blus, L.J. and Prouty, R.M. 1979. Organochlorine pollutant and population status of least terns in South Carolina. Wilson Bull. 91 : 62-71.

Blus, L.J., Henry, C.J., Lenhart, D. J. and Cromartie, E. 1976b. Effects of heptachlor treated cereal grains on Canada geese in the Coumbia basin. In: Management and biology of Pacific fly way Geese: A symposium. (Ed) R.L. Jervis, and J.C. Bartonek, OSU Book Store Inc., Opregan., pp 105-116.

Buck, W.B. 1970. JAMA, J. Am. Med Assoc. 156: 1434.

Buck, W.B.1975. J .Am.Vet. Med. Assoc. 166: 222.

Chakrabarty, A., Pal, S., Das, A. K., Sukul, P., Bhattachayya, A. and Adityachoudhury, N. 1996. Monitoring of endosulfan residues in market fish sample. Pesticide Research Journal 8 (2) : 164-167.

Deka, S.C., Barman, N. and Baruah, A.A.L.H. 2004. Monitoring of pesticide residues in feed, fodder and butter in Assam. Pesticide Research Journal 16 (1) : 86-89.

Dhaliwal, G.S. and Kalra, R.L. 1977. Indian J. Ecol. 4 : 13-22.

Dikshit, T. S. S., Kumar, S. N., Raizada, R. B. and Srivastava, M. K. 1989. Organochlorine insecticide residues in cattle feed. Bull. Environ. Contam. Toxicol. 43: 691-696.

Flickinger, E.L.1979. Effect of aldrin exposure on snow geese in Texas rice field. J. Wlldl manage. 43: 94-101.

Gupta, A., Parihar, N.S. and Singh, V. 1997. HCH and DDT residues in bovine milk and milk powder. Pesticide Research Journal 9 (2): 235-237.

Gupta, A., Singh, B., Parihar, N.S. and Bhatnagar, A. 2000. Monitoring of HCH and DDT residues in certain animal feed and feed concentrates. Pestology 24 (12) : 47-49.

Gupta, P., Dubey, J.K., Patyal, S.K. and Nath, A. 2001. Contamination of mother's milk with pesticide residues. Pesticide Research Journal 13 (2) : 207-212.

ICMR, 1993. Surveillance of food contamination in India. Council of Medical Research, New Delhi. pp.117.

Indraningsih, McSweeney, C.S., Ladds, P.W., 1993. Residues of endosulfan in the tissues of lactating goats. Australian Veterinary J., 70 (2): 59-62.

Kalra, R.L. and Chawla, R.P. 1983. Studies on pesticide residues and monitoring of pesticide pollution. Final Technical Report. PL 480 Project, Ludhiana. pp.230.

Kalra, R.L. and Chawla, R.P. 1985. Pesticidal contamination of foods in the year 2000 A.D. In : Proc. of Indian National Science Academy B52 (1) : 188-204.

Kalra, R.L., Kaur, H., Sharma, S. and Kapoor, S.K. 2001. Surveillance of DDT and HCH residues in infant formula samples and their implication on dietary exposure: A multicenter study. Pesticide Research Journal 13 (2) : 147-151.

Kang, B. K., Singh, B., Chahal, K.K. and Battu, R.S. 2002. Contamination of feed concentrates and green fodder with pesticide residues. Pesticide Research Journal 4 (2) : 308-312.

Kannan, K., Tahabe, S., Romesh, A., Subramanian, A. and Tatsukawa, R. 1992. Persistent organochlorine residues in food stuff from India and their implication on human dietary exposure. J. Agric. Food. Chem. 40: 518-524.

Kaphalia, B.S. and Seth, T.D. 1982. Organochlorine pesticides contamination in some species of fodder grasses. Environ. Pollut. Series B.3 : 231-237.

Kapoor, S.K. and Kalra, R.L. 1988. Residues of HCH in milk after its oral administration or dermal application to Indian buffalo, Bubalus bubalis (L.). Pestic. Sci. 24 : 193-204.

Kapoor, S.K. and Kalra, R.L. 1997. Transfer of HCH isomers from feed into milk of Indian Buffalo (Bubalus bubalis L.). Pesticide Research Journal .9 (1): 72-78.

Kathpal, T.S., Kumari, B., Singh, S. and Singh, J. 2004. Multi-residue analysis of bovine and human milk in cotton growing belt of Haryana. In Book: Pesticide: Environment and Food Security. Eds. P, Dureja, D.B.Saxena, Jitender Kumar, Madhuban Gopal, Shasi Bala Singh and R.S.Tanwar. Society of Pesticide Science, India, New Delhi. pp. 140-148.

Kathpal, T.S., Singh, G., Yadav, G. S., Dhankar, J. S. and Singh, A. 1992. Monitoring of milk and milk products for DDT and HCH contamination. Pesticide Research Journal 4 (2) : 123-131.

Kumar, N.R. and Nath, A. 1996. Monitoring of bovne milk for DDT and HCH. Pesticide Research Journal 8 (1): 90-92.

Laxminarayana, V. 1980. Paper presented at the meeting of the ICAR expert committee to review the pesticide residue problems in the country and to formulate a need based programme to be implemented, held in Ludhiana.

Mukerjee, I. and Gopal, M. 1993. Organochlorine pesticide residues in dairy milk in and around Delhi. Journal of AOAC International, 76 (2) : 283-286.

Nag, S.K. and Raikwar, M.K. 2002. First Annual Report of Lal Bahadur Shastri Young Scientist Scheme "Monitoring of pesticide residues in animal feed, fodder and milk with special reference to Bundelkhand region" submitted to ICAR, New Delhi.

Nag, S.K. and Raikwar, M.K. 2003. Second Annual Report of Lal Bahadur Shastri Young Scientist Scheme "Monitoring of pesticide residues in animal feed, fodder and milk with special reference to Bundelkhand region" submitted to ICAR, New Delhi.

Nag, S.K., Mahanta, S.K., Raikwar, M.K. and Bhadoria, B.K. 2004. Excretion of residues through milk and performance of goats following oral administration of endosulfan. Small Ruminant Research(Communicated).

Nag, S.K. and Shah, N.K. 1999. Residual persistence of endosulfan in fodder sorghum. Pestology 23 (11) : 52 – 55.

Nag, S.K. and Shah, N.K. 2001. Endosulfan residue and its dissipation in Lucerne (Medicago sativa L.). Pesticide Research Journal 13 (1): 109-111.

Nag, S.K. and Shah, N.K. 2002. Residues and efficacy of endosulfan against pest complex of fodder cowpea. J. Ent. Res. 26 (2) : 133-139.

Nornnha, A.B.C. 1978. Studies on pesticide residues in food. M.Sc. Thesis, University of Bombay.

Pierson, D.A., Hoffman, J.S., Nord, P.J., Gebhart, J.E. and Frank, C.N. 1982. Distribution of chlorinated pesticides in animal feed components and finished feeds. J. Agric. Food. Chem. 30: 187-189.

Prasad, K.S.N. and Chabara, A. 2001. Organochlorine pesticide residues in animal feeds and fodders. Indian Journal of Animal Science 71(12) : 1178-1180.

Raha, P., Agarwal, N. R. and Samanta, S. 1999. Organochlorine pesticide residues in mother's milk. In Book: Green Pesticides, Crop Protection and Safety Evaluation. Eds. N. P. Agnihotri, S. Walia. and V. T. Gajbhiye. Society of Pesticide Science, India, New Delhi. pp. 231-234.

Raikwar, M.K., Nag, S.K., Banerjee, T. and Shah, N.K. 2003. Persistence behaviour of endosulfan in fodder maize. Pesticide Research Journal. 15 (2) : 186-190.

Raikwar, M.K., and Nag, S.K. 2004. Dissipation of carbendazim residues in fodder sorghum. Indian J. of Agricultural Sciences 74 (4) : 227-229.

Regupathy, A. and Kuttalam, S. 1992. Monitoring of HCH and DDT residues in certain avian eggs in Tamilnadu. Pesticide Research Journal. 4 (2) : 149-153.

Sandhu, T.S. 1979. Pesticide residues in food. Paper presented at the IDA's seminar on quality control of milk held in New Delhi from Nov. 9-10.

Sandhu, T.S. 1980. Pesticide residues in foods. Indian Dairyman. 32: 61-63.

Saxena, D.B., Sharma, K.K. and Kalpana 2002. Status of pesticide residues in food commodities : Indian scenario. Lecture given in the Summer School on "Pesticides : Chemistry and Modern Methods of Residue Analysis" held at GAU, Anand from 28th May to 17th June, 2002.

Shah, P.G., Patel, B.K., Raj ,M.F. and Patanwadia, R.D. 1992. Monitoring of HCH and DDT residues in ghee and butter samples in Gujarat. Pesticide Research Journal 4 (2) :117-121.

Shastry, M. S. 1983. Monitoring of pesticide residues in animal feeds and animal products. Pesticide, December issue. pp. 36-38.

Singh, P.P., Battu, R.S. and Kalra, R. L. 1988. Insecticide residues in wheat grain and straw arising from their storage in premises treated with BHC and DDT under malaria control programme. Bull. Environ. Contam. Toxicol. 40: 696-702.

Singhal, K.K. and Mudgal, V.D. 1990. Transfer of organochlorine pesticide (DDT) from feed to milk. Indian J. Dairy Sci. 43 (3) : 348-350.

Stickel, L.F., Stickel, W. H., McArthur, R.D. and Hughes, D. L. 1979a. Chlordane in Birds: a study of lethal residues of and loss rates. Toxicol Occupat Med. pp. 387-396.

Stickel,W.H., Reichel, W.L. and Hughes, D. L.1979b. Endrin in Birds: lethal residues and secondary poisoning. Toxicology Occupational Med. pp.397-406.

Surendara Nath, B., Unnikrishanan, V., Gayathri, V., Chitra, P.S. Preeja, C.N. and Rama Murthy, M.K. 1998. Organochlorine pesticide residues in animal tissues and their excretion through milk. J. Food Sci. Technol., 35 (6) : 547-548.

Surendara Nath, B., Unnikrishanan, V., Preeja, C.N. and Rama Murthy, M.K. 2000. A study on the transfer of organochlorine pesticide residues from the feed of the cattle into their milk. Pesticide Research Journal 12 (1) : 68-73.

Unnikrishanan, V., Surendara Nath, B., Gayathri, V., Sampath. K.T. and Rama Murthy, M.K. 1998. Organochlorine pesticide residues content in feed and feedstuff. Indian J. Dairy & Biosciences. 9. 59-64.

Van Houweling, C.D., Bixler, W. B. and Mc Dowell, J.R. J.Am. Vet. Med. Assoc., 171 : 1153.

Vasanthi. D., Kuttlam. S., Jayakumar, R., Vijayalakshmi, K and. Chandrasekaran, S. 2003. Monitoring of bovine milk samples for chlorinated pesticides. Pesticide Research Journal 15 (2) : 193-194.

Wiemeyer, S.N. Swineforf, D.M., Spitzer, P.D. and McLain, P. D. 1978. Organochlorine residues in New Jersey Osfrey effs. Bull. Environ. Contam. Toxicol. 19 : 56-63.

Wilbur, S.R. 1978. Turkey vulture egg shell thinning in California, Florida and Texas. Wilson Bull. 90: 642-643.

Williams, S. and Mills, P.A. 1964. Residues in milk of cows fed rations containing low concentrations of five chlorinated hydrocarbon pesticides. Journal of AOAC, 47 (6) : 1124-1128.

Witt, J.M., Whiting, F..M., Brown, W.H. and Stull, J.W.J. 1966. Contamination of milk from different routes of animal exposure to DDT. J. Dairy Sci. 49 : 370-380.

23
ANTIQUALITY FACTORS IN FEEDS

Brijesh K Bhadoria

Prevalent farming system in Indian subcontinent normally includes small-scale crop and livestock making livestock an integral part of mixed farming system in India. Consequent upon, India holds one of the largest livestock population embracing 232million cattle, 95 million buffaloes, 124 million goats, 59million sheep and 843 million poultry engaging 79 million rural families in milk production for their livelihood[1] amounting 2/3 of national GNP. The huge livestock population demands 1057mt green and 588mt dry fodder against the supply of 395mt and 452mt respectively with cropped area 6.9×10^6 ha (Planning Commission 2001). The limited land resources for forage and food production due to geometrical increase in Indian livestock and human population seriously warrants for another green revolution for livestock if current human and animal nutritional standards are to be maintained. The deficit fodder supply for the animals is further exacerbated with the availability of nutritionally low-grade roughage as straw of cereals. The prevalence of high Yielding Dwarf Varieties (HYDV) of cereal crops making them deprived of this roughage too and the forest grazing resources are also dwindling @ $1.5 \mathrm{X} 10^6$ ha /year. There is hardly scope for any expansion for the fodder cultivation and there is a serious threat to reorient livestock production. In such scenario Animal nutritionists are thus compelled to explore the new avenue to bridge this yawning gap of demand and supply with use of non-edible and non competitive unconventional forages, shrub and tree fodder and increase the basic resource. Shrubs and trees are one solution to feed problem, however it is interesting enough, that the farmers have traditionally used these sources to feed their animals, based on experience and convenience and was regarded as one of the practical means of animal rearing and neglected, inadequately understood aspect of feeding system of ruminants in developing countries. Therefore in the recent years there has been growing trend in many regions throughout the developing word to identify the potentially important feed resources among shrub and tree leaves for their utilization with scientific approaches.

Apart from nutritional consideration, in the consumption of plants as food is based on many other chemical constituents which are responsible for taste and aroma, a complex response from tongues and nostrils and forming a chemical communication system between plant and animal. These chemicals in plants are produced in great variety to combat environmental vagaries, invasion of pathogens and herbivores. All these phytochemicals of diverse range are called "secondary metabolites or compounds "or such compound are also called as allelochemicals or anti nutritional factors in nutritional science. It is widely accepted that secondary compound mediate interaction between plant and other organism in the environment[2]. Many a times rejection or selection of any nutritious plant depends on the presence of these disagreeable chemicals / toxins. There are more than 240000 known structure of secondary metabolites, and many more are waiting for their turn to be identified, encompassing classes of compound that have anti nutritional and toxic effect on mammals. The significance of secondary compounds in tropical forage plant is higher than that of temperate pasture plants on which much of animal production is based. Plants of tropics are always in contact with greater diversity of climatic shocks, more frequent attacks of herbivores and pathogens than those of temperate plants and to survive such an environment, a correspondingly higher level and variety of protective compounds are expected.

In turn these secondary compounds pose challenge in foraging environment and unconcealed problem of toxicity to mammalian herbivores. It is one end of a continuum of effects that include the syndrome of aversion responses, reduced intake, or digestibility, induced deficiencies and mortality ,due to unknown reason. Many a times there may be simple aversion from consumption but in the event of compulsion due to scarcity of feed or starvation the animal faces toxicity or health problem. However more frequently animal will reject such plant entirely , but voluntary intake will be low as may also be digestibility and animal performance .

A stream of publications continued to flow on all aspects of anti-nutrition constituents in feed and fodder and I propose to review briefly a few which were found interesting or significant to animals with their determination techniques.

Factors causing hepatotoxicity and neurotoxicity -Alkaloids are the most physiologically active group of the compounds causing mainly neurological or hepatotoxicity in mammals[3-4] and are chemically defined as molecules of phytochemicals containing nitrogen in carbon ring structure. . It is noteworthy that these nitrogenous compounds are not the part of protein but are produced from amino acids only. More than thousands type of structurally different alkaloids have been investigated from higher plants and micro-organisms and have shown the ability to change in biochemistry of the other organism on their ingestion. These are widely distributed and quite often found in plants of Solanaceae, Convolvulaceae, Euphorbiaceae, Boraginaceae , Legumonaseae, Astraceae and Compositeae[5] family. The occurrence of alkaloids in grasses have not been reported much but slowly and slowly the researches are exhibiting their presence in them. The subfamilies Fesctuceae, Avenaceae, Panicaeae and Andropgonceae have been reported to contain pyrrolizidine alkaloids.

Pyrrolizidine alkaloids–Among the livestock pyrrolizidine alkaoids (PA) toxicity is common though accidentally. Approximately 6000-7000 plant species contain PA and the problems due to these are alike in human and animals through out the world. The pyrrolizidine nucleus contain two five membered ring linearly fused with nitrogen, More than 200 PAs have been identified and their structure determined. The literature exhibits that Crassocephalaum, Echinaceae and Homogyne (Astraceae) Cordia (Ehretiaceae)Hunggonia (Linaceae) Schinusus (Ponaceae) Castenosperum ,sp Angylocalyx, Loncocarpus sp. Xanthocercus sp Aexa sp.Swansinone sp Deris eliptica (leguminoceae) Ipomea sp, Calystegia sp Convolvulus sp,(Convolvulaceae), Morus sp(Moraceae), Omphalea diandra, Endosoermum sp. (Euphorbiaceae),Eugenia jambolana (Myratecaea) Atropa baladona, scapolia carniolica ,Solenum sp. Datura alba Physalis sp Mandragora offincicarum, Hyscymus niger(Solanaceae) have been shown to contain PAs[6-8] (Table 1).The significant role of PA in ruminant nutrition is their interaction with vitamin A and Copper metabolism[9]. Because of the consumption of plant containing the indication of PA appears in sheep as excessive liver copper concentration followed by haemolytic crisis of copper toxicity, the condition is referred as toxemic jaundice, haemolytic jaundice, and haematogenous copper toxicity. Further Vitamin A, also accumulated in liver and transported in association with protein synthesised in liver. The effect of PA on animal causing depressed liver and blood vit.A due to a) PA inhibits the synthesis of protein in liver to transport with Vit. A. b) PA inhibits vit. A absorption. c)PA impairs the ability to take Vit.A. Pyrrolizidine alkaloid hepatotoxicity depends on the extent to which alkaloids are converted to pyrrolic metabolites in liver. The PAs are well known for their hepatotoxic effects and for nutrient interaction. Chronic exposure of sheep to Echum and Heliotropium sp. containing PA with low acute toxicity leads elevated copper concentration in liver hemolytic crisis of Cu toxicity-[8-9]. Though the mechanism of elevation of Cu concentration is not yet fully known. The condition of copper concentration in liver is not restricted but it is prevalent in monogastric animals also[10]. The mono-gastric and poly gastric animals(ruminants) both are equally susceptible for PA poisoning. However various animal species have different susceptibility to PA. Sheep are relatively resistant towards the hepatoxicity of PA. They can tolerate an intake of several times of their body weight. Goats are slightly more susceptible than that of sheep. The susceptibility depends on lack of PAs absorption, degradation of PAs in rumen, lack of hepatic fermentation of pyrrole and conjugation and excretion of PA and pyrrole. Shull (1976)[11] reported that susceptible species had high rate of liver pyrrole production while resistant species had low rate. Consumption of a moderate amount i.e. 10% of animal's body weight of rag wrot(Senecio jacobeae) by cattle will cause the death due to chronic liver diseasewhereas sheep can consume 20 more time than cattle.

The PAs pass to milk of animals and also in human beings but amount is very low and not adequate to cause hazard in them. PAs poisoning of grazing livestock can largely be eliminated through application of sound livestock management technique Plant containing PA are normally not consumed by the animals in presence of adequate feed. An alternative approach is to manipulate animal metabolism. One way is feeding sulphur containing amino acid feeding to supply sulphhydryl group to conjugate with pyrrole. The synthetic antioxidant like BHT or BHA or ethoxyquin have shown protective activity against PA[12-13].

Piperidine alkaloids- Their structures are having six membered ring with N, example Conicum maculatum. They effect on nervous system. The piperdine alkaloid toxicity is indicated by the symptoms of acute weakness, incoordination, dilation of pupil, coma, failure of respiratory system and death.

Pyridine alkaloid- possess pyrdine nucleus as in nicotine from Tobacco (Nicotiana sp.) Nicotine. The toxicity produced by consumption of Nicotiana sp and teratogenic defects in foetus, rapid respiration, staggering , weakness in limbs, followed by death[13].

Indole Alkaloids are one of the most important livestock poisoning alkaloids. This class is indicated by ergot alkaloids mainly, which is of fungus origin, because of the infected grains feed with Cleviceps and producing ergot amine, an alkaloid[14]. Thus creating ergot poisoning in livestock by consumption of ergot infected grains or grasses containing ergotised seed head. The symptoms of ergot poisoning are convulsion, incoordination, lameness, difficult breathing, excessive salivation, diarrhoea, dry gangrene, abortion, high neonatal mortality reduced lactation[14]. All these effects are not seen in all types of animal. They are species specific and also dependant of ergot source, amount of consumption, period of exposure, age and stage of production. The animals can be saved by removing the animals from the field with ergot infected plants are common.

Sophisticated techniques are available for the analysis of pyrrolizidine alkaloids. Before that some processing is needed.

Crush the plant material, Extract it with 1N NaOH and $CHCl_3$, Acidify wioth 1N H_2SO_4 re-extract with $CHCl_3$ and test by any of the technique.

GLC, Detector N/P temp 250^0 C, Column Methyl Silicon WCOT DB-1,Oven Temp 90-170 ,Carrier gas He

Advanced analytical such as GC-MS (Gas Chromatograph- Mass Spectroscopy) are being used to detect and identify the pyrrolizdine alkaloids but there is a need for simple and handy methodology for common technician in field for selecting possible toxic plant and extraction of alkaloids from plants.

Field test[15]:-

App.1g of plant or dried material is ground with ascorbic acid solution and filter then warm on water bath add aq. Nitropruside reagent then add Ehlrich reagent a magenta colour is obtained for positive alkaloids. Test for basic pyrrolizidine alkaloids Crush the plant material and extract with chloroform for 2-3 times and heat on water bath with o-chloranil then add Ehlrich reagent. Emergent color indicates the presence of pyrrolizidine alkaloid.

Thin layer Chromatography

The thin layer chromatography is one the most common and easily applicable technique. Standard size silica gel G plate can suitably be run on CMA(60:10:1)and CM containing 0.15M LiCl . The spots are visualized by o-chloranil and Ehlrich reagent.

Table 1. Characterization of animal species by susceptibility to PA toxicity and in vitro pyrrole production

Species	Susceptibility	In vitro pyrrole production rate
Cow	High	High
Horse	High	High
Sheep	Low	Low
Goat	Low	?
Rat	High	High

Table 2. Plants known for Proanthocynidines (PA)

S.No	Plant	Name of Alkaloid	LD_{50} (mg Kg^{-1})
1	Compositae	Seneciphylline	77
	Senecio jacobeae	Senecionine	85
		Jacobine	77
	Senecio vulgaris	Senecionine	
		Seneciphylline	77
		Restrorsine	38
	Senecio longifolius	Riddelline	85
		Senecionine	38
	Leguminoseae	Seneciphylline	105 (mouse)
	Crotolaria		
	spectabilis	Monocrotoline	175
	C. retusa	Spectabiline	220
	Boraginaceae	Retusine	NA
	Heliotropium		
	europium	Heliotrine	300
		Lasiocarpine	72
		Europine	1000
	Echiam	Supinine	450
	plantagineum	Echiumine	NA
		Echiumidine	200

Estrogenic problems

Many a times animals are encountered by the problems of reproduction due to the presence of oestrogenic substances in feeds and fodder. These are referred as phyto-oestrogens. Phyto-oestrogens, a group of plant poly phenols have been shown to have both oestrogenic and anti-oestrogenic properties. They are structurally similar to endogenous mammalian hormone oestradiol and possess good binding to oestrogen b receptor enabling them to behave as oestrogenic and anti-oestrogenic. Plant estrogens have widespread effects in a number of populations to livestock and human poulation[16-17] Though the sub clinical effects of phytoestrogens are not visible until these are observed carefully. These in fact are the silent and unobserved problems of the livestock causing severe loss in the livestock industry. The effects of phytoestrogens are some times devastating as they are concerned directly with the reproduction in female ruminants The estrogenic effects includes infertility syndrome, failure into conceive, prolapsed uterus, dystocia, and permanent infertility. Although the cattle have relatively low circulating concentration of oestradiol so it is expected that estrogenic effects would be more (Adam 1995) yet cattle are less susceptible towards the estrogenism due to isoflavonoids however they develop infertility accompanied by swelling of the vulva, discharge of cervical mucus, enlargement of the uterus and behavioural abnormalities and irregular oestrus. Sheep suffer from clover disease indicated by low lambing rate, prolapsed of uterus, dystocia, enlargement of bulbo- urethral glands and permanent infertility. It is clear from the available data that isoflavonoids enter in bloodstream within 15-20 minutes after ingestion[18-19]. The concentration of phyto-oestrogen in plasma of 0.2 to.03 nmol/ml blood (50-800ng/ml)[20] is achieved in 70-80 kg adult by consumption of 50mg isoflavonoid/d. These level exceeds the circulating level of oestradiol which ranges from 0.14-0.28pmol /ml (40-80-pg/ml)[21]. Oestrogens have strong binding affinity in serum protein In contrast to phyto-oestrogens which have considerably weaker affinity for protein binding hence theoretically greater opportunity for isoflavonoids to act biologically than that of endogenous oestrogen[22]. Phytoestrogens may have additive effects when present in feed in adequate amount for growth promotion.

The factors responsible for these oestrogenic activity of forages include isoflavonoids, coumstans, and lignan. The isoflavone has C6-C3-C6 and coumstane are coumarin like lactone and the lignans are also flavonoidal derivatives. Phyto-oestrogen have type of chemical structure which can bind estrogen receptor and the position of OH groups in molecule plays important role in activity. The biological activity of coumstans is 1/1000 and isoflavonoid 1/10000 of steroidal oestrogen[23]. Coumestrol, 4'methylcoumestrol, and genistein, biochanin A, formonentein and daidzein and pratensein are important phytoestrogen. There are more than 200 types of isoflavonoids reported from leguminous and non leguminous forages.

Besides these lignans another type of phyto-oestrogen, are present in wide variety of plants. The highest amount of lignans have been detected in linseed, barleys, rye grass and cereals. The first bioactive lignan found in mammals was from the human urine[24] and its chemical nature with molecular structure was proved as enterolactone[25]. In fact two primary lignans enterodiol and enterolactone are formed by the action of bacteria action on lignan precursors present in the intestine[26]. The principal lignan precursor identified so far in plants secoisolariciresinol of course this is not oestrogenically active per se but biologically metabolite, referred to as "mammalian lignan" Like other Phyto-oestrogens these also play important role in oestrogenic disease [27-30]. However biological effect of lignan in relation to ruminants health have received little attention so far. The determination of concentration of precursors in food is quite cumbersome to analyse but estimates have been made for several feeds by indirect analytical method using in vitro fermentation to approximate the likely yield of mammalian lignan[31].

Table 3. Lignans precursors in feeds

Feed	Total lignans mg/kg
Line seed meal	675
Line seed flour	572
Lentil	179
Soyabean	8.6
Oat bran	6.5
Wheatbran	5.7
Oats grain	2.3

Table 4. In vitro metabolism of various plant lignan and potential precursors of enterolactone and enterodiol

Compound	Metabolite
Matairesinol	ENL(62%)
Secoisolariciresinol	ENL+END (72%),ENF
Pinoresinol	ENL+END (55%) ENF & other minor metabolites
Syringaresinol	ENL+END(4%),dehydroxy and demethylated of ENL &END anolouges
7'-Hydroxymatairesinol	ENL +7'OHENL (23%)
Arctigenin	ENL (4%)
Isolariciresinol	Mostly unchanged
Lariciresinol	ENL+END main metabolite and minor ENF

The isoflavonoids assay furnishes the valuable guide for the judicious utilization of the pasture and forages. Since these are the group of the phenolics hence poses some difficulty in pin pointing the type of the isoflavonoids. However phytoestrogens can be extracted with polar solvents like alcohol or methanol and by the use of UV or floroscent light can be assayed chemically if they are in high concentration. Coumstanes are normally 10 times low in concentration than that of phytoestrogens of isoflavonoidal nature. Therefore, then create more difficulty in estimation. But a semi quantitative assay by TLC is possible with suitable reference. Chang and Yoder[33] have developed a crude chemical method for determination of isoflavonoiid content of plants. The method was crude not able to fractionate the type of isoflavonoid. A separate method to measure the genistein was developed by Currow[34]. Now days the predominant method of analysis in general is HPLC. The main advantage is its ease of use. It is not time consuming and does not require pre-treatment and sample after extraction needs to be cleaned up and followed by injection to analyse. The main problem which is encountered is sensitivity and gain adequate resolution. Since phytoesrogen are usually low and commonly UV detectors or Photo Diode Array (PDA) are used but recently Coulometric Electrode Array (CEA) detectors is getting popularity especially for mammalian lignan work in biological fluid. CEA is porous flow though graphite electrode having high surface area allowing the process of electrolysis, resulting in highly reproducible total peak area (coulombs) [35-36]. The technique has significant advantage in the detection of phenolics owing to sensitivity, selectivity and linear response of electrochemical detectors. It has unique property of Coulometric electrode resolution of co-eluting solute can be achieved on the basis of small differences in their oxidation reduction behaviour. In1995 Franke etal [37] developed a method for analysis of isoflavone in plants and successively extended to milk to obtain more precise data on Phyto-oestrogens like daidazine, genistein, formonentine, biochanine-A and coumestrol and the metabolite such as equol and o-deslesmethylangolensin were analysed by HPLC after solid phase extraction(SPE c.18)follwed by hydrolysis by gucouronidase /sulphatase at 37^0. Then samples were charge on HPLC C_{18} RPS column attaché guard column with gradient elution at a flow rate at 0.8ml/minute mobile phase first than water and detector was UVPD A 260nm and 280 and 342 for coumesrol. The detecting limit was 5-78nM (for injection 20ml.) flavone was used as internal detector. HPLC is the common technique for its assay now a day. Gas chromatography has been also used by some workers.

Bioassay

Increase in uterine weight of immature female mice has been quantitative method most commonly used until recently. But this method have given confused results too(166,128),122)Mice and guinea pigs are not very reliable. The ruminants have very different way It has been observed some animals prefers high estrogenic diet some do not. Diet selection in such lab animals result confusion. To over come directly sheep are used to assay in field conditions. Which include milk secretion; teat length and their vaginal and uterus response are considered in bioassay. Cyanogenic glycosides- The HCN toxicity in the animals is well known due to presence of cyanogenic glycosides present in many plant families. They liberate HCN either by enzymatic or acid hydrolysis on ingestion. Cyanogenic glycosides contain mono or disaccharide b- linked nitrile moiety and liberation of nitrile group as HCN gas in biological system causing the death. The critical level of HCN is 200ppm and in low concentration consumption for longer duration may cause goiter to the animal because the detoxification of the cyanide in system the production of sulfur to form thiocynate takes place. The toxic symptom in animals appear by problem in respiration. The HCN in the forages could be determined by the simple procedure using alkaline picrate The weighed quantity of crushed plant tissue is mixed in test tube with a few drops of chloroform and filter paper strip (10x 0.5cm) moist with sodium picrate solution is hanged over treated tissue with the help of tight stopper. After 24 hr the yellow colour of strip changes to red depending on quantity of HCN liberated. The colour of strips are eluted with distilled water and absorbance is recorded on spectrophotometer to quantify the amount of HCN.

Toxic Amino acids-All the amino acids formed and present in the plants do not occur in the protein. Some of them are toxic to the animals and human beings. The mimosine toxicity from Leuceana leucocephala is well known in the animal. Indigofera species are important range legume forage in tropics but contain an amino acid Indospecin , b-N –oxalyl –L-a-b-diaminopropionic acid. It cause weight loss. Neurological problems and teratogenic effects in animals.

Polyphenolics - The group of phenolics commonly referred as tannins , are always encountered by the ruminants either by choice or under compulsion. These are in fact are polyphenolics possessing affinity to bind with protein an. There is great variation in the molecular structure and molecular weight of these substances. The proteiophilic nature of these compounds vary depending on their molecular size, weight and orientation of the molecules. More precisely In 1981 Horvath[38] defined them as " any phenolic compound of sufficiently high molecular weight containing sufficient hydroxyl groups and other suitable groups (i.e., carboxyl groups) to form effectively strong complexes with protein under particular environment". Because of their ability to interact with protein by precipitating salivary protein they reduce the voluntary intake, digestibility, and make the feed unpalatable or immobilizing the enzymes[39]. Tannins also diminish the permeability of the gut walls by reacting so that the outer layer of the gut[40] so that the passage of the nutrients through the gut is diminished . In(1969) Donelly and Anthony[41] reported that tannin level required for the rejection is 20 mg /g dm. The ability to form complexes with minerals could also be added to this definition. The tannins may also form the complexes with starch and cellulose The enigmatic behaviour of tannin lies in its negative and positive role of in biological systems[43-44]. Tannins in high concentration reduce intake, digestibility of protein, carbohydrates and minerals and finally[45-47]. In low and moderate concentration of tannin not only prevent bloat but also increase the flow of non- ammonia nitrogen and essential amino acids from rumen [48-51].The inconsistent relationships of tannins with different nutritional attributes makes complicated the subject in research in nutritional toxicology.

Tannins are usually categorised in two groups : Hydrolyzable Tannins (HT) and Condensed tannins (CT) or Proanthocyanidin. Hydrolysable tannins are the ester of gallic acid or ellagic acid and sugars. Hydrolysable tannins are more susceptible to enzymatic hydrolysis than PA and are usually soluble in water. Hydrolysable tannins are further classified on the basis of products of hydrolysis such as gallotannins yeilds gallic acid and glucose, ellagitannin yields ellagic acid and glucose [48].

Codensed tannins or Proanthocyanidin are the polymers of flavan- 3-ols interlinked through the interflavan carbon bond which is not susceptible to hydrolysis. Many a times hydrolysable tannins also undergo condensation reaction and produce condesed HT. Therefore the term condensed tannin is potentially confused and the term proanthocyanidin is used to define condensed tannin derived from flavonoidal nuleus/ rings. Further the nomenclature for PA is derived from the acids, catalyzed oxidation reaction that produces red colour due to anthocyanidins on heating with acidic alcohols[49]. The most common anthocyanidin produced are cynidin and delphinidins from the corresponding proanthocyanidins. There are some hydrolysable tannin like catechin gallates which consist of gallic acid esterified to catechin showing properties of hydrolysable and condensed tannin both and are toxic to some ruminal bacteria[44]. More recently gallic acid ester of proanthocyanidin have been discovered [50].

Isolation and quantification of soluble phenolics are essential to judge the nutritional and ecological effects[51-53]. However the quantitative estimation is generally made colorimetrically though it has many problems[52-54]. Equating the phenolics with tannins is also a problem because many phenolics that react with the analytical reagents are not phenolics by strict definition as they do not interact with proteins but they can be converted to tannins by oxidative polymerisation. Therefore it is necessary to estimate the phenolics and tannins in addition their biological effects. Despite the fact there numbers of methods available for determining the tannins and phenolics no single method give satisfactory results in context to nutritional effects because the chemical properties involved in reactivity of polyhenols or precipitation assay may differ from the properties that underlie their nutritional effects.

To estimate polyhenolics accurately is easy but enigmatic task. The sample preparation has large influence on the determination of tannins fresh samples are preferred due to low complex formation, oxidative polymerisation and high solubility in suitable solvent. If the storage is required, freezing is always preferred for preserving the samples, because above 40^0 C enzymes may still function to oxidize the plant constitutes and at temperature more than 60 ^{0}C there would be polymerization due to heat The very first problem with Proanthcyanidin is its extraction problem which is often over looked. However the extraction may be improved by fine milling and in hot condition at 70-80^{0}c. But there is always substantial amount of PA left in fibrous residue. Hence distribution should be assayed. High molecular weight proanthocyanidin remains completely insoluble in organic solvents.

Folin - Dennis and Folin – Ciocaleteau's reagent (1927)[57] is the most common reagent for the phenolics. The Vannilin–HCl [58] and the Butanol –HCl reactions[59] are the most prevalent procedure for the tannin estimations. The Folin reaction is based on reduction of phosphomolybdic acid by phenols in the presence of aqueous alkali. This methods determines the total free phenolic OH groups and therefore is suitable for total soluble phenolics. This reagent has a flaw of interfering with the number of plant metabolites[60-61]. The Vannilin –HCl reagent is specifc for flavan –3-ols and proanthocyanidins based on of phenolic aldehyde (Vannilin) and and phloroglucinol structure of flavan –3-ol and proanthcyanidin while Butanol -HCl reaction is specific to proanthcyanidin and flavan –3,4-diols. Lack of suitable standards limit the usefulness of all the colorimeteric procedures .Although the commonly used standards are tannic acid ,catechin and tannins isolated from the plants for Folin – Ciocaleteau's reagent , Vannilin –HCl reagent and Butanol –HCl reactions. In plants thus there is either under- or over estimations of phenolics, causing great deviation in tannin concentration reported in literature .

The combination of Gravimetric and colorimetric methods developed by Reed(1985). The method is based on ability of trivalent ytterbium to selectively precipitate the polyphenols from plant extract. In this method no standard is required. The yield of soluble phenolics by formation of insoluble Yb-oxalate some times misleads.

The protein interaction methods are often quoted as more realistic for determining the tannin contents in plant tissue due to their closeness to the biological effects[62] .The methods are based on the amount of protein reacted with the phenolics. In these methods the Bovine serum albumin solution is treated with phenolics solution to form the protein phenolic complex, in which phenolic content and amount of protein are colormetrically estimated .The recent radial diffusion protein precipitation assay scores over this protein precipitatipon method. However, these procedures also depend on standards. The most common standard used is tannin acid .The usefulness of the protein precipitation method lies in their indication of ability of plant phenolics to form the protein complex but less useful to quantify the tannin content than the colorimetric methods.

The investigations on anti-nutritional constituents encompasses a wide range of multidiscipline research endeavour, It requires right from correct identification of forage species by considerable knowledge of botany, plant chemistry, nutritional biochemistry and physiology. The isolation and characterization of toxin/anti-nutritional factor is first step after identification of plant, Because of the fact management techniques must be built open accurate prediction of variation in toxin level associated with plant sp., growth stage and environmental changes, which is them requires the development of accurate and sanative analytical techniques for such measurements. The analytical method selected is therefore dependent on reorganization, of structural likely to be common, to all other class.

Bibliography

Adams N.R. Sanders MR. And Ritar A.J. (1988) Aust. J.Agric. 39:71

Adlercuretz, H & Mazur W.1997, 29,95-120

Adlercuretz, H, Markkanen H.,and Watanabw S. (1993) Lancet 342,1209-1210

Allison M.J. In "Effects of Poisonous plants in livestock (Ed, Keeler R.F Vankempn, L.F. and James)101-118 Acedemic Press NY

Anderson R.A. and Todd J.R.;(1991),. Tobbaco Sci12:107

Astanov K.A., Kushmura Y.K.and Sadykova A.S. (1985) In "Alkaloids: Chemical and biological Perspectives" Vol2, 105-148 John Willey USA

Barry T.N. and Duncan S.J.(1984) Br. J. Nutr. 51:485

Barry T.N. and Maneley T.R. (1989) Br.j.Nutri.51:493

Bate –Smith E.C.(1973) Phytochemistry 12; 1809

Bate-Smith E.C. (1973) , Phytochemistry 14 :1107 –1112

Bate-Smith E.C. (1981) , Phytochemistry 20 :211-216

Bickoff E.M. (1968) Oestrogenic constituents of forage plants Review series 1/1968 CAB UK

Bove F.J. (1970). The story of Ergot S.Karger N.York

Broadhuurst R.B.and Jones W.T. (1978). J. Food Sci. Agric.29:788

Bull L.B.,Dick A.T. Keast J.C. and Edgar S.Aust.J.Agri.Res. 7:281(1956) ,5

Cheeke P.R. and Shull L.R. (1985) Natural toxicants in feeds and poisonous plants. Avi Publication Conneectiicut USA

Cheng E. and Yoder L.(1958), Proc. Iowa Acad, Sci 65-,220-223

Curnow D.H. (1954), Biochem J. 58,283-287

Donelly E.D. and Anthony W.B. (1969) Crop Sci . 10:200-202

Egan A .R.and UlyattM .J. , (1980). J. Agric .Sci 94: 97

FAO (2004) year Book Food Agriculture Organisation UN

Fenny P.P. and BostockH.(1968). Phytochemistry 7:871

Folin O. and CiocaleteauV.(1927) J.Biol.Chem.73:627

Franke A.A., Custer L.J.,Carmenata M.C., and Narala K. (1995) Proceed. Soc. Exp. Bio. Med 208, 18-26.

Gamache P.H. and Acworth I.N. (1998). Proceed. Soc. Exp. Bio. Med. 217, 110-117 Haggerman A.E. 1987, J. Chem Ecol 13:437

Harbone J.B. (1976). Function of flavonoid .In chemistry and biochemistry of plant pigments ed T.W. goodwin vol 1 pp734 Acedamic press N york

Haslam E., (1989). Plant Polyphenols –vegetable tannins Revisited Cambridge University Cambridge UK

Haslam E. (1982). Proanthcyanidin ; In J.B. harbone and T.J. Mabry (Ed) The flavonoids :Advances in Research Chapman and Hall London

Heinonen S., Nurmi T. Liukknonn K. Poutanen K. Wâhâlâ K.Deyama T. Nishubi S and Adlercuretz, H, (2001) J.agric. food Chem,49, 3178-3186.

Howorth P.J.(1981) The nutritionaland ecologicalsignificanse of .Acer tanninsand related polyphenols M.S. Thesis Cornell University Itheca Newyork

Keeler R. F. and Crow (1984) Cornell Vet. 74, 50-59

Liggins J., Grimwood R., and Bingham S.A. (2000). Anl. Biochem 287,102-109

Lookhart G.L. (1980). J. Agric. Food.Chem.28: 666

Martin J .S. and Martin M.M.(1982). Oecologia 54:295

Mattock A.R. (1988) Recent advances in Pyrrolozidine Alkaloids 3rd International Symposium on Poisonous Plants held at Uttah Iowa state USA (Ed J,F. Keeler, M.P. Hegatary, E.M. Bailey, and P.R. Cheeke) pp161-168

Mattock A.R. and Rudukes (1988). The detection of potential toxic pyrrolizidine Alkaloids under field condition. 553-5553rd International Symposium on Poisonous Plants held at Uttah Iowa state USA

Mazur W., Wähälä K., rasku S., Salakka A., Hase T. and Adlercuretz, H (1998) Brt.J.Nutri. 79, 37-45

Mc Nabby W .C. Waghorn G .C , and Shelton I .D., (1993) Br. J. Nutr 70:647

Miranda C.L., Carpenter H.M., Cheeke P.R. and Butler D.R. 1981 Chem. Bio. Interaction 37, 95-107

Mitjavila S., Llacombe C. ,Carrera G., and Derache R. (1977) J.Nutri.107, 2113-2120

Moghaddam M. F. and Cheeke P.R. (1989) Toxicology letters 55, 425

Morton M.S., Ferrerira A. Moleerio L., Correrla R., Blacklock N., Chan P.S.F., Cheng C., Lloyd S., Wu C.P., and Griffith K (1997), Cancer Letter 114, 145-157

Muller Hearvey I., McAllan A.B. , Theodoru M.K. and Beever D.E. (1988). Proc. of a workshop at ILCA Addis Ababa Ethopia Dec.7-10- 1987 ILCA Adis Ababa p97

Nash R.J. Wattson A. and Asano N. (1997). Polyhydroxy alkaloids that inhibits glycosidase In "Alkaloids: Chemical and biological Perspectives"Vol 11 Ed William Pelletier, Prggmon press UK

Nurmi T. and Adlercuretz, H (1999) Anal. Biochem 274, 210-217

Pietinen P., Stumpf K.,Mannistu S. Mannistos S., kalaja V. ,Uusitupa M.and Adlercuretz, H Cancer Epidemiology Biomarker and Prevention 10:339-334

Porter L.J. (1994) Flavans and Proanthocyanidins In J.B. harbone (Ed) the flavonoids Advances in Research Since (1986) p23Chapman and Hall London

Reed J.D (1997) Ecological Biochemistry of secondary plant compound in herbivore nutrition 221-223 Proceedings of XVIII International Grassland Congress held at Winnipeg Canada 8-17 July (Ed. J.G. Buchanan, L.D. Bailey and P. Mc Caughey)

Reed J.D. ,Soller H. Wooward A. (1990), Anim. Feed Sci Technol30:39

ReedJ.D. ,HovarthP .J. Allen M.S. and Van Soest P.J. (1985). J.Sci Food Agric.36:255

Rosenthal G.A. and janzen R.G. (1979) Herbivores: their interaction with secondary metabolites 718 pp Academic press NY

Rowland I.R.., Wiseman H., Sanders T., Adlercuretz, H, and Bowey E., (1999) Biochem. Soc. Trans. 27, 304-208

Setchell K.D.R. and Adlercuretz, H, (1988) Mammalian lignan and Phyto-oestrogens : recent studies in their formation , metabolism and biological role in health disease In " Role of gut flora in toxicity and cancer pp315-45 (Rowland I.R Editor) Acedemic Press NY

Setchell KDR, and Cassidy A.(1999) J.Nutri. 129suppl.758s-767s

Sharma O.M.P. Adlercuretz, H., Strandberg J.D.,Zirkin B.R. Coffee D.S. and Ewing L.L. (1992) , J. Steroid Biochem. Mole.Bio. 43:557

Shull L.R., Buckmaster G.W. and Cheeke P.R. (1976), J. Anim. Sci 43,1247-1253

Singleton V.L.and Rossi J.A.; (1965); Am.J. Ecol. 16:144

Swain T (1979). Tannins and Lignins In G.A. Rosenthall and D.H. Janzen (ed) Herbivores, their interaction with secondary plant metabolites p657 Academic Press NewYork

Tempol A.S. (1982). J. Chem. Ecol 8:1289

Thompson L.U. Robb P. Serraino M. and Cheng F. (1991) Nutrition and Cancer 16, 43-52

Waghorn G .C., Ulyatt M. J, John A. and Fisher M .T., (1987) L. Br. J. Nutr; 57:115

24
EXTRUSION TECHNOLOGY

G.V.N. Reddy And Y. Ramana Reddy

Once ingredients are ground and mixed, they can be fed as a mash or subjected to further processing that usually involves heat or heat and pressure in combination. The most common forms of this thermal processing encountered in the feed industry are pelleting, roasting, steam flaking and extrusion/expansion. Extrusion processing has been used in the preparation of human foods for more than 50 years (Ferket, 1991). Extrusion is a highly flexible process for various raw materials, wide range of moisture contents (10-40%), feed ingredients, cooking temperatures (80 to 200°C) and residence times (10 to 270 seconds). An extruder is considered as high temperature short time (HTST) bioreactor that transforms a variety of raw ingredients into modified intermediate and finished products. The successful use of extrusion processing in the feed industry includes pet foods, aquatic sinking and floating foods, full fat soya, baby pig and calf feeds and slow release urea products for ruminants.

Extrusion Processing

Extrusion cooking is a process by which moistened, expandable feed materials are plasticized in a tube by the combination of moisture, pressure, heat and mechanical shear. The material to be extruded is fed from a holding bin, through a mixing cylinder and into the extruded barrel. The extruded barrel houses a series of locks, dies and orifices with greater and greater restrictions from inlet to outlet. The material being extruded is subjected to increasing pressure, friction and attrition as it passes through the extruder barrel such that the material temperature is raised to 135 to 160°C at pressures of 15 to 40 atmospheres in as little as 30 seconds. As the extruded material exits the extruder barrel, the sudden drop in pressure results in violent expansion as steam escapes from the product. Loss of steam reduces moisture content of the extruded material by as much as 50 per cent depending on initial moisture content. From the nutritional standpoint of view, of view desired effects of extruders are shearing and gelatinization of starch, denaturation and shearing of protein, destruction of microorganisms and some toxicants, restructuring of tactile components and dehydration (Smith, 1975).

Extrusion Cookers

Extruder cookers are classified as of single and twin-screw designs. The single screw cooking extruder has been the heart beat of the dry expanded pet and aquatic food industry. Single screw extruders are used to make virtually all the extruded soybeans in livestock feeding. The capacity of the extruder varies from 30 to 15,000 kg/hr with total KW of 11 to 500. The length and diameter ratios vary from 5 to 18. Twin-screw technology involves much higher capital costs which are about 1.5 to 2.5 times higher than single screw extruder of comparable hourly production capacity. The capacity of the extruder ranges from 0.5 to 15,000 kg/hour. The length and diameter ratio varies between 7 and 50. In both the extruder cookers, the final product characteristics are affected by the screw and barrel profile, screw speed, processing conditions (temperature, moisture etc.) raw material characteristics and die/knife selection.

In the extrusion chamber of both single and twin-screw extruders, there are three processing zones viz. feeding, kneading and final cooking zone. In the feeding zone the incoming material is compressed to expel the trapped air. Water is injected into the barrel to facilitate textural and viscosity development and to enhance conductive heat transfer. In the kneading zone of the cooking extruder, the compression that started earlier is continued and the flow channels of extruder screw have a higher degree of fill. Pressure starts building up in the kneading zone, where discrete particles of material begin to agglomerate. At the end of the kneading zone, the extrudate most typically reaches its maximum compaction. In the final cooking zone amorphorizing and texturizing occur. Temperature and pressure reach their peak and maximum compression of the extrudate occurs. The extrudate is then expelled from the extruder die to form the desired final product texture, density, colour and functional properties.

Extrusion cookers are further classified as wet and dry cooking extruders. Dry extruders are used in processing low moisture highly expanded starch products, and in processing whole soybeans to full fat soy flour for both food and feed industries. In dry extrusion there is no preconditioning of the ingredients with steam or moisture before entering the extruder barrel. All the heat produced by the dry extrusion process is generated by the mechanical energy applied to the ingredients via the screws, steam locks and the barrel wall. Longer barrels can now provide increased capacity of cooker. Dry extruders generate heat and pressure mechanically as a result of frictional and shear forces produced within the extruded barrel. With dry extruders, the highest reduction in trypsin inhibitor activity (TIA) appears to occur at a temperature range of 138 to 150°C. Most standard dry extruders are manufactured in such a way that the speed of rotation of the main shaft is around 550 revolutions per minute (R.P.M). Wet cooking extruders are more complex with precision metering system for steam or water injection into either the conditioner and/or the extruder barrel. Preconditioning is a very important part of the extrusion process. Preconditioning is known to enhance flavor development and aid in the final product texture (Huber, 1990). After extrusion, the product should be dried and cooled. The advantages of extruded feed is to make them free from pathogen free with further additions of flavour and colours, reduction of toxins, improved palatability, control of growth inhibitors and allergens, improved handling/less dusting and to inhibit effect of the release of ammonia on extruder starch and urea products.

Effect of Extrusion Cooking on Feed Components

Carbohydrates - In the extrusion cooking of starchy foods or cereal grains gelatinization of starch occurs resulting in irreversible destruction of crystalline structure of starch granules and the surface of every molecule made available to enzymes (amylases). Gelatinization enhances the ability of starch to absorb more water leading to improved digestibility and feed conversion efficiency in non-ruminants and ruminants (McElroy and Glass, 1956). The degree of gelatinization of starch depends on variation in physico-chemical properties including structure of granules, viscosity, solubility, macromolecule modifications and lipid complex formation (Asp and Bjorck, 1989). In addition, during the extrusion process fibre content and composition in high fibre formulations, soluble fibre increases by approximately 3% and carbohydrate content increases by 4-5%.

Proteins - The short time/high temperature (STHT) extrusion cooking of oilseeds is one of the methods to reduce the degradability of proteins without affecting their quality. Protein degradability of highly degradable protein sources such as groundnut, soybean and sunflower cakes (Yugandhar Kumar et al., 1994) and protein concentrates consisting of sunflower cake, niger cake and tobacco seed cake (Prasad Reddy and Anjaneya Prasad, 1985) was reduced by extrusion cooking technology. Extrusion processing of lupin seeds decreased the protein degradation in the rumen of sheep, thereby increased the intestinal digestibility of proteins in fattening lambs (Pajak et al., 2001). The amount of nitrogen which escapes rumen degradation was more and digestibility of escaped protein increased due to denaturation of heat labile trypsin inhibitor in extruded whole soybean fed dairy cattle (Stern et al., 1985). In extrusion cooking, temperature, pressure, moisture, swelling time and shear forces applied must be carefully coordinated to achieve a change in the folding of tertiary and quaternary structure of the proteins (texturing) and to make unfold again at low pH value (pH 2-3) in the stomach and further down in the small intestine. However, over heating is detrimental to protein as it reduce protein digestibility.

Fats - Extrusion has little effect on fat, but fats have an important physical function in the extrusion process. Extrusion cooking of oilseeds results in rupture of cells and release of more oil into the system to act as lubricant and tend to limit expansion. However, high fat content of oilseeds limits thermal and mechanical effects by reducing the shearing forces and heat elevation inside the extruder during extrusion cooking (Melcion et al., 1988). To overcome this, it is advisable to associate oilseeds with starch rich cereal grains.

Anti-nutritional factors - Enzyme inactivation (protease inhibitors, lipase and lipoxygenase) in feeds and feed ingredients during extrusion cooking contributes to the stability of feed and its acceptability after extended storage. Extrusion of faba (Vicia faba L.) bean at temperature of 85°C with 23% moisture was most effective in reducing the anti-nutritional factors like trypsin inhibiter activity, polyphenols and haemagglutinin activity, and increasing the protein digestibility (Prakrati Rajwat et al., 1999). Extrusion cooking of soybeanat HTST helps in retaining the nutritional value and also in reducing the anti-nutritional trypsin inhibitor factor as much as 90% (Naik and Gleason, 1988). Extrusion cooking results in the reduction of gossypol content and glucosinolate contents in cottonseed-soya mixture and rapeseed-soya mixtures, respectively (Cheng, 2003). Extrusion cooking is more effective in reducing trypsin inhibitors (95%), chymotrypsin inhibitors (64%), polyphenols (54%) and haemagglutinins (98%) in field beans (Pisum sativum L.). Lately, extrusion cooking and expander extrusion technology has been used to detoxify neem kernel (Azadirachta indica) cake (Joji Reddy, 2003) and rape seed (Brassica sp.) cake (Narasa Reddy, 2003[a]).

Vitamins and minerals - Most of the vitamins are destroyed during extrusion processing of feeds due to temperature, moisture and pressure. In addition, other parameters such as raw materials used, flow rate, screw speed, energy input, die open area, shear, redox reactions drying temperature and duration also influence the stability of vitamins (Schlude, 1987; Coelho, 1994; Rokey and Huber, 1994). The most sensitive vitamins to the extrusion process are A, E, C, B_1 and folic acid, where as the other B complex vitamins (B_2, B_6, B_{12}, niacin, calcium-pantothenate and biotin) are very stable. With an expander vitamin E alcohol, menadione and ascorbic acid were the least stable vitamins. These vitamins lost 20% of their activity at the lowest expander temperature and shortest residence time. At highest temperatures and longest resident times vitamin D, vitamin E acetate, B_{12} ascorbyl phosphate and choline chloride lost only slight activity and retained 80% of their original activity.

Extrusion processing of barley, corn gluten meal, soybean meal and wheat reduced the total P and Fe content marginally (Cheng, 2003).

Effect of Extrusion Processing on Animal Performance

Poultry - Extrusion of poultry feeds offers several advantages over conventional pelleted and mash feeds. According to Peisker (1994) expanders increase starch gelatinization, increase fat stability, allow more fat to be added, increase metabolizable energy, decreased microbial contamination and increase the soluble fibre. Extrusion processing also helps in inclusion of by-products as value added ingredients, and in producing hygienic feeds (Cheng, 2003). Fancher et al. (1996) reported improved growth and feed conversion in male turkeys fed expanded diets as compared to diets that were pelleted only. Smith et al. (1995) found that there was no difference in true metabolizable energy due to expansion, although expansion increased feed conversion in broilers. It would seem that the use of shear force by an expander would allow increased nutrients to be accessible which were previously bound within cellular material (Armstrong, 1993; Peisker 1994; Fancher et al., 1996). Work in Kansas state university has shown that increased amino acid bio-availability may occur when corn or soybean meal is expanded under different cone pressures. Birds that were fed expanded pelleted feeds had numerically higher plant yield (thigh and breast). In another study, the average body weight of birds receiving expanded-pelleted feed was significantly improved and the feed conversion ratio was significantly better (Wicker, 1995). Extruded soybeans increased the egg production and feed conversion in laying hens as compared to control soybean diets.

Swine - Hygienic pig feeds with high degree of gelatinization without using excess heat can be prepared by extrusion processing with prior conditioning technology. Dry extrusion of food waste, amended animal feed, reduced the load of potential pathogenic bacteria and risk of infectious diseases in animals and humans (Kelly and Walker, 1999). The extrusion process denatures the protein and inactivates allergens and growth inhibitors. The pig stomach will receive extruded vegetable protein similar to that of an animal protein. This results in transition between sow milk and dry feed using less expensive source of protein.

Extrusion improved energy and N digestibility of high tannin sorghum grains but not growth performance in nursery pigs (Noland et al., 1976). Extrusion of corn did not affect N utilization or lysine in nursery pigs but increased energy value (DE and ME) as compared to ground corn (Herkelman et al., 1990). In extruded barley-soybean mixture, the digestibilities of DM, GE, starch, and N at the terminal ileum were increased by 12, 12, 16 and 11 per cent, respectively (Fadel et al., 1988). Hancock et al. (1991[a]) reported that substitution of extruded for hammer milled sorghum did not affect ADG but increased efficiency of gain by 5% in finishing pigs. This increased gain/feed was accompanied by increase of 8 and 23% digestibilities of DM and N, respectively. Replacing soybean meal and soy oil with extruded soy beans also improved efficiency of gain by 5%, but the greatest efficiency was with extruded sorghum plus extruded soybeans in pigs (i.e., a 10% improvement vs. the control). Improved protein utilization by nursery pigs was demonstrated when dry roasting was replaced by extrusion processing (Hancock et al., 1990[a]; 1991[c]). Also ADG for pigs fed low-inhibitor extruded soybeans was 14% greater than that of pigs fed commercially prepared soybean meal plus soybean oil. Finally Hancock et al., (1992) reported that extrusion improved gain/feed by 4, 9, 6 and 3 per cent in finishing pigs fed corn-, sorghum-, wheat- and barley-based diets, respectively compared to simply grinding and cereals in a hammer mill.

Hancock et al. (1991[b]) believes that National Research Council's (NRC) value for ME of extruded soybeans is probably too low. Their data showed a 6% increase in dry matter digestibility and a 14% increase in nitrogen digestibility compared to non extruded soybeans. This disparity in nutritional value of heat-processed soy products was further evidenced by Kim et al. (2000), where the ileal digestibilities for lysine in growing pigs were 83, 67, 86 and 88% for soybean meal, roasted soybeans, extruded soybeans, and soybeans processed with an extrusion aid (sodium sulfite). Unfortunately the new NRC (1998) still categorizes all full fat soy products as "heat processed seeds" although it seems a differentiation among the processes used to create full fat soy products.

The advantage of extrusion cooking/expanding of corn-soybean meal based diets on DM digestibility (%), nitrogen digestibility (%), gross energy availability (%) ADG and feed efficiency over mash and pelleting in pigs was reviewed by Cheng (2003).

Ruminants - Extrusion cooking of deoiled salseed meal (DOSSM) was found to be an effective method to improve the utilization of nutrients in sheep, where energy value of DOSSM was increased by 23% (Anand Kumar Reddy et al., 1985). Various oil seeds such as soybean (Faldet et al., 1992), rapeseed (Doreau et al., 1987), sunflower (Mc Guffey and Schingoethe, 1982), cottonseed (Stults et al., 1988) and peas (Walhain et al., 1992) were processed by extrusion cooking process prior to inclusion in the rations of dairy cows. Extrusion processing of oil seeds like soybean has a favorable impact on milk production as well as milk composition (Scott et al., 1991) and also meat production in beef cattle (Albro et al., 1993). The increased energy value of extruded soybeans have been credited to disruption of the soybean fat globules, which improves accessibility to lipase enzymes (Hancock et al., 1990[b]). The same disruption could also contribute to improved protein digestibility because limited protein denaturation increases their susceptibility to enzymatic attack. In addition to reducing protein degradability, extruded oil seeds are a good source of protected fat, which partly voids digestive interaction (Subub et al., 1996), modifies the profile of fatty acids adsorbed in the duodenum and thus modifies the fatty acid profile of milk fat (Kim et al., 1993) or adipose tissue (Rule and Beitz, 1986). Extrusion cooking of pea + rapeseed blends resulted in increased flow of amino acids to the intestines and also an increased proportion of C 18:1, C 18:2 and C 18:3 fatty acids in the milk fat (Chapoutot and Sauvant, 1997). Further, the denaturation of biologically active proteins (conglycinin and beta conglycinin) in soybean seeds, which have antigenic properties, by thermal treatment, led to lower anti-soy titres thereby improved digestive function in pre-ruminant calves (Sissons et al., 1979, 1982).

Extrusion Technology for Slow Release Urea Products

NPN substances like urea and some dietary proteins are rapidly degraded by rumen microorganisms leading to high levels of ammonia in the rumen. Efforts are made to inhibit the release of ammonia rapidly in the rumen, since not all the ammonia produced in the rumen is utilized for protein synthesis by the microbes. Several slow release urea products as alternative to vegetable protein supplements have been developed. Extrusion cooking of mixtures of cereals with urea increased the level of urea that can be used safely in dairy, beef and sheep rations. This method was developed at Kansas State University by Helmer et al. (1970). A mixture of finely ground grain (corn, sorghum, barley etc.) and urea was expanded through a cooker extruder under moisture, temperature and pressure that causes starch to gelatinize, slows the release of ammonia in the rumen by temporarily binding the urea and also causes simultaneous release of energy and ammonia for efficient microbial protein synthesis in the rumen. The product was called Starea' by Bartley and Coworkers. Starea was approximately equal to soybean meal and products with protein equivalents of 44, 50 or 70 per cent of soybean meal have been developed as protein supplements for lactating cows (Helmer et al., 1970; Stiles et al., 1970).

Slow release urea products (Salurea 50, Salurea 70 and 90) were developed at the Department of Animal Nutrition, College of Veterinary Science, Tirupati under the leadership of Anjaneya Prasad by extrusion cooking of deoiled sal seed (Shorea robusta) meal, an unconventional energy supplement, and urea (Konda Reddy et al., 1979, 1981; Seshi Reddy and Prasad 1988[c]; Anjaneya Prasad et al., 1982). Other unconventional and conventional energy supplements like tapioca (Manihot esculenta) flour, mango seed (Mangifera indica) bajra (Pennisetum americanum) and Ragi (Eleusine coracana) have also been used with urea at different proportions for development of slow release urea products (Nageswara Rao et al., 1985; Bala Subramanyam, 1981; Chalapathi Rao, 1985;

Srinivasa Rao et al., 1997[a,b]). These products could replace expensive groundnut cake nitrogen from 50-72 percent in concentrate mixtures of ruminants (Prasad et al., 1982; Rao et al., 1985; Seshi Reddy and Prasad 1988[a,b]; Srinivasa Rao et al., 1997[a,b]).

Expander Extruder Technology

This is a system, which combines the features of expanding (application of moisture, pressure and temperature to gelatinize the starch portion) and extruding (pressing the feed through constrictions under pressure). They require less energy and maintenance input. Conveying is combined with shearing (kneading) dissipative heating, pressuring and expanding of the material through a ring gap. They always operate at a similar stressing profile over the length of the barrel and provide for relatively high throughput. Throughput ranges from 1.5 to 40tons/hr. The installed driving power is between 75 and 315 KW. Normally pressure is allowed to rise to 15-100 bars. For most products the length diameter ratio (L/D) of the expander is equal to 7.

The different ingredients of the diet to be expander - extruded have to be proportioned as per formula into100 kg batches using appropriate scales. The ingredients requiring grinding will be ground in a hammer mill. The ground ingredients will come to mixer through screw conveyor and bucket elevator and hopper above the mixer. The ingredients that do not require grinding will be directly added to the mixer. Molasses will be pumped from the tank to preheating tank, where it will be heated upto 70°C. The heated molasses will be sent to the mixer through a dosage tank as per formula. The micro-ingredients (vitamins, antibiotics etc.) will be made into a premix by diluting with ground grain or bran and required quantity of premix will be added to the mixer directly. Later, all the ingredients will be mixed for about 10 minutes. While mixing, the mash at 12-13% moisture and room temperature will be reconstituted with required quantity of water to get 17-18% moisture in the mixer itself and then sent to the hopper above the expander-extruder from which, it passes through screw in which it attains 90-95°C by the time it comes out of the die openings. Otherwise, the mash without reconstitution can be sent to hopper and steam will be added to get required moisture while the feed is passing through the screw of expander-extruder. The pellets coming out of the expander-extruder will be cooled and collected into sacs.

Rise in temperature is due to friction force that occurs in the barrel. Thus the feed not only undergoes a short term temperature increase but the feed particles have also experienced a shear force. Exposure to high temperature occurs for a short time so that destruction of heat sensitive nutrients appears to be minimal under standard conditions. Presumably, these factors may lead to an improvement in bioavailability of previously hard to digest feed components, while decreasing the microbial content of the feed (Peisker, 1994; Armstrong, 1993; Fancher et al., 1996). Further, the cost of processing of complete diet using expander extruder will be reduced by about 25% compared to conventional steam pelleting, since the former can be processed without steam.

Effect on roughages - Five crop residues (groundnut haulms, soy straw, bajra straw, castor straw and palm press fibre) were processed by chopping, grinding, expander extruder processing and steam pelleting to study the physical characters and nutritive value (Reddy 2003[a]; Narasa Reddy, 2003[b]).

Expander extruder processing of ground material increased the bulk density by 15 (soybean straw) to 103% (bajra straw). However, expander extruder processed pellets were less dense compared to steam pelleting due to less compaction in the former. These differences in bulk density among the residues may be attributed to differences in particles size, shape, fibre characters and compactness of the molecules. Castor straw absorbed water at the time of reconditioning but oozed out at the time of pelleting with expander extruder due to presence of pith and hence, could not be processed with expander extruder. It requires addition of concentrates for processing with expander extruder. Pelletability with expander extruder processing was good with groundnut straw and soybean straw due to the presence of more leafy material in these straws (Reddy 2003[a]; Narasa Reddy, 2003[b]).

Expander extruder processing significantly ($P<0.05$) increased the dry matter intake and digestibilities of nutrients in sheep compared to ground and chopped crop residues but comparable to that of steam pelleting (Narasa Reddy, 2003[b]). TDN was significantly ($P<0.05$) higher on expander extruder processing and steam pelleting compared to chopping and grinding on all the crop residues.

Effect of expander extruder processed complete diets on animal performance

The expander extruder processed diets recorded 6.9% higher dry matter intake and digestibilities of dry matter, organic matter and crude protein and hence, the animals were on better plane of nutrition (Reddy and Reddy, 2003[b]). These rations had better rumen fermentation pattern. Expander extrusion processing was used to improve the nutrient utilization of sugarcane bagasse (Narasa Reddy et al., 2002) and maize cobs (Narasa Reddy and Raj Reddy, 1999) based complete rations in male calves.

Effect on growth - Expander extruder processed diet containing 40% maize cobs recorded 13% higher ADG with 6.8% less DMI/kg gain and 6%

less cost of feed/kg gain (Narasa Reddy and Raj Reddy, 1999) while that containing 40% sugarcane bagasse recorded 14.8% higher ADG with 17.6% less DMI/kg gain and 16.9% less cost of feed/kg gain compared to respective mash diets in Ongole bull calves (Narasa Reddy et al., 2002).

Effect on milk production - Expander extruder processed diet containing 28.5% sorghum straw recorded 6.8% higher milk yield with 12.8% less DMI and 6.1% less cost of feed/kg milk yield in crossbred cows while that containing 28.5% maize cobs recorded 5.6% higher FCM yield with 19.4% DMI/kg FCM and 33.3% less cost of feed/kg FCM production in Murrah buffaloes compared to respective mash diets (Reddy et al., 2001). The expander extruder processed diets containing maize cobs/cotton stalks/sunflower heads (28.5%) recorded significantly 9-30% higher milk yield with 20-33% less cost of feed/kg milk production in Murrah buffaloes compared to conventional ration containing green grass, paddy straw and concentrate mixture in on-farm situation (Reddy et al., 2001). Expander extruder processed complete feed based on forest grass supported 10.68 kg milk yield/d in cows which was 11.4% higher than on conventional feed. This diet also increased milk yield in goats by 0.1 l/d (Badve, 2003).

Effect on meat production - Complete diet containing cotton straw/maize cobs/sunflower heads (40%) maintained ADG of 102 to 121g in Nellore lambs and 71-81g in local kids which was 14-21% higher in lambs and 10-24% higher in kids compared to conventional diet (Reddy and Linga Reddy, 2003). The cost of feed/kg gain was reduced by 13-20% in both the species. Expander extruder processed complete diets containing bajra straw/castor straw recorded higher ($P<0.05$) ADG in lambs compared to mash. However, expander extruder processing and steam pelleting recorded similar performance in buffaloes and lambs. The results of feeding expander extruded complete rations on the performance of different species of ruminants have been recently reviewed by Reddy and Reddy (2003[b]).

Extrusion Processing of Aquatic Feeds

Extrusion cooking is one of the most promising methods to produce high quality aquatic feeds. Production of aquatic feeds fell into one of four production categories: floating feeds, sinking feeds, slow sinking feeds and soft moist feeds. Extruders are also capable of producing sinking floating and soft moist foods. The ability to control the density of a finished product allows the production of floating or sinking aquatic feeds that are tailored for particular species of aquatic animals. Floating aquatic feeds are in the density range of 320 to 400 g/l. They are expanded pellets varying in diameter from 1.5 to 10 mm. Typical floating feeds are extrusion cooked at the high temperature and lower moisture levels and expands upon exiting the diet approximately 125 to 150% of the original hole size (Anjaneya Prasad, 2003).

Sinking aquatic feeds are typically in the density range of 400 to 600g/l. These products are generally 1.5 to 4.0 mm in diameter and predominantly are used for shrimp feeding. Slow sinking aquatic feeds are in the density range of 390 to 410 g/l. These products sink in salt water. These types of feeds are being used in the salmon raising industry. The technology of producing soft moist feeds is very similar to producing floating aqua feeds on the extruder (Anjaneya Prasad, 2003).

Aqua feeds can be manufactured through extrusion processing that hit precise targets in terms of size, durability, density and nutritional composition at a competitive price. Twin-screw extrusion technology can be used to process ultra-high fat aqua feeds with fat levels above 17% (Rokey and Huber, 1994).

Extrusion Technology in Manufacturing Pet Foods

Dry expanded pet foods are produced through extrusion-cooking process and are typically composed of a mixture of ground cereal grains such as wheat, corn or sorghum and soybean meal as well as milk products, fats and oils, salt and color. In addition, micro-ingredients such as vitamins, minerals, amino acids, antibiotics and enzymes are added to pet food formulae and extrusion process allow the addition of liquids of micro ingredients on the final product of pet foods (Gilbert, 1997). Addition of amylase enzymes to the conditioner in the extrusion processing of dog foods increases throughput by 20-30% without increasing the extruder energy requirement, drying need or changing the kibble texture, shape, hardness or bulk density, thereby saving extrusion cost upto 5-10% (Ziggers, 2002).

In conclusion, extrusion processing is widely used in preparation of variety of pet foods and aquatic feeds and to some extent, to manufacture specialty items used in livestock feeding (e.g. soy preparations for newly weaned pigs). The extrusion processing holds a great promise as a method to improve the nutrient utilization of feed ingredients/complete diets in ruminants, pigs and poultry. However, the extrusion technology that produces feeds to meet the market demand must also have high operating efficiency at the lowest costs. Then only this technology is useful in the manufacturing of livestock and poultry feeds.

Bibliography

Albro, J.D., Weber, D. W. and Delcurto, T. 1993. Comparison of whole, raw soybeans, extruded soybeans, or soybean meal and barley on digestive characteristics and performance of weaned beef steers consuming mature grass hay. J. Anim. Sci. 71:26.

Ananda Kumar Reddy, Anjaneya Prasad, D. and Prabhakara Rao, Z. 1985. Effect of extrusion cooking deoiled salseed meal on the utilization of nutrients by sheep. Agricultural wastes, 13:179-187.

Anjaneya Prasad, D. 2003. Extrusion/expansion application in the feed industry. In: short term course on 'Feed Processing Technology' held at ANGRAU, Rajendranagar, Hyderabad. pp.102-108.

Anjaneya Prasad, D., Prabhakara Rao, Z., Ramachandra Reddy, R., Rama Prasad, J. and Kodanda Rami Reddy, S. 1982. Studies on replacement of groundnut-cake nitrogen by extruded deoiled salseed-meal urea product (Salurea-70). Indian. J. Anim. Sci. 52:379-383.

Armstrong, H. 1993. Nutritional implications of expanded feed. Feed Mix. 1: 26-27.

Asp, N.G. and Bjorck, I.1989. Extrusion cooking, 99:399.

Badve, V. C. 2003. Complete feeds for economical milk and meat production. Paper present at workshop on 'Present Status of Feed Technology and Future Strategies', held at ANGRAU, Hyderabad, from July, 22nd to 23rd, 2003. pp. 101-107.

Balasubramanyam, K. 1981. In vitro and in vivo evaluation on extruded mangoseed meal, deoiled salseed meal and urea products (70% crude protein). M. V. Sc. thesis submitted to APAU, Rajendranagar, Hyderabad.

Chalapathi Rao, A. S. 1985. Development and evaluation of extruded bajra flour and urea product. M. V. Sc. thesis submitted to APAU, Rajendranagar, Hyderabad.

Chapoutat, P. and Sauvant, D. 1997. Nutritive value of raw and extruded pea-rapeseed blends for ruminants. Anim. Feed Sci. Technol. 65: 59-77.

Cheng, J. 2003. Extrusion technology and its application in the feed industry. 11th Annual ASA South-east Asian Feed Technology and Nutrition 'workshop held at Hanoi, Vietnam from July 28th to August 1st, 2003.

Coelho, M. 1994. Comparison with pelleting and extrusion. Vitamin stability in expanders. Feed Management 45: 10-15.

Doreau, M., Chillard, Y., Voisin, A., Michalet-Doureau, B., Bauchard, D. and Legaycarmier, F. 1987. Utilization des graines oleagineuses extrudees dans l' alimentation du ruminant. In: uisson-extrusion, Nantes, France, 16-17 September, 1986. INRA Publ., Versailles (Ed.), Les Coloqus des l' INRA, No: 41, pp: 259.

Fadel, J. D., Newman, C. W., Newman, R. K. and Graham, H. 1988. Effects of extrusion cooking of barley on ileal and fecal digestibilities of dietary components in pigs. Can. J. Anim. Sci. 68:891.

Faldet, M. A., Son, Y.S. and Satter, L.D. 1992. Chemical, in vitro and in vivo evaluation of soybeans heat treated by various processing methods. J. Dairy Sci. 75:789.

Fancher, B., Rollins, D. and Trimbee, B. 1996. Feed processing using the annular gap expander and its impact on poultry performance. J.A.P.R. 5: 386-394.

Ferket, P. R. 1991. Technological advances could make extrusion an economically feasible alternative to pelleting. Feedstuffs 63(9):1.

Gilbert, R. 1997. New extrusion developments for pet food manufacturer. Feed Tech. 2:16-17.

Gilbert, R. 1998 Extruded legumes provide greater nutritional value. Feed Tech. 2:16-18.

Hancock, J.D., Hines, R. H., Fitzner, G. E. and Gugle, T. L. 1991[a]. Effect of extrusion processing on the nutritional value of sorghum and soybeans for finishing pigs. p 113. Proc. 17th Biennial Grain Sorghum Utilization Conference, February 17-20, 1991, Lubbock, TX.

Hancock, J. D., Hines, R. H. and Gugle, T. L. 1991[b]. Extrusion of sorghum, soybean meal, and whole soybeans improves growth performance and nutrient digestibility in finishing pigs. p. 92. Kansas State Univ. Swine Day, Kansas Agric. Exp. Sta. Rep. Prog. No. 641.

Hancock, J. D., Hines, R. H., Richert, B. T. and Gugle, T. L. 1992. Extruded corn, sorghum, wheat, and barley for finishing pigs. p. 130. Kansas State Univ. Swine Day, Agric. Exp. Sta. Rep. Prog. No. 667.

Hancock, J. D., A. J. Lewis, P. G. Reddy, D. B. Jones, M. A. Giesemann and B. J. Healy. 1990[a]. Processing method affects the nutritional value of low-inhibitor soybeans for nursery pigs. p. 52. Kansas State Univ. Swine Day, Kansas Agric. Exp. Sta. Rep. of Prog. No. 610.

Hancock, J. D., Lewis, A. J., Reddy, P. G., Jones, D. B. and Giesemann, M. A. 1991[c]. Extrusion processing of low-inhibitor soybeans improves growth performance of nursery pigs fed protein-adequate diets. p.40. Kansas State Univ. Swine Day, Kansas Agric. Exp. Sta. Rep. of Prog. No. 641.

Hancock, J. D., Bramel Cox, P.J., Smit, K.R., Healy, B. J., Klopfenstein, C. F. and Witt, M. D. 1990[b] J. Anim. Sci. (suppl.1), 90:320.

Helmer, L.G., Bartley, E. E. and Deyoe, C. W. 1970. Feed processing VI : Comparison of starea, urea and soybean meal as protein sources for lactating dairy cows. J. Dairy Sci. 53: 883-887.

Herkelman, K. L., Rodhouse, S. L., Veum, T.L. and Ellersieck, M. R. 1990. Effect of extrusion on the ileal and fecal digestibilities of lysine in yellow corn in diets for young pigs. J. Anim. Sci. 68:2414.

Huber, G. R. 1990. Preconditioning and related extrusion processing issues. American Association of Cereal Chemists Extrusion short course.

Joji Reddy, K. 2003. Estimation of certain toxins of neem (Azdirachta indica) seed cake and its effect on sheep. Paper presented at workshop on 'Present Status of Feed Technology and Future Strategies', held at ANGRAU, Hyderabad, from July, 22nd to 23rd, 2003. pp. 44-54.

Kelley, T. R. and Walker, P. M. 1999. Bacterial concentration reduction of food waste amended animal feed using a single screw dry extrusion process. Bioresourse Technol. 67: 247-253.

Kim, I. H., Hancock, J.D. and Hines, R. H. 2000. Influence of processing method on ileal digestibility of nutrients from soybeans in growing and finishing pigs. Asian-Aus. J. Anim. Sci. 13:192.

Kim, Y. K., Schingoethe, D. Y., Casper, D. P. and Ludens, F. C. 1993. Supplemental dietary fat from extruded soybeans and calcium soaps of fatty acids for lactating diary cows. J. Dairy Sci. 76: 197.

Konda Reddy, P., Bhaskar Rao, S. and Anjaneya Prasad, D. 1979. Evaluation of extruded salseed meal urea treated products by in vitro techniques. Proceedings of the All India Symposium (UNDP/ICAR) held at Karnal from May 21st to 23rd. pp.45-48.

Konda Reddy, P., Bhaskar Rao, S. and Anjaneya Prasad, D. 1981. Development and evaluation of extruded deoiled salseed-meal urea products (salurea-50 and salurea-70) by in vitro and in vivo methods. Indian J. Anim. Sci. 51:604-610.

McElroy, W. D. and Glass, B. 1956. In symposium on 'Inorganic Nitrogen Metabolism'. John Hopkins Press, Baltimore.

McGuffey, R. K. and Schingoethe, D. J. 1982. Whole sunflower seeds for high producing dairy cows. J. Dairy Sci. 64:1479.

Melcion, J. P., Zernicki, W. and Conan, L. 1988. L' aliment extrude colza-pois: une nouvelle matiere premiere. ev. Alement. Anim. 36:417.

Nageswara Rao, K., Anjaneya Prasad, D. and Krishna, N. 1985. Development and nutritional evaluation of extruded Tapioca flour and urea products (Tapurea-70). Cheiron. 14: 104-112.

Naik, G. and Gleason, J. E. 1988. An improved soy processing technology to help alleviate protein malnutrition in India. Food and Nutrition Bulletin, 10:45-49.

Narasa Reddy, G. V. 2003[b] Effect of processing of crop residues on physical characteristics and nutrient utilization in sheep. Paper present at workshop on 'Present Status of Feed Technology and Future Strategies', held at ANGRAU, Hyderabad, from July, 22nd to 23rd, 2003. pp.115-121.

Narasa Reddy, G. V. 2003[a]. Detoxification of rapeseed (Brassica sp.) meal and its effect on animal health and performance. Paper present at workshop on 'Present Status of Feed Technology and Future Strategies', held at ANGRAU, Hyderabad, from July, 22nd to 23rd, 2003. pp. 23-43.

Narasa Reddy, G. V. and Raj Reddy, M. 1999. Effects of feeding extruded complete diet containing maize cobs in ongole calves. Indian J. Anim. Nutr. 16:210.

Narasa Reddy, G. V., Joji Reddy, K. and Nagalakshmi, D. 2002. Effect of expander extruder processed complete diets containing sugarcane bagasse on growth and nutrient utilization in ongole bull calves. Indian J. Anim. Sci. 72:406.

Noland, P. R., Campbell, D. R., Jr.Gage, R. K., Sharp, R. N. and Johnson, Z. B. 1976. Evaluation of processed soybeans and grains in diets for young pigs. J. Anim. Sci. 43:763.

NRC. 1998. Nutrient Requirements of Swine (10th Ed.). National Academy Press, Washington, DC.

Pajak, J. J., Kowalczyk, J., Zebrowska, T., Kowalik, B. and Dlugolecka, Z. 2001. Effect of extrusion-cooking temperature on the nutritive value of lupin seeds in fattening lambs. J. Anim. Feed Sci. 10 (suppl.2):357-362.

Peisker, M. 1994. Influence of expansion on feed components. Feed Mix. 2: 26-31.

Prakrati Rajwat., Kushwah, A. and Kushwah, H. S. 1999. Effect of extrusion cooking variables on antinutritional components and in vitro protein digestibility of faba bean. Indian J. Anim. Nutr. 16:301-305.

Prasad, D. A., Rao, Z. P., Reddy, R. R., Prasad, J. R. and Reddy, S. K. 1982. Studies on replacement of groundnut cake nitrogen by extruded deoiled salseed meal urea product (salurea - 70). Indian J. Anim. Sci. 52:379.

Prasada Reddy, E. and Anjaneya Prasad, D. 1985. Effect of extrusion cooking, heat or formaldehyde treatment of protein concentrate on nutrient digestibility and nitrogen balance in growing crossbred calves. Cheiron, 14:47-52.

Rao, K. N., Prasad, D. A. and Krishna, N. 1985. Development and nutritional evaluation of extruded tapioca flour and urea product (tapurea-70). Cheiron, 14:104-112.

Reddy, M. R. and Reddy, G. V. N. 2003[b]. Processing of complete diets for ruminants and their effect on animal performance. In: short term course on 'Feed Processing Technology' held at ANGRAU, Rajendranagar, Hyderabad. pp.215-233.

Reddy, G.V.N., Joji Reddy, K. and Nagalakshmi, D. 2001. Effect of feeding expande-extruder processed complete diet containing of maize cobs on performance of buffaloes. Indian J. Anim. Nutr. 18:8-14.

Reddy, G. V. N. and Linga Reddy, J. 2003. Effect of cotton stalks based complete diet on growth and carcass characteristics in sheep and goat in field condition. Indian J. Anim. Nutr. 20: 97-100.

Reddy, G. V. N. 2003[a]. Effect of processing of crop residues on physical characteristics and nutritive value. In: short term course on 'Feed Processing Technology' held at ANGRAU, Rajendranagar Hyderabad. pp. 199-214.

Rokey, R. and Huber, G. 1994. Feed Manufacturing Technology - IV. pp. 479.

Rule, D. C. and Beitz, D. C. 1986. Fatty acids of adipose tissue, plasma, muscle and duodenal ingesta of steers fed extruded soybeans. J. Am. oil. chem.. Soc. 63:1429.

Schlude, M. 1987. Extrusion Technology for the food industry. p. 23. Elsevier Science Publishing Co. NY, USA.

Scott, T. A., Combs, D. K. and Grummer, R. R. 1991. Effects of roasting, extrusion and particle size on feeding value of soybeans for dairy cows. J. Dairy. Sci. 74:2555.

Seshi Reddy, B. and Prasad, D. A. 1987. Effect of extruded deoiled salseed meal and urea (salurea-90) on nitrogen utilization in Nellore brown weathers. Indian J. Anim. Nutr. 4:39-43.

Seshi Reddy, B. and Prasad, D. A. 1988[a]. Nutrient utilization and nitrogen metabolism in calves fed different levels of extruded deoiled salseed meal urea (salurea-90). Indian J. Anim. Nutri. 5:1-6.

Seshi Reddy, B. and Prasad, D. A. 1988[b]. Comparison of nutrient utilization from groundnut cake, urea and Salurea-90 in crossbred bullocks. Indian J. Anim. Nutri. 5:7-13.

Seshi Reddy, B. and Prasad. D. A. 1988[c]. Optimisation of conditions for extrusion cooking of deoiled sal seed meal and urea complexation into salurea - 90. Indian J. anim. Nutr. 5:110-115.

Sissons, J.W., Smith, R. H. and Hewitt, D. 1979. The effect of giving feeds containing soya-bean meal treated or extracted with ethanol on digestive processes in the preruminant calf. Br. J. Nutr. 42:477.

Sissons, J. W., Smith, R. H., Hewitt, D. and Nyrup, A. 1982. Prediction of the suitability of soya-bean products for feeding to preruminant calves by an in vitro immunochemical method. Br. J. Nutr. 47:311.

Smith, P. A., Firman, J. D. and Dale, N. 1995. Effects of feed processed in an annular gap expander on subsequent broiler performance. Poultry Sci. 74: (abst.)145.

Smith, O. B. 1975. Textured vegetable proteins. World soybean Research Conference, University of Illinois.

Srinivasa Rao, M., Rama Prasad, J., Prabhakara Rao, Z. and Srinivasa Rao, D. 1997[a]. Development and Evaluation of ragurea-70 product. Indian J. Anim. Nutr. 14: 89-92.

Srinivasa Rao, M., Rama Prasad, J., Prabhakara Rao, Z. and Srinivasa Rao, D. 1997[b]. valuation of extruded ragurea-70 product as protein supplement in growing cattle. Indian J. Anim. Nutr. 14: 154-157.

Stern, M. D., Santos, K. A. and Satter, L. D. 1985. Protein degradation in rumen and amino acid absorption in small intestine of lactating dairy cattle fed heat-treated whole soybeans. J. Dairy Sci. 68:45-56.

Stiles, D. A., Bartley, E. E., Deyoe, C. W. and Pfost, H. B. 1970. Feed processing III: Effect of an extrusion processed mixture of grain and urea (starea) on nitrogen utilization in cattle and on urea toxicity. J. Dairy Sci. 53:1436.

Stults, J. A., Nipper, W. A., Adkinson, R. W., Chandler, J. E. and Achacoso, A. S. 1988. Protein solubility, in vitro ammonia concentration and in situ disappearance of extruded whole cottonseed and other protein sources. J. Dairy Sci. 71:3323.

Subub, A. M. H., Rowan, T. G. and Lawrence, T.L.J. 1996. Effect of heat or formaldehyde treatment on the rumen degradability and intestinal tract apparent digestibility of protein in soya bean meal and in rapeseed meals of different glucosinolate content. Anim. Feed Sci. Technol. 57:257.

Walhain, P., Foucart, M. and Thewis, A. 1992. Influence of extrusion on ruminal and intestinal disappearance in sacco of pea (Pisum sativum) proteins and starch. Anim. Feed Sci. Technol. 38:43.

Wicker, D. B. 1995. The effects of annular gap expansion on broiler feeds. In:proc. of 22nd Annual Carolina Poultry Nutrition Conference, North Carolina. pp.45-63.

Yugandhar Kumar, M., Rama Prasad, J. and Krishna, N. 1994. Effect of heat, formaldehyde or extrusion cooking on rumen protein degradability of rapidly degradable protein supplements in crossbred cattle. Indian J. Dairy Sci. 47:459.

Ziggers, D. 2002. Save on extrusion costs by using enzyme. Feed Tech. 6:12-13.

25
CODEX ALIMENTARIUS : FOOD SAFETY & QUALITY CONTROL

Arun Verma

Food safety and quality assurance are the two essentials of consumers protection and effective food control system for human and animal life of any country.

Consumers expect protection from hazards occurring along the entire food chain,(often described as the farm-to-table continuum). Protection will only occur if all sectors in the chain operate in an integrated way, and food control systems address all stags of this chain.

Potential Hazards of food safety include improper use of supplement and unscientific processing procedures. Food safety and quality are adversely affective due to following reasons:

- Improper agricultural practices
- Poor hygiene at all stages of food chain
- Lack of preventive operational control in food processing and preparation
- Misuse of chemical, biological, metabolites, hormones, drugs and supplements for increasing growth and profit.
- Adulterants and immitants in processed food and feed.
- New entrants in this are GMO, allergens, and antibiotics.

Food Control System

In UN terms food control is mandatory regulatory activity of enforcement by national or local authorities to provide consumer protection and ensure that all foods during production, handling, storage, processing, and distribution are safe, wholesome and fit for human consumption; conform to safety and quality requirements; and are honestly and accurately labeled as prescribed by law.

An ideal food control system should include effective enforcement of mandatory requirements, along with training and education, community outreach programmes and promotion of voluntary compliance. The introduction of preventive approaches such as the Hazard Analysis Critical Control Point System (HACCP) have resulted in industry taking greater responsibility for and control of food safety risks. Thus an integrated approach will improve consumer protection, effectively and also stimulate agriculture and food processing industry to promote healthy growth and also trade.

Access of countries to food export markets will continue to depend on their capacity to meet the regulatory requirements of importing countries.

World Authorities in Business of Food safety and Quality Assurance.

The need for technical assistance in strengthening food control systems in developing countries is well recognized. FAO and WHO are the two main specialized agencies of the United Nations involved in food quality and safety technical cooperation programmes with developing countries.

i) Food and Agricultural Organization FAO

FAO assistance in food control and food standards is a major activity and is delivered at global, regional, and country levels. Published manuals of food quality control cover a range of different aspects of food control systems and are used internationally. Meetings, seminars and workshops are conducted in all regions of Africa, Asia and the Pacific, Latin America and the Caribbean, Eastern Europe the Near East and North Africa. Technical assistance is provided in many areas such as the following:

- Establishing or strengthening national food control systems and infrastructure;
- Assistance in preparation of food law and regulations;
- Workshops on developing national strategies for food control;
- Assistance in establishing or improving food analysis capabilities;
- Assessing the implications of SPS and TBT Agreements
- Provide training in food inspection, analysis and food handling;
- Providing training of trainers in HACCP;
- Providing training in management of food control systems; and
- Assistance in strengthening National Codex Committees

ii) World Health Organization

WHO has in recent years substantially increased the priority of its food safety activities at international and regional level. The Organization also provides technical assistance at international, regional and country levels. Under its decentralized structure, WHO is divided into six regions, with Regional Offices responsible for providing assistance to Member States in developing and strengthening their National Food Safety Programmes. Regional Offices currently undertake a range of capacity building initiatives designed to safeguard consumer health. The nature and extent of these activities is influenced by available resources, but includes the following:

- Developing regional and national food safety policy and strategies;
- Preparation of food legislation, food regulations and standards and codes of hygienic practice;
- Implementation of food inspection programmes;
- Promoting methods and technologies designed to prevent food borne diseases, including the application of the HACCP system;
- Developing or enhancing food analysis capability;
- Development and delivery of hygiene training and education programmes;
- Establishing healthy markets and enhancing the safety of street food; and
- Promoting the establishment of forborne disease surveillance activity.

iii) World Trade Organizations: SPS and TBT Agreements

a) SPS and TBT Agreements

The conclusion of the Uruguay Round of Multilateral Trade Negotiations in Marrakech led to the establishment of the WTO on 1 January 1995 and to the coming into force of the Agreement on the Application of Sanitary and Phytosanitary Measures (SPS) and the Agreement on Technical Barriers to Trade (TBT). Both these Agreements are relevant in understanding the requirements for food protection measures at the national level and the rules under which food is traded internationally.

The SPS Agreement confirms the right of WTO member countries to apply measures to protect human, animal and plant life and health. The Agreement covers all relevant laws, decrees, regulations, testing, inspection, certification and approval procedures and packaging and labeling requirements directly related to food safety. Member States are asked to apply only those measures for protection that are based on scientific principles only to the extent necessary and not in a manner which may constitute a disguised restriction on international trade. Thus the Codex standards serve as a benchmark for comparison of national sanitary and phytosanitary measures. While it is not compulsory for Member States to apply Codex Standards, it is in their best interests to harmonize their national food standards with those elaborated by Codex.

The TBT Agreement requires that technical regulations on traditional quality factors, fraudulent practices, packaging, labeling etc. imposed by countries will not be more restrictive on imported products than they are on products produced domestically. It also encourages use of international standards.

iv) Good Agricultural Practices (GAP)

Practices of primary food producers (such as farmers and fishermen) those are necessary to produce safe and wholesome agricultural food products conforming to food laws and regulations.

v) Good Manufacturing Practices (GMP)

Conformance with codes of practice, industry standards, regulations and laws concerning production, processing, handling, labeling and sale of foods decreed by industry, local, state, national and international bodies with the intention of protecting the public from illness, product adulteration and fraud.

PART-II

Codex Alimentarius & HACCP

A. Codex Alimentarius Commission

The Eleventh Session of the Conference of FAO in 1961 and the Sixteenth World Health Assembly in 1963 both passed resolutions to establish the Codex Alimentarius Commission. The two bodies also adopted the Statutes and Rules of Procedure for the Commission.

The Codex Alimentarius Commission (CAC) is an intergovernmental body that coordinates food standards at the international level. Its main objectives are to protect the health of consumers and ensure fair practices in food trade. The CAC has proved to be most successful in achieving international harmonization in food quality and safety requirements. It has formulated international standards for a wide range of food products and specific requirements covering pesticide residues, food additives, veterinary drug residues, hygiene, food contaminants, labeling etc. Codex work has created worldwide awareness of food safety, quality and consumer protection issues and has achieved international consensus on how to deal with them scientifically through a risk based approach. As a result there has been a continuous appraisal of the principles of food safety and quality at the international level. There is increasing pressure for the adoption of these principles at the national level.

a) The Statutes provide the legal basis for the Commission's work and formally reflect the concepts behind and reasons for its establishment. Article1 of the Statutes provides the Commission with its purposes, terms of reference and objectives:

Article 1 The Codex Alimentarius Commission shall be responsible for making proposals to and shall be consulted by the Director General of the Food & Agriculture Organization (FAO) and the World Health Organization (WHO) on all matters pertaining to the implementation of Joint FAO/WHO Food Standards Programme the purpose of which is:

- Protecting the health consumers and ensuring fair practices in the food trade;
- Promoting coordination of all food standards work undertaken by international governmental and non-governmental organizations;
- Determining priorities and initiating and guiding the preparation of draft standards through and with the aid of appropriate organizations;
- Finalizing standards elaborated under (c) above and after acceptance by governments publishing them in a Codex Alimentarius either as regional or world wide standards together with international standards already finalized by other bodies under (b) above wherever this is practicable;
- Amending published standards, after appropriate survey in the light of developments.

Article 2 defines eligibility for membership of the Commission, which is open to all Member Nations and Associate Members of FAO and WHO. In 2002 membership comprised 167 countries representing 97 percent of the world's population.

b) The Rules of Procedure of the Codex Alimentarius Commission described and formalize working procedures appropriate to an intergovernmental body. They provide for:

- Conditions of membership of the Commission;
- The appointment of Commission officers including the chairperson, three vice-chair persons, regional coordinators and a secretary, and prescribe their responsibilities;
- The establishment of an executive committee to meet between Commission sessions to act on behalf of the Commission as its executive organ;
- The frequency and operation of Commission sessions;

- The nature of agendas for Commission sessions;
- Voting procedures;
- Observers;
- Preparation of Commission records and reports;
- Establishment of subsidiary bodies;
- Procedures to be adopted in the elaboration of standards;
- Allocation of a budget and estimates of expenditure; and
- Languages to be used by the Commission

Currently, the Commission meets every two years alternately at FAO headquarters in Rome and at WHO headquarters in Geneva. Between sessions of the Commission the Executive Committee act on behalf of the Commission. Plenary sessions of the Commission are attended by as many as 500 people. Representation at sessions is on a country basis. National delegations are led by senior officials appointed by their governments. Delegations may and often do include representative of industry, consumers organizations and academic institutes. Countries that are not yet members of the Commission sometimes attend in an observer capacity.

A number of international governmental organizations and international NGOs also attend in an observer capacity. Although they are "observers" the tradition of the Codex Alimentarius Commission allows such organizations to put forward their points of view at every stage except in the final decision, which is the exclusive prerogative of Member Governments.

To facilitate continuous contact with member countries the Commission in collaboration with national governments has established Codex Contact Points and many member countries have National Codex Committees to coordinate activities nationally.

Interest in Codex Alimentarius activities has been growing steadily since the Commission began and the increasing involvement of developing countries in its work has been a highlight of the progress made as well as a vindication of the foresight shown by the founders of the Commission.

The SPS and TBT agreements of the WTO have accorded additional status to the work of Codex. Codex standards are explicitly recognized as reference in international trade disputes.

c. The Commission Operations

Compiling the Codex Alimentarius

One of the principal purposes of the Commission is the preparation of food standards and their publication in the Codex Alimentarius.

The legal base for the Commission's operations and the procedures it is required to follow are published in the Codex Alimentarius - Procedural Manual currently in its twelfth edition. Like all other aspects of the Commission's work the procedures for preparing standards are well defined open and transparent. In essence they involve:

- The submission of a proposal for a standard to be developed by a national government or a subsidiary committee of the Commission;
- A decision by the Commission or the Executive Committee that a standard be developed as proposed. "Formal Criteria for the Establishment of Work Priorities and for the Establishment of Subsidiary Bodies" assist the Commission or Executive Committee in their decision making and in selecting or creating the subsidiary body responsible for steering standards through development;
- The preparation of a proposal draft standard is arranged by the Commission Secretariat and circulated to Member Governments for comment;
- Comments are considered by the subsidiary body that has been allocated responsibility for the development of the proposed draft standard and this subsidiary body may present the text to the Commission as a draft standard;
- If the commission adopts the draft standard it is sent to the governments a number of times in a step procedure, which if completed satisfactorily results in the draft becoming a Codex standard. In an accelerated procedure, the number of steps required for the development of a standard varies from a maximum of eight to a minimum of five. In some circumstances steps may be repeated. Most standards take a number of years to develop;
- Once adopted by the Commission a Codex standard is added to the Codex Alimentarius.

d. Procedural Manuals

A "Format for Codex Commodity Standards and their Content" is provided in the Procedural Manual of the Codex Alimentarius. It includes the following categories of information:

- Scope - including the name of the standard;
- Description, essential composition and quality factors-defining the minimum standard for the food;

- Food additives - only those cleared by FAO and WHO may be used;
- Contaminants;
- Hygiene and weights and measures;
- Labeling - in accordance with Codex General Standard for the labeling of Pre-packaged Foods; and
- Methods of analysis and sampling.

e. General Standards to Cover All Types of Foods

In addition to commodity standards the Codex Alimentarius includes general standards, which have across the board application to all foods and are not product specific. There are general standards or recommendations for:

- Food labelling;
- Food additives;
- Contaminants;
- Methods of analysis and sampling;
- Food hygiene;
- Nutrition and foods for special dietary uses;
- Food import and export inspection and certification systems;
- Residues of veterinary drugs in foods; and
- Pesticide residues in foods.

The Commission and its subsidiary bodies are committed to revision of Codex standards and related texts as necessary to ensure they are consistent with and reflect current scientific knowledge. Each member of the Commission is responsible for identifying and presenting to the appropriate committee any new scientific and other relevant information that may warrant revision of existing Codex standards or related texts. The procedure for revision follows that used for the initial preparation of standards.

f. Structure of the Codex Alimentarius

This is in 16 volumes having following subjects covered in this

- Volume 1A - General requirements;
- Volume 1B - General requirements (food hygiene);
- Volume 2A - Pesticide residues in foods (general texts);
- Volume 2B - Pesticide residues in foods (maximum residue limits);

- Volume 3 - Residues of veterinary drugs in foods;
- Volume 4 - Foods for special dietary uses (including foods for infants and children);
- Volume 5A - Processed and quick frozen fruits & Vegetables;
- Volume 5B - Fresh Fruits and vegetables;
- Volume 6 - Fruit Juices;
- Volume 7 - Cereals, pulses (legumes) and derived products and vegetable proteins;
- Volume 8 - Fats and oils and related products;
- Volume 9 - Fish and fishery products;
- Volume 10 - Meat and meat products; soups and broths;
- Volume 11 - Sugars, cocoa products and chocolate and miscellaneous products;
- Volume 12 - Milk and milk products;
- Volume 13 - Methods of analysis and sampling.

The volumes contain general principles, general standards, definitions, codes, commodity standards, methods and recommendations. The content list is well organized for ease of reference for example:

Volume 1A - General Requirements

1. General Principles of the Codex Alimentarius;
2. Definitions for the Purpose of Codex Alimentarius;
3. Code of Ethics for International Trade in Foods;
4. Food labelling;
5. Food Additives-including the General Standard for Food Additives;
6. Contaminants in Food-including the General Standard for Contaminants and Toxins in Foods;
7. Irradiated Foods;
8. Food Import and Export Food Inspection and Certification Systems.

Published volumes of the Codex Alimentarius are available in English, French and Spanish and individual standards are available on the World Wide Web and CD-ROM.

g. Subsidiary Bodies

Under its Rules of Procedure the Commission is empowered to establish two kinds of subsidiary body:

- Codex Committees, which prepare draft standards for submission to the Commission.
- Coordinating Committees through which regions or groups of countries coordinates food standards activities in the region including the development of regional standards.

A feature of the committee system is that with few exceptions each committee is hosted by a member country which is chiefly responsible for the cost of the committee's maintenance and administration and for providing its chairperson.

h. General Subject Committees are so called because their work has relevance for a wide range of foodstuffs. General subject Committees are sometimes referred to as "horizontal committees".

- Committee on General Principles, hosted by France
- Committee on Food Labeling, hosted by Canada
- Committee on Methods of Analysis and Sampling, hosted by Hungary;
- Committee on Food Hygiene, hosted by the United States
- Committee on Pesticide Residues, hosted by the Netherlands;
- Committee on Food Additives and Contaminants, hosted by the Netherlands;
- Committee on Import/Export Inspection and Certification Systems, hosted by Australia;
- Committee on Nutrition and Foods for Special dietary Uses, hosted by Germany (a General Committee for the purpose of Nutrition);
- Committee on Residues of Veterinary Drugs in Food, hosted by the United States;
- Committee on Meat and Poultry Hygiene, hosted by New Zealand.

Among other things these Committees develop all embracing concepts and principles applying to foods in general specific foods or groups of foods; endorse or review relevant provisions in Codex commodity standards and based on the advice of expert scientific bodies develop major recommendations pertaining to consumers health and safety.

i. Commodity Committees have responsibility for developing standards for specific foods or classes or food. In order to distinguish them from the "horizontal committees" and recognize their exclusive responsibilities they are often referred to as "Vertical Committees.

- Committee on Fats and Oils, hosted by the United Kingdom;
- Committee on Fish and Fishery Products, hosted by Norway;
- Committee on Milk and Milk Products (formerly the FAO/WHO Committee of Government Experts on the Code of Principles of Milk and Milk Products) hosted by New Zealand;
- Committee on Fresh Fruits and Vegetables hosted by Mexico;
- Committee on Cocoa Products and Chocolate hosted by Switzerland;
- Committee on Sugars, hosted by the United Kingdom;
- Committee on Processed Fruits and Vegetables hosted by the United States;
- Committee on Vegetable Proteins, hosted by Canada;
- Committee on Cereals, Pulses and Legumes, hosted by the United States:
- Committee on Natural Mineral Waters hosted by Switzerland.

Commodity Committees convene as necessary and go into recess or are abolished when the Commission decides their work has been completed. New committees may be established on an adhoc basis to cover specific needs for the development of new standards.

Host countries call meetings of Codex subsidiary bodies at intervals of between one and two years according to need. Attendance at some Codex committees is almost as large as that drawn by a plenary session of the Commission.

j. Coordinating Committees have no standing host countries. Meetings are hosted by countries of a region on an adhoc basis and in agreement with the Commission. There are six Coordinating Committees i.e. one each for the following regions:

- Africa
- Asia
- Europe
- Latin America and the Caribbean
- Near East
- North America and Southwest Pacific.

k. Task Forces (ad hoc Intergovernmental Task Forces)

In order to expedite work on specific subjects the Commission also establishes time limited ad hoc intergovernmental task forces whose mandate normally does not exceed five years. The first three task forces were established in 1999 and dealt with:

- Foods derived from biotechnology (hosted by Japan)
- Animal Feeding (hosted by Denmark)
- Fruit and Vegetables Juices (hosted by Brazil).

l. Member Countries Acceptance of Codex Standards

The harmonization of food standards is generally viewed as a prerequisite to the protection of consumer health as well as allowing the fullest possible facilitation of international trade. For that reason the Uruguay Round Agreements on the Application of Sanitary and Phytosanitary Measures (SPS) and Technical Barriers to Trade (TBT) both encourage the international harmonization of food standards.

Harmonization can only be achieved when all countries adopt the same standards. The General Principles of the Codex Alimentarius specify the ways in which member countries may "accept" Codex standards. Forms of acceptance vary somewhat depending on whether the standard is a commodity standard a general standard or concerns levels for pesticide or veterinary drug residues or food additives. Generally, however the proposed forms of acceptance are full acceptance, acceptance with minor deviations and free distribution. The ways of acceptance are clearly defined in the General Principles are their suitability in the light of experience is subject to review by the Codex Committee on General Principles.

The Codex Alimentarius also contains the Recommended International Code of Practice for Control of the Use of Veterinary Drugs, which has the express aim of preventing the use of drugs that create a hazard to human health.

There are also a number of so-called codes of technological practice, which are intended to ensure that the processing, transport and storage of foods produced to Codex standards are such that consumers receive end products that are wholesome and of the expected quality. Codes of technological practice exist for:

- Food for infants and children
- The packaging and transport of fresh fruit and vegetables
- Storage and transport of edible oils and fats in bulk
- Processing and handling of quick frozen foods.

m. Organizational Structures of National Food Control System

Strengthening Organizational Structures for National Food Control Systems

Given the wide scope of food control systems there are at least three types of organizational arrangements that may be appropriate at the national level. These are:

- A system based on multiple agencies responsible for food control - Multiple Agency System;
- A system based on a single, unified agency for food control - Single Agency System;
- A system based on a national integrated approach - Integrated System.

a) Multiple Agency System

While food safety is the foremost objective, food control systems also have an important economic objective of creating and maintaining sustainable food production and processing systems. In this context food control systems play a significant role in the following:

- Ensuring fair practices in trade;
- Developing the food sector on a professional and scientific basis;
- Preventing avoidable losses and conserving natural resources; and
- Promoting the country's export trade.

Food control systems may also be fragmented between national, state and local bodies and the thoroughness of implementation depends upon the capacity and the efficiency of the agency responsible at each level. Thus consumers may not receive the same level of protection throughout the country and it may become difficult to properly evaluate the effectiveness of interventions by national, state or local authorities.

While multiple food control agencies may be the norm they suffer from serious drawbacks including:

- Lack of overall coordination at national level;
- Frequent confusion over jurisdiction and resultant inefficiencies in performance;
- Differences in levels of expertise and resources and hence uneven implementation;
- Conflict between public health objectives and the facilitation of trade and industry development;

- Limited capacity for appropriate scientific inputs in decision making processes;
- Lack of coherence leading to over-regulation or time gaps in adequate regulatory activity; and
- Reductions in the confidence of domestic consumers and foreign buyers in the credibility of the system.

During the preparation of a national food control strategy it is important to consider the type and size of the organization(s) that are necessary to implement the strategy. It is often not possible to have a single unified structure or an integrated food control system due to various historical and political reasons. In such cases, it is necessary for the national food control strategy to clearly identify the role of each agency to avoid duplication of effort and to bring about a measure of coherence among them. It should also identify areas or segments of the food chain, which require special attention and need additional resources for strengthening.

b) Single Agency System

The consolidation of all responsibility for protecting public health and food safety into a single food control agency with clearly defined terms of reference has considerable merit. It acknowledges the high priority that Government places in food safety initiatives and a commitment to reducing the risk of food borne disease. The benefits that result from a single agency approach to food control include:

B. Hazard Analysis and Critical Control Point (HACCP)

HACCP is a system that identifies, evaluates and controls hazards, which make a food unsafe for human consumption. HACCP is a systematic approach for the control of food safety throughout the commodity system of food chain. Before HACCP most of the food systems were based on end product testing which does not assure 100% safety. It required a good understanding of the relationship between cause and effect in order to be more proactive. HACCP is a key element in Total Quality Management HACCP

- Good Manufacturing Practices (GMP)
- Good Hygienic Practices (GHP)
- Good Agricultural Practices(GAP)
- Good Storage Practices(GSP)

Good Agricultural Practices

Land use for crop, horticulture, fodder and pasture production should be fit and free of problems and not contaminated with heavy metals, industrial affluent or biological waste. Farmers should also control production so that pest and disease of plants and animals do not contaminate food or feed.

Good Agricultural practices include Good Hygienic Practices(GHP). This became more significant in animal products like milk, meat and egg. Good Storage Practices(GSP) should be followed when commodity is stored on farm. GSP related guidelines are covered in Food Hygiene Basic Texts(CODEX) there also four ISO procedures that cover storage of cereals & pulses (ISO 6322 series).

Good Manufacturing Practices(GMP)

- Establishment and design facility : Structure location of processing plants, design to minimize contamination, maintain cleanliness disinfection, environmental facilities etc.
- Control Operation : Time, temperature humidity, potable water equipment maintenance etc.
- Maintenance of Sanitation - Throughout the GMP
- Personal Hygiene : Handlers awareness of hygiene
- Transportation : To prevent contamination and deterioration of quality, controlled temperature containers etc.
- Training : All handlers should be trained in HACCP paraphernalia.

Product Information & Consumer Awareness

Basic Principles of HACCP : Seven Principle

i) Conduct a hazard analysis
ii) Determination of critical control/points
iii) Establish critical limits
iv) Establish a monitoring system
v) Establish a procedure for corrective action when monitoring at CCP indicates a deviation from a established critical unit.
vi) Establish procedures for verification to confirm the effectiveness of the HACCP Plan.
vii) Establish documentation concerning all procedures and records appropriate to these principles and their application.

Developing a HACCP Plan

There are 12 tasks to develop HACCP Plan.

i. Establish HACCP team
ii. Describe the product
iii. Identify the products intended use
iv. Draw up the commodity flow diagram
v. On site confirmation of flow diagram
vi. Identify and analyse hazards (Principle I)
vii. Determine the critical control point (Principle II)
viii. Establish critical limit for each CCP(Principle I)
ix. Establish a monitoring procedure (Principle I)
x. Establish corrective action (Principle 5)
xi. Verify the HACCP Plan (Principle 6)
xii. Keep Records (Principle 7)

Food safety and standard bill 2005 (Ministry of Food processing and Industries).

A Draft Bill was proposed by the Ministry, which has following provisions. Comments from various organizations NOGs and public are awaited for improving the Draft before putting for final approaval. Under this following provisions are included:

(i) Food safety and Standard Authority of India (FSSAI)
(ii) General principles of food safety
(iii) General provisions as to articles of food
(iv) Special responsibility of food safety
(v) Analysis of articles of food and enforcement of act
(vi) General provisions relating to import and export
(vii) Offence and penalties
(viii) Adjudication and food appellate tribunal

Schedule I

(i) Prevention of food adulteration act 1954
(ii) Fruit products order 1955
(iii) Milk and Milk products order 1992
(iv) Meat food order 1973

(v) The Vegetable oil product control order 1947

(vi) The solvent extraction oil, de-oiled meal and edible flour and control order 1967.

(vii) Infant milk substitute, feeding bottle, infant foods (regulation of production supply and distribution Act 1992.

(viii) Any other order under essential commodities Act 1955 relating to food

Index